PROGRESS IN CYSTIC FIBROSIS RESEARCH

PROGRESS IN CYSTIC FIBROSIS RESEARCH

MARGARET A. HARRISON
EDITOR

Nova Biomedical Books
New York

For permission to use material from this book please contact us:
Telephone 631-231-7269; Fax 631-231-8175
Web Site: http://www.novapublishers.com

Library of Congress Cataloging-in-Publication Data

ISBN 1-59454-232-5

Published by Nova Science Publishers, Inc. ✣ New York

Contents

Preface

Cystic fibrosis (CF) is a genetic disease at once tragic and theoretically puzzling. Predominantly found in Caucasian and Semitic populations, its incidence in the United States is 1 in approximately 3000 births. The global population of cystic fibrosis sufferers has been estimated to be about a quarter of a million persons, many of whom will never be accurately diagnosed during their lifetime. Chapter I examines recent research findings and clinical trial results that offer a new specification of the linkage between genetics and disease in the case of CF: a linkage involving the transport of reduced glutathione (GSH). Chapter II discusses how Cystic fibrosis (CF) is characterised by defective epithelial transport. In the intestine this affects both absorption and secretion. Bile acid dysfunction has been well described in CF suggesting that the handling of bile acids by the intestine is affected by the disease. Metabolic alkalosis in association with low serum electrolyte concentration (hyponatremia, hypochloremia, and hypokalemia) is well known complication of cystic fibrosis (CF) in infancy. The records of 109 children diagnosed as having CF before the age of 12 months, in the period from 1990 to 2002, were reviewed to ascertain the prevalence of the electrolyte depletion with metabolic alkalosis as a major presenting manifestation of CF in our region and to define the possible risk factors for its occurrence and is reported in Chapter III.

Cystic fibrosis (CF) is the most frequent genetic disease affecting Caucasian populations. In cystic fibrosis, as a result of chronic pulmonary infections and digestive malabsorption, an imbalance between the production of reactive oxygen species and their inactivation by protective systems is observed. This imbalance may cause impairment of cell metabolism and oxidative injury. The aim of the study presented in Chapter IV was to examine whether the antioxidant status in cystic fibrosis patients with pancreatic insufficiency provided sufficient protection against oxidative damage to protein and lipids. Chapter V discusses how auxological abnormalities are frequently observed in Cystic Fibrosis (CF), as well as in other chronic pediatric diseases. In 20% of CF children the height is subnormal (at least -2 SDS) and bone age and puberty onset are delayed by a mean of 2 years. Final height tends to be below both the population mean and the target stature, owing to a decreased growth spurt. With respect to their mothers CF girls experience menarche approximately 1 year later and their menarcheal delay may be related to both genotype and disease severity. Other factors that may be implicated in the pathogenesis of growth and puberty retardation in CF are undernitrition, chronic hypoxia and respiratory acidosis.

Chapter VI reviews the genetic defect characterising cystic fibrosis (CF) and how it leads to a failure to produce mature cystic fibrosis transmembrane regulator (CFTR) protein that plays a crucial role in regulating fluids and electrolytes in lung secretions, this results in impaired mucociliary clearance and is likely to play an important role in reducing the effectiveness of the innate immune response to pathogens. The consequence is recurrent endobronchial infection and inflammation that leads to progressive respiratory disease. Chapter VII explains how Cystic fibrosis (CF) is a common autosomal recessive disease in the Caucasian population. Although more than 900 mutations have been reported, the most common mutation, deltaF508, accounts for about 70% of all CF mutant alleles in Northern Europeans. The disease frequency in Hispanic population is much less and deltaF508 mutation accounts for about 50% of CF alleles in Hispanic population.

More women with cystic fibrosis (CF) now reach reproductive age and wish to become pregnant. Although women with CF have reduced fertility, many of them can become mothers. A pregnancy ought to be carefully planned since several studies have shown that pregnancy is well tolerated if good medical care is provided, and the woman with CF is in a stable good condition Women with CF should be advised against pregnancy after lungtransplantation. This subject is discussed in length in Chapter VIII. Chapter IX reports a study to evaluate the effect of short-term ibuprofen therapy on interleukin-8 (IL-8) cytokine levels in sputum-producing patients with cystic fibrosis (CF), a double-blinded, placebo-controlled study was performed in a crossover manner, consisting of two 14-day periods. The method used was pharmacokinetic analysis, done by high-performance liquid chromatography before start. The conclusion was short-term high-dose ibuprofen treatment did not result in significantly decreased IL-8 concentration in sputum of CF patients with relatively advanced pulmonary disease. A multicenter approach may be necessary for further evaluation of the place of ibuprofen in the anti-inflammatory treatment of CF patients.

Cystic fibrosis (CF) used to be considered a paediatric disease, as most patients died before school age. However, factors such as diagnosing at an earlier age, improved nutritional treatment, and more effective early use of anti-obstructive and antimicrobial therapy have resulted in improved clinical status and survival as discussed in chapter X. The improved survival during the last decades, especially among the very young patients with CF, has totally changed the attitude towards the disease. But, the fact that fewer CF patients die early in life make long time survival predictions more and more difficult to carry out. Modern CF care emphasises preventative care to further improve survival and quality of life for individuals diagnosed with CF. In order to maintain adherence with life long treatment, patients may need support to build up self-esteem to stand up to the fact of being different, having to carry out daily treatment and take enzymes with every meal. Assessing the results of the offered CF care and estimating the future population and its demography are important in order to evaluate treatment regimens and to calculate future needs of health care resources. It is of great importance that resources match the growing adult population, otherwise the improving survival rate can not be expected to continue.

In: Progress in Cystic Fibrosis Research
Editor: Margaret A. Harrison, pp. 1-28
ISBN 1-59454-232-5

Chapter I

Cystic Fibrosis: The First Identified Glutathione Transport Disease

Valerie M. Hudson
Brigham Young University

Abstract

Cystic fibrosis (CF) is a genetic disease at once tragic and theoretically puzzling. Predominantly found in Caucasian and Semitic populations, its incidence in the United States is 1 in approximately 3000 births. The global population of cystic fibrosis sufferers has been estimated to be about a quarter of a million persons, many of whom will never be accurately diagnosed during their lifetime. Average life expectancy in the United States has risen to about 32 years of age, but the median age at death for the most common mutation pair, delF508/delF508, remains about 23 years of age even with the most advanced care. The life expectancy of females with cystic fibrosis tends to be a few years shorter than the life expectancy of males. Proximate cause of death in about 95% of cases is respiratory failure [1].

The very real tragedy of CF does not belie the theoretical puzzlement it causes researchers. How, exactly, do CF mutations (one thousand and counting), give rise to the unique pathophysiology of CF? It has been known since 1989 that CF mutations cause the anion efflux channel created by the CFTR protein in the cell membrane to be missing or defective. What is the relationship of that channel dysfunction to the three hallmarks of CF disease: thickened mucus, chronic and exuberant inflammation, and ineffective pathogen clearance by the immune system? Theories abound, but the mechanism remains notably underspecified.

In this essay, we will examine recent research findings and clinical trial results that offer a new specification of the linkage between genetics and disease in the case of CF: a linkage involving the transport of reduced glutathione (GSH).

Key words: cystic fibrosis, glutathione, s-glutathiolation, s-nitrosoglutathione, inflammation, immune response, mucolysis

Not Just a Chloride Channel

The CFTR channel has a long-standing nickname: "the chloride channel." Indeed, much CF research and theorizing revolves around the efflux, or lack of efflux of the chloride anion from CF cells. Theories relating chloride, sodium, and water movements are central to the current understanding of CF [2].

However, it is possible that this emphasis on chloride has been less than helpful. Pharmaceutical modification of chloride or sodium concentrations, such as through the use of amiloride, has not been shown to reverse CF symptoms [3]. There is more to the theoretical picture than chloride alone.

New research demonstrates that there are other anions of possible clinical relevance whose efflux is affected by CFTR mutation. Two that are receiving attention at this point in time are bicarbonate and reduced glutathione (GSH). Though we will concentrate on glutathione in this essay, bicarbonate's importance in regulation of pH has attracted the attention of several research teams whose work will undoubtedly be tracked with care by CF clinicians and patients [4,5].

It was the work of two Canadian researchers, Paul Linsdell and John Hanrahan, that first brought to the attention of the CF research community in 1998 that cellular efflux of GSH was significantly reduced by dysfunction of the CFTR channel [6]. In the subsequent five and a half years, other research teams have moved swiftly to confirm and extend those findings. Using cell lines of CF lung epithelia, Gao et al. were also able to demonstrate significantly reduced efflux of GSH [7]. Ilana Kogan and colleagues found this same diminished GSH efflux with a variety of CFTR mutants, including G551D, R347D, K464A, and K1250A [8,9], and through the use of sophisticated tests were able to confirm that purified CFTR protein alone directly mediates nucelotide-dependent GSH flux and not via other associated chloride transport proteins. Brian Day and colleagues also found a 50% reduction in lung epithelial lining fluid (ELF) GSH levels in uninfected CFTR knockout mice [10]. Finder et al. have uncovered a 49% reduction of GSH in in bronchoalveolar lavage fluid from CF patients [11].

In short, these research teams discovered that CF mutations cause a primary and profound glutathione transport malfunction. Would such a significant decrease in GSH efflux cause disease? The answer is yes.

GSH, GSH Transport, and Health

Unless one is actually working in the field of glutathione research, it is not uncommon to find oneself relatively uninformed about its several pivotal roles in health and disease. But even a cursory glance at the over 60,000 abstracts on glutathione or GSH compiled on PubMed can serve to propel the uninitiated into a broader understanding of this ubiquitous and physiologically essential tripeptide.

GSH is synthesized by the cells of the body from the amino acids glutamine, glycine, and cysteine, with cysteine serving as the rate-limiting component. Meister states that an adult human male will synthesize approximately 10 grams of GSH per day [12]. In addition to synthesis, glutathione is available in small amounts in the human diet, and there exist specific co-transporters of intact glutathione in the mammalian jejunum [13, 14-17].

Organ systems, and even cell types, differ according to the *level of total glutathione* (GSH+GSSG, the latter being glutathione disulfide) and the *glutathione redox ratio* (GSH:GSSG) found therein. In systems openly exposed to oxidants, such as the lung or cornea, or devoted to detoxification, such as the liver, the level of total glutathione may be quite high, and the redox ratio also quite high [18]. But even within such systems, differences may be found between various cell types; for example, monocytes have, in general, higher levels of total glutathione than neutrophils [19].

Let us now turn to a discussion of glutathione's functions. We will divide this discussion into four parts: 1) glutathione as an antioxidant; 2) glutathione's role in mucus viscosity; 3) glutathione as an immune system modulator; and 4) glutathione's relationship to the NO system of the body.

Glutathione as an Antioxidant

Glutathione's sulfur-hydrogen, or thiol, group is a potent reducing agent, and GSH can be considered the one of the body's most important water-soluble antioxidants. Antioxidant defenses in humans are comprised of both enzymatic and non-enzymatic defenses; some defenses operate intracellularly and others have additional extracellular functions. The antioxidant enzymes are glutathione peroxidase, superoxide dismutase, and catalase. There are two types of non-enzymatic antioxidants, the water soluble and the fat soluble. The water soluble antioxidants are reduced glutathione and ascorbic acid; the fat soluble are alpha-tocopherol and the carotenoids. The enzymatic antioxidants are lodged within the cellular membranes (though there is a free plasma glutathione peroxidase [348]); in contrast the water soluble antioxidants (as free molecules) are present in the cytosol of the cells, though some, including GSH, are also present in the extracellular environment. The fat soluble antioxidants are found within the lipid membranes. Each antioxidant defense system protects the cells from oxidative damage in its own sphere of action, and a deficiency in any category puts the cell at risk for oxidative damage. It should be noted that GSH is a precursor for the function of glutathione peroxidase. In addition to its cellular functions, GSH is also present in extracellular epithelial fluids, such as the epithelial lining fluid (ELF) of the lung, blood plasma, semen, saliva, and so forth, where antioxidant action is similarly useful.

GSH provides powerful antioxidant protection to body systems heavily exposed to reactive oxygen species (ROS), such as the lung [20,21]. For example, the normal level of extracellular GSH in the lung epithelial lining fluid (ELF) is 140 times the normal level of extracellular GSH in blood plasma, and it is probable that the lung, under oxidative stress, becomes a net importer of circulating GSH [22] In addition, under conditions of oxidative or nitrosative stress, vulnerable proteins may undergo s-glutathiolation, wherein GSSG binds to protein, thus protecting it, and also allowing for that binding to be reversed when the stress has passed [23]. However, it would be wrong to view GSH only or even most importantly in terms of its antioxidant properties when considering its importance in lung defense.

Glutathione and Maintenance of Proper Mucus Viscosity

A second property of reduced glutathione that should not be overlooked is its promotion of mucolysis. Because of its chemistry, GSH, like N-acetylcysteine (NAC), is able to cleave disulfide bonds, which serves to reduce the viscoelasticity of mucus when the glutathione system is functioning normally [24,25]. Furthermore, reduced glutathione plays a role in establishing the volume of periciliary fluid, and also affects mucus hydration through its indirect relationship with epithelial sodium channels (ENaC), topics we will explore in a later section.

Glutathione and Immune Function

A third property of reduced glutathione is to regulate inflammation and immune response. This regulation is carried out in a number of ways, which will be discussed below. Generally speaking, however, the main mechanism of regulation is by redox potential. Since GSH is synthesized by virtually every cell in the body, a redox equilibrium is established within each of these cells, and the efflux of GSH from the cells establishes an extracellular redox equilibrium as well. Both intracellular and extracellular redox equilibria vary: extracellularly, the equilibrium varies by bodily system, as noted above; and intracellularly, the equilibrium varies by cell type. As noted previously, the intracellular GSH level of monocytes is three times that of neutrophils [19]. The redox potential, expressed by the ratio GSH:GSSG influences many sensitive cellular systems and functions. Indeed, as we shall see, inflammation, immune response, and cell viability, among other things, are intimately tied to this ratio. If, as we will hypothesize in a later section, CF leukocytes and lymphocytes (along with other cells possessing anion channels redundant to the CFTR) are prone to chronic alteration of the GSH:GSSG ratio, immune response will be profoundly affected.

Glutathione and the Nitric Oxide System

NO, an important factor in cell signalling, pathogen killing, ciliary beat function, and smooth muscle relaxation, is profoundly affected by GSH system function. In the extracellular compartment, GSH combines with NO to form s-nitrosoglutathione (GSNO). In healthy systems, GSNO is easily cleaved and is not only an important reservoir of GSH, but also an important reservoir of NO. GSH also appears to bear a relationship to the expression of iNOS [26-31]. NO in turn affects expression of gamma-glutamylcysteine synthetase, the rate-limiting enzyme for GSH synthesis, apparently to counteract NO cytotoxicity [32-35].

The Effects of Glutathione Transport Dysfunction in Cystic Fibrosis

In order to more fully discuss the effects of glutathione transport dysfunction in cystic fibrosis, two levels of analysis must take place. First, we must understand the consequences of CFTR mutation on total levels and redox ratios of glutathione in three compartments:

- CF cells whose primary means of effluxing GSH is the CFTR;
- CF cells that have other anion efflux channels redundant to the CFTR;
- The extracellular milieu in CF.

Second, since glutathione transport dysfunction has not been, generally speaking, a topic of research in cystic fibrosis, we must investigate what medical science knows about the effects of GSH deficiency in these three compartments in disease conditions other than CF for insights into what we might expect in CF as a result of this dysfunction.

Glutathione in the Three Compartments in CF

Research on glutathione status in CF is very new. Only a few research findings can be referenced. Nevertheless, what currently exists provides a basis for partial understanding.

In CF cells whose primary means of GSH efflux is the CFTR, such as bronchial epithelial cells, normal total levels of glutathione (GSH+GSSG) have been found [36]. (Indeed, it may be very difficult for such cells to suffer depletion of GSH, which may have ramifications for appropriate apoptosis in these cells.) However, there is currently no research concerning the GSH:GSSG ratio in these CF cells.

Second, in CF cells that possess redundant anion efflux channels to the CFTR (RACP cells, meaning Redundant Anion Channel Present), in particular the MRP family of channels (and GS-X pumps more broadly), depletion of total levels of glutathione has been found. Cells with such characteristics would include hepatocytes, leukocytes, erythrocytes, and lymphocytes, among others. Tirouvanziam found substantially lower levels of GSH in sputum neutrophils from CF patients compared to GSH levels in blood neutrophils, which also correlated with cell death rates [37]. Lands and colleagues found that total glutathione levels of the peripheral blood lymphocytes of CF persons were, in general, depressed [38]. Again, no studies of GSH:GSSG ratio have been conducted for this compartment. However, upregulation of MRP1 in CF erythrocytes has been noted [39].

Third, more plentiful research is available on glutathione status in the extracellular milieu in CF, especially in the lung ELF, but also in blood plasma. A noted previously, Brian Day and colleagues found a 50% reduction in lung epithelial lining fluid (ELF) GSH levels in uninfected CFTR knockout mice [10], and Finder et al. found a 49% reduction of GSH in in bronchoalveolar lavage fluid from CF patients [11]. Roum et al. found a profound deficit of GSH in CF lung ELF, with levels dropping to 5-10% of normal. Roum and colleagues also investigated GSH:GSSG ratios in CF lung ELF, and also found a large decrease, from a norm of over 9:1 in healthy persons to approximately 3:1 in CF patients [40]. In blood plasma,

Brown et al. found a 50% decrease in total GSH, which was replicated by Roum et al. in a later study [41]. Roum et al. also found decreased GSH:GSSG ratio in CF blood plasma [40].

Emphasizing that transport of GSH is the issue, not synthesis or any other aspect of the glutathione system, studies have found normal synthesis of GSH in CF, and normal or even elevated levels of glutathione peroxidase, glutathione reductase, γ-glutamyl transpeptidase, and γ-glutamylcysteine transferase [42,43,17,44,45].

Glutathione Deficiency and Pathophysiology

The clearest way to demonstrate the importance of a properly functioning GSH system is to detail what scientific research tells us about the effects of GSH deficiency, even when studies have not been conducted concerning CF per se. We will discuss three main categories of known effects of GSH deficiency: impaired antioxidant capability, decreased mucolysis, and abnormal immune response, including decreased nitric oxide production and availability.

A) Impaired Antioxidant Capability

When a key antioxidant such as GSH is deficient in the extracellular compartment and in RACP cells, direct damage from oxidants increases greatly. In addition, glutathione deficiency in leukocytes (a type of RACP cell) has been shown to cause increased release of hydrogen peroxide [46]. Oxidant damage to lung epithelial cells from a diminished extracellular antioxidant screen reduces lung function, causing fibrosis and permitting greater adhesion of bacteria [20,21,47-49]. When GSH is deficient, other antioxidants may be consumed in higher-than-normal amounts to handle the increased oxidant burden. Thus, GSH deficiency is often accompanied by lower levels of alpha-tocopherol and ascorbate, and decreased activity of glutathione peroxidase, catalase, and superoxide dismutase, all of which are reversible when GSH level is normalized [50]. New research also points to the direct role of GSH in neutralizing HOCl, one of the deadliest oxidants to be found in the respiratory milieu, with the reaction being

$2GSH + HOCl \rightarrow GSSG + H_2O + HCl$ [51].

GSH deficiency also causes oxidant damage to the liver [52-62] and pancreas [63-65], resulting in impaired function of these organs, including reduced bile flow [54,59,61,66], and is associated with the onset of diabetes mellitus [67-73], rheumatoid arthritis [74], peripheral nerve damage [75], and myocardial injury [76]. GSH deficiency results in intestinal mucosal injury and chronic inflammation of the gut [77-82], decreased absorption of nutrients such as calcium [83], and general cachexia and growth retardation [84-87]. GSH deficiency also causes greater lipid peroxidation, which, in turn, causes cell damage [88-94]. (As peroxidation of arachidonic acid yields especially damaging metabolites, it is noteworthy that CF persons have been found to have threefold more arachidonic acid and threefold less DHA in the cell membrane than normal persons [95], and that the cytotoxicity of arachidonic acid is enhanced by GSH depletion [96]. The metabolism of arachidonic acid also entails the production of free radicals by virtue of the lipooxygenase and cyclooxygenase pathways, further increasing oxidant burden. For example, 8-isoprostane in breath condensate of CF persons is elevated three-fold above normal controls [97].

Loss of GSH antioxidant capability in the extracellular milieu has secondary effects, as well. One such effect is oxidant-derived inactivation of the anti-protease system [98-100]. Such inactivation produces its own cascade of harmful effects due to unbound neutrophil elastase (NE). In the lung, these include, as Barbero notes in a review of the scientific literature, "cleavage of fibronectin, lung elastin, immunoglobulins and immune complexes, complement receptors in neutrophils, and other receptors on T-cells and B-cells. Furthermore, NE inhibits ciliary beating and stimulates mucus production from goblet cells and facilitates P. aeruginosa adherence. Finally, by cleaving receptors for interleukin (IL)-1 and IL-2 or the T cell antigen receptor, it may hypothetically inhibit message transmission and immune recognition. Thus, besides destruction, [free NE] may lead to acquired immune suppression" [101]. GSH depletion has also been linked to increased levels of collagenase [102].

Other secondary effects of the loss of GSH antioxidant protection in the extracellular milieu include degradation of lung surfactant, both via oxidant damage and through the inability of the body to maintain appropriate levels of phosphatidycholine under conditions of GSH deficiency [03-105]. This in turn may be related to the linkage between GSH depletion and reduced lung surface tension [106]. S-glutathiolation protection of vulnerable proteins will also be reduced. Though it is intriguing to note that GSH depletion also leads to free radical-induced respiratory muscle fatigue, which contributes to respiratory failure in patients with lung disease [107], and that more generalized skeletal muscle fatigue also results from GSH depletion [108], since muscle cells are generally non-RACP cells, it is not clear whether these findings would be pertinent to the case of CF. However, it is relevant to the CF case to note that GSH depletion, by increasing airway inflammation, has been hypothesized to lead to the development of asthma [109].

When GSH in the ELF is deficient, the body decreases enzymatic activity transforming GSSG back into GSH, and instead further oxidizes GSSG into chloramines, long-lived oxidants capable of profound injury to the lung [110,111]. (For illustration, chloramines are the agent of lung damage when ammonia and bleach are mixed.) Oxidation products also serve to inhibit the enzymatic activities of glutathione reductase, essential in recycling of GSSG into GSH [112,113], and we would expect this inhibition in RACP cells. Oxidation appears to decrease gamma-glutamylcysteine transferase (g-GCT) activity, as well [114], and this would affect both RACP and non-RACP cells.. These secondary effects, by damaging the integrity of lung tissue, increasing epithelial permeability, and further disrupting the GSH antioxidant system, allow for increased adhesion of pathogens [115]. Regulation of neutrophil adhesion is also affected by GSH depletion [116]. GSH depletion also causes oxidation of protein thiols, protein denaturation and aggregation, increases in insoluble proteins [117], all of which can serve to initiate stress responses in cells, such as induction of heat shock protein 70 (HSP70) [118,119] and stress-activated protein kinases [120], as well as disruption of other types of cell signalling [121], repair processes [122], protein synthesis [123-125], and even mitochondrial energy production [126]. GSH depletion also causes other cell structure alterations, including increased DNA damage [127], loss of junctional and cytoskeletal integrity [128,129], and abnormal cellular bodies [130-132]. We would hypothesize that these cellular effects would be seen in the RACP cells of CF patients.

It should be noted that glutathione deficiency in the ELF has been associated not only with cystic fibrosis, but also with such pulmonary diseases as acute respiratory distress syndrome (ARDS) [133], chronic obstructive pulmonary disease (COPD) [20], idiopathic interstitial pneumonia (IIP) [134], idiopathic pulmonary fibrosis (IPF--of non-smokers) [135], idiopathic respiratory distress syndrome (IRDS) [106], and diffuse fibrosing alveolitis (DFA) [136] A deficiency has also been found in the lungs of HIV-positive patients [137,138].

B) Impaired Ability to Maintain Proper Mucus Viscosity

Extracellular GSH deficiency impairs maintenance of proper mucus viscosity, as GSH facilitates cleavage of disulfide bonds in mucus [139]. Increased viscoelasticity of mucus further inhibits ciliary beating, and also allows for increased opportunity for bacterial colonization of the lung. [140-144]. Interestingly, GSH depletion has also been shown to provoke mucin secretion by tracheal epithelial cells [145], and increased NFkappaB due to GSH deficiency stimulates mucus oversecretion by epithelial cells in the presence of Pseudomonas aeruginosa [146]. However, since these are not RACP cells, these observations are only interesting if it is the case that despite their normal levels of total glutathione, CF epithelial cells have a significantly decreased GSH:GSSG ratio. Given the high amount of oxidant stress in CF, in part due to chronic and progressive extracellular GSH deficit caused by the CFTR mutation, this alteration might occur. If so, then it is also interesting to note that GSH deficit also precludes IFN-gamma inhibition of Na+ and fluid absorption [147,148], and perhaps NO regulation of ENaC, as well [149,150]. As noted above, oxidative stress due to GSH depletion leads to an increase in free NE, which also stimulates mucus secretion [151].

C) Abnormal Immune Response

Though GSH is well known for its antioxidant properties, and somewhat less well known for its role in maintaining proper mucus viscosity, it is not as widely known for the key role it plays in immune system regulation. Because RACP cells include leukocytes and lymphocytes, the literature in this area should be pertinent to the case of CF. The following discussion is not comprehensive, but rather serves to outline the broad parameters of the topic.

First, as noted in the introduction, the redox status of GSH is the primary mechanism by which this regulation takes place. GSH deficiency in immune system cells (which are RACP cells) triggers inflammation, and chronic GSH deficiency in these cells leads to chronic and exaggerated inflammation. Cellular GSH deficiency is related directly to increased transcription of NFkappaB [152-159]. NFkappaB codes for the inflammatory cytokines, and a deficit of either the water soluble or fat soluble antioxidants increases NFkappaB activity, which is a critical early event in the pathogenesis of many lung diseases [160]. This mechanism is demonstrated in HIV-infected macrophages, wherein there is increased activity of NFkappaB due to decreased GSH synthesis. Consequently, there is a progressive increase of inflammatory cytokines as the disease progresses (and as GSH continues to be diminished). Increasing the redox potential of infected macrophages correlates with a decrease in inflammatory cytokines, as well as a decrease in HIV replication [161-163]. The concept of cellular redox potential is particularly germane to immune cell function due to its influence on NFkappaB activity. Diseases that have a chronic inflammatory component, whether affecting a single organ (e.g., hepatitis), or as systemic inflammation (as in AIDS), will manifest GSH deficiency either in the affected organ or systemically, respectively. These deficits can occur due to insufficient GSH synthesis or transport, or consumption in pathological oxidative reactions that outpaces replenishment.

Accordingly, the cytokine profile of GSH deficiency includes elevated levels of AP-1 [155,156,158,159], TNF-alpha and its by-products [154,164-167], IL-1-induced MCP-1 [155,168], and IL-8 [158,164,169]. GSH also appears to exert some regulation over HIF-1alpha [157], regulates chemokine receptor expression [170], and appears to increase levels of IL-1a [171]. This cytokine profile leads to increased recruitment of neutrophils and macrophages [172,173], and, in general such a profile would produce chronic inflammation even in the absence of pathogen challenge.

However, under conditions of chronic GSH deficiency in RACP cells and in the extracellular milieu, the inflammation is for naught. GSH deficiency in neutrophils and macrophages decreases effectiveness of bactericidal action of these cells. There are several reasons for this: first, GSH deficiency in such cells produces premature apoptosis, both because GSH depletion is a necessary step in apoptosis, perhaps because GSH depletion is associated with the activation of sphingomyelinases [174], and because GSH deficiency allows for greater oxidant damage to these cells [46,175-186]. Second, GSH deficiency causes neutrophils to suffer microtubule damage, impaired release of lysosomal enzymes, depressed leukotaxis, and in general, decreased phagocytosis [46,187-189]. Third, premature apoptosis in a context of enhanced recruitment of neutrophils by cytokines causes increased spillage of toxic compounds and DNA into the extracellular milieu [190]. Such spillage promotes increased viscosity of secretions, increased oxidant and elastase burden, the establishment of a positive feedback loop to IL-8 production and further neutrophil recruitment, and, in general, an increased opportunity for pathogenic lung colonization [190]. Fourth, GSH appears to regulate the oxidative burst of neutrophils, with GSH deficiency leading to decreased burst activity [191]. The interplay of GSH and NO in bactericidal action will be discussed in a separate section below.

The immune response also becomes abnormal under conditions of chronic GSH deficiency because of an alteration of Th1/Th2 response. Depletion of GSH in antigen-presenting cells (APC, also a RACP cell) decreases interferon-gamma (IFN-gamma) and enhances Th2-associated humoral immunity responses at the expense of cell mediated immune response [147,192,193]. This alters the ability of APC to function normally, in part because GSH reduction of disulfide bonds is necessary for proteolysis of the antigen [147]. This interference of signalling between the APC and the T cells prevents proper T cell response [147,194,195]. Other cell signalling involving T cells may also be adversely affected [196]. As noted previously, IFN-gamma signalling is dysregulated by GSH depletion [148]. Extreme depletion of GSH in APC as well as in T cells has been shown to diminish both T cell proliferation and IL-12 production, as well as increasing apoptosis of T cells [147,195,197-207]. B cell and fibroblast proliferation also appears related to intracellular GSH level [208,209]. Activation and cytolytic activity of T cells and B cells is decreased with GSH depletion [193,210-214]. Again, this appears to be the result of cell structure abnormalities due to GSH depletion [215]. Movement towards a Th2 response has been associated with a negative outcome in many diseases [216-219].

D) Decreased Nitric Oxide Production and Availability

In the extracellular compartment, GSH deficiency will result in less extracellular GSNO, an important source of NO. In RACP cells (and perhaps non-RACP cells if depressed intracellular GSH:GSSG ratios were present in them), a variety of noteworthy consequences result. GSH deficiency has been shown to decrease iNOS expression and decrease levels of S-nitrosoglutathione (GSNO), which two phenomena may be interrelated [26-31]. NO and GSH appear to regulate cell energy metabolism [220,221], and NO stimulates enhanced expression of gamma-glutamylcysteine synthetase, the rate-limiting enzyme for GSH synthesis, apparently to counteract NO cytotoxicity [32-35]. GSNO is not only a reservoir of readily accessible NO, it is also a reservoir of easily accessible GSH, which becomes important under conditions in which cells become depleted of GSH through cytoprotective activities. Indeed, there appears to be a balance between GSH and GSNO, which under conditions of GSH depletion, favors cleavage of GSNO [222]. The balance appears to determine whether NO will be cytotoxic or cytoprotective [223-225]. Depletion of GSH markedly increases cell susceptibility to the harmful effects of peroxynitrite (ONOO-), leading to cytostasis and apoptosis [226-233]. In addition, under conditions of GSH depletion and resulting lower levels of GSNO (which is formed both intracellularly and extracellularly) and oxygen radical release from inflammatory cells, NO is readily transformed into nitrites and nitrates [234,235]. ONOO- has also been shown to inactivate glutathione reductase [113]. As NO is important in bactericidal action, lowered levels of NO significantly depress such action, leading to increased infection with organisms such as Pseudomonas aeruginosa [149]. GSH depletion reduces smooth muscle relaxation in response to NO, producing in the lung a tendency towards generalized bronchoconstriction [236,237]. NO also appears to regulate both the CFTR channel and a non-CFTR Cl- channel, and a decrease in NO leads to a decrease in conductance [238,239]. NO also appears to regulate ENaC sodium absorption via cGMP, with decreased NO leading to loss of the signal to downregulate sodium absorption [149,150]. Trans-epithelial potential difference, being regulated in part by sodium absorption, is thus seen to be regulated by iNOS, with decreased iNOS leading to increased potential difference [149]. Last, ciliary beat function is regulated by NO, with depletion of NO leading to impaired ciliary function [150].

Clinical Trials of GSH Use in CF Patients

If GSH transport plays a role in the pathophysiology of cystic fibrosis, then it is natural to ask whether rectification of this problem might provide therapeutic benefit to CF patients. There are various approaches that have been discussed in the literature:

Reinstatement of Cellular Glutathione Transport

One approach, advocated by the research team that includes Henry Forman and John Tomich, is to create a synthetic peptide that will create a channel in the cell membrane allowing glutathione efflux [240]. Though at least several years away from clinical trials, reinstatement of transport in this manner would arguably have great therapeutic significance.

Increased Synthesis of GSH through Cysteine Donors

As noted previously, cysteine is the rate-limiting component of GSH synthesis in the body. The use of cysteine donors, such as n-acetylcysteine (NAC) or special whey powders (e.g., Immunocal), will boost synthesis of GSH. Such an approach should not be overlooked, but increased synthesis will not solve the transport difficulties caused by CF mutation. The use of cysteine donors may well be complementary, however, to other approaches that tackle the transport problem more directly.

Exogenous Augmentation of GSH

Provision of GSH to the extracellular milieu could be therapeutic in CF. First, increasing the total level of glutathione and the redox ratio in the extracellular compartments of interest, expecially the lung, would decrease oxidant damage and also promote proper mucus viscosity. Second, ample extracellular GSH can rectify any chronic GSH deficit in RACP cells, with immune system cells of most interest here. Such rectification could help dampen the chronic exuberant inflammation characteristic of CF, as well as increase the efficacy of pathogen clearance. GSH augmentation has usually taken place in one of three ways: intravenous administration, oral administration, and aerosolized administration. Given that CF patients would have to use GSH on a daily basis as a maintenance therapy, the usefulness of IV administration is highly questionable. However, both oral administration and aerosolized glutathione deserve a more detailed discussion.

Oral Administration of GSH

There have been no clinical trials of oral glutathione in CF patients. We urge such trials, as alleviation of aspects of gastrointestinal symptoms in CF, as well as thinning of lung mucus, have been reported anecdotally by CF patients with use of oral glutathione. Some have argued that uptake of intact GSH by transporters in the human jejunum, though present, as noted previously, is not very effective. However, such studies have not considered long term use by a patient group with such a unique pathology involving cellular efflux of glutathione.

Aerosol Administration of GSH

There have been ten in vivo trials of aerosolized glutathione, with three of those trials focussing on CF patients [241-250]. In the first CF trial, whose principal investigator was James Roum, unbuffered GSH was administered for three days, b.i.d., each dose being 600 mg, to 7 CF patients [247]. Roum found the treatment well tolerated, and also that superoxide anion release by ELF inflammatory cells was significantly reduced. In the second trial, whose PI was Matthias Griese, 17 CF patients received buffered GSH (pH 7.0) over a 14 day period, with the maximum dose being 450 mg t.i.d [249]. Griese found restoration of normal levels of total glutathione in the ELF, with ELF total glutathione still doubled over baseline levels after twelve hours. Though inhalation was immediately followed by a transient drop in FEV1, this was spontaneously reversed in less than one hour, and the treatment was well tolerated. By the end of the trial, peak expiratory flow, FEV1, and FVC had all increased significantly by 6-7%. However, number of neutrophils, total protein, fraction of carbonyls and reduced thiols, and lipid peroxide content of BAL fluid remained unchanged. The third trial was controlled, with 10 CF patients on treatment and 9 on placebo with the PI being Clark Bishop [250]. Dosage was 66 mg/kg/day, divided into 4 doses given every 3-4 waking hours apart of buffered glutathione (pH approximately 6.0). Bishop also found the treatment to be well tolerated, and found peak flow to be significantly increased, and in an ancillary compliant analysis found cough to be signficantly decreased. FEF25-75 tended toward significant improvement, as well.

Other Approaches

Other approaches include aerosol administration of GSNO, which provides not only NO, but GSH as well to the lung compartment [251]. Complements to glutathione-centered approaches include support of a healthy glutathione system, which demands appropriate levels of riboflavin, selenium, magnesium, ascorbate, and E. Still other approaches include coaxing the expression of MRP-type channels at the apical surface of lung epithelia, through the use of agents such as colchicine [252]. These channels would then provide natural glutathione efflux.

Conclusion

Cystic fibrosis is, among other things, the first identified glutathione transport disease. Though cystic fibrosis is certainly multi-factorial, the pathophysiology of this disease appears to be linked, at least in part, to CFTR mutation-derived glutathione transport dysfunction. This new perspective on cystic fibrosis suggests possible therapeutic interventions that might offer significant amelioration of symptoms. In three small scale clinical trials of aerosolized glutathione in CF patients no adverse events were noted, and in two of the three trials, significant improvement in one or more measures of lung function were found even with as little as two weeks' use. This encouraging beginning deserves follow-up, with large scale, multi-center clinical trials, examining not only aerosolized glutathione, but oral glutathione as well. Such a small and inexpensive intervention may well turn out to make a large difference in the lives of CF patients.

References

[1] Skach, W. R. *Cystic fibrosis: methods and protocols*. Humana Press; Totowa, NJ 2002.

[2] Boucher, R. C. New concepts of the pathogenesis of cystic fibrosis lung disease. *Eur. Respir. J. Jan* 23(1):146-158; 2004.

[3] Roomans, G. M. Pharmacological approaches to correcting the ion transport defect in cystic fibrosis. *Am. J. Respir. Med.* 2(5):H13-31; 2003.

[4] Coakley, R. D.; Grubb, B. R.; Paradiso, A. M.; Gatzu, J. T.; Johnson, L. G.; Kreda, S. M.; O'Neal, W. K.; Boucher, R. C. Abnormal surface liquids p++ regulation by cultured cystic fibrosis bronchial epithelium. *Proc. Natl. Acad. Sc. USA*. Dec 23, 100(26):16083-16088; 2003.

[5] McShane, D.; Davies, J. C.; Davies, M. G.; Bush, A.; Geddes, D. M.; Alton, E. W. Airway surface p++ in subjects with cystic fibrosis. JOURNAL?

[6] Linsdell P and JW Hanrahan, "Glutathione Permeability of CFTR," *Am. J. Physiol. - Cell Physiol*. 44(1): C323-C326, 1998 July.

[7] Gao L, Kim KJ, Yankaskas JR, Forman HJ, "Abnormal glutathione transport in cystic fibrosis airway epithelia," *Am J Physiol Lung Cell Mol Physiol* 1999 Jul;277(1):L113-8.

[8] Kogan I, Ramjeesingh M, Kidd J, Li C, Wang Y, Bear CE, "Characterization of glutathione permeability through the CFTR channel pore," *Ped Pulmonol* 2002 Oct; 24:189-90.

[9] Kogan I, Ramjessingh M, Li C, Kidd JF, Wang Y, Leslie EM, Cole SPC, Bear CE, "CFTR directly mediates nucleotide-regulated glutathione flux," *EMBO*, 2003 May 1; 22(9):1981-9.

[10] Velsor LW, van Heeckeren A, Day BJ, "Antioxidant imbalance in the lungs of cystic fibrosis transmembrane conductance regulator protein mutant mice," *Am J Physiol Lung Cell Mol Physiol* 2001 Jul;281(1):L31-8

[11] Finder, J. D.; Engman, C. L.; Kagan, V. E.; Tyurina, Y. Y. Brondoalveolar lavage fluid from patients with cystic fibrosis have diminished levels of reduced glututione. *Ped. Pulm. Supplement* 25; A158; 239; 2003.

[12] Meister, A. Glutathione metabolism. *Methods Enzymol* 251:3-7; 1995.

[13] Buhl R et al., "Augmentation of the Antioxidant Screen of the Epithelial Surface of the Lower Respiratory Tract by Aerosol Administration of Glutathione," *Proc. Natl. Acad. Sci.* USA 87:4063-67, 1990 June.

[14] Iantomasi T et al., "Glutathione transport system in human small intestine epithelial cells," *Biochim. Biophys. Acta* 1330(2): 274-83, 1997 December 4.

[15] Hunjan MK and DF Evered, "Absorption of glutathione from the gastro-intestinal tract," Biochim. *Biophys. Acta* 815(2): 184-8, 1985 May 14.

[16] Favilli F et al., "Effect of orally administered glutathione on glutathione levels in some organs of rats: role of specific transporters," Br. J. Nutr. 78(2): 293-300, 1997 August.

[17] Hagen TM et al., "Bioavailability of dietary glutathione: effect on plasma concentration," *Am. J. Physiol.* 259 (4 Pt 1): G524-9, 1990 October.

[18] Vina, J.; Bannister, J. V.; Bannister, W. H. *Glutathione: metabolism and physiological functions*. CRC Press: Boca Raton, FL; 1990.

[19] Pietarinen-Runtti P, Lakari E, Raivio KO, Kinnula VL, "Expression of antioxidant enzymes in human inflammatory cells," *Am J Physiol Cell Physiol* 2000 Jan; 278(1):C118-25.

[20] Rahman I, MacNee W, "Lung glutathione and oxidative stress: implications in cigarette smoke-induced airway disease," *Am J Physiol* 1999, 277 (Lung Cell Molecular Physiol 21): L1067-L1088.

[21] Kelly FJ, "Glutathione: in defence of the lung," *Food Chem Toxicol* 1999 Sep-oct; 37(9-10):963-6.

[22] Cantin A. M.; North S. L.; Hubbard R. C.; Crystal R. G.; "Normal alveolar epithelial lining fluid contains high levels of glutathione," *J Appl Physiol* 1987, 63:152-157.

[23] Klatt, P.; Lamas, S. Regulation of protein function by S-glutathiolation in response to oxidative and nitrosative stress. *Eur. J. Biochem.* Aug 267(16):4928-4944; 2000.

[24] Noszal B, Visky D, Kraszni M, "Population, acid-base, and redox properties of N-acetylcysteine conformers," *J Med Chem* 43(11):2176-82, 2000 Jun 1

[25] Ziment I, "Acetylcysteine: a drug that is much more than a mucokinetic," *Biomed Pharmacother* 42(8):513-9, 1988.

[26] Chen G, Wang SH, Warner TD, "Regulation of iNOS mRNA levels in endothelial cells by glutathione, a double-edged sword," *Free Radic Res* 2000 Mar;32(3):223-34

[27] Kang KW, Pak YM, Kim ND, "Diethylmaleate and buthionine sulfoximine, glutathione-depleting agents, differentially inhibit expression of inducible nitric oxide synthase in endotoxemic mice," *Nitric Oxide* 1999 Jun;3(3):265-271.

[28] Vos TA, Goor H, Tuyt L, Jager-Krikken A, Leuvenink R, Kuipers F, Jansen PL, Moashage H, "Expression of inducible nitric oxide synthase in endotoxemic rat hepatocytes is dependent on the cellular glutathione status," *Hepatology* 1999 Feb;29(2):421-426.

[29] Wang F, Wang LY, Wright D, Parmely MJ, "Redox imbalance differentially inhibits lipopolysaccharide-induced macrophage activation in the mouse liver," *Infect Immun* 1999 Oct;67(10):5409-5416.

[30] Davidson CA, Kaminski PM, Wolin MS, "NO elicits prolonged relaxation of bovine pulmonary arteries via endogenous peroynitrite generation," *Am J Physiol* 1997 Aug;273(2 Pt 1):L437-444.

[31] Singh SP et al., "The chemistry of the S-nitrosoglutathione/glutathione system," *Proc. Natl. Acad. Sci., USA*, 93:14428-14433, 1996 December.

[32] Moellering D, McAndrew J, Patel RP, Cornwell T, Lincoln T, Cao X, Messina JL, Forman HJ, Jo HJ, Darleyusmar VM, "Nitric oxide-dependent induction of glutathione synthesis through increased expression of gamma-glutamylcysteine synthetase," *Archives of Biochemistry and Biophysics* 1998 Oct 1;358(1):74-82.

[33] Li H, Marshall ZM, Whorton AR, "Stimulation of cystine uptake by nitric oxide:regulation of endothelial cell glutathione levels," *Am J Physiol* 1999 Apr;276(4 Pt 1):C803-11.

[34] Kuo PC, Abe KY, Schroeder RA, "Interleukin-1-induced nitric oxide production modulates glutathione synthesis in cultured rat hepatocytes," *Am J Physiol* 1996 Sep;271(3 Pt 1):C851-862.

[35] Levonene AL, Laasko J, Vaskonen T, Mervaala E, Karppanen H, Lapatto R, "Down-regulation of renal glutathione synthesis by systemic nitric oxide synthesis inhibition in spontaneously hypertensive rats," *Biochem Pharmacol* 2000 Feb 15;59(4):441-443.

[36] Gao L, Kim KJ, Yankaskas JR, Forman HJ, “Abnormal glutathione transport in cystic fibrosis airway epithelia,” *Am J Physiol Lung Cell Mol Physiol* 1999 Jul;277(1):L113-118.

[37] Tirouvanziam RM, Tjioe I, Moss RB, Parks DR, Herzenberg LA, Wine JJ, “Multiparameter study of CF blood and lung leukocytes using 3-laser, 11-color cytometry,” *Ped Pulmonol* 2001 Oct; 22:271-272.

[38] Lands LC, Grey V, Smountas AA, Kramer VG, McKenna D, "Lymphocyte glutathione levels in children with cystic fibrosis," *Chest* 1999 Jul;116(1):201-205.

[39] Abraham EH, Sterling KM, Kim RJH, Parker HW, Boyle WE, "Expression of CFTR and of DF508 CFTR in the reb blood cell membrane," abstract presented at the 13th

Annual European Cystic Fibrosis Conference, June 2000, Stockholm, Sweden, abstract 14.

[40] Roum JH, Buhl R, McElvaney NG, Borok Z, Crystal RG, "Systemic deficiency of glutathione in cystic fibrosis," *J Appl Physiol* 1993 Dec;75(6):2419-2424.

[41] Brown RK, Wyatt H, Price JF, Kelly FJ, "Pulmonary dysfunction in cystic fibrosis is associated with oxidative stress," *Eur Respir J* 1996;9:334-339.

[42] Hagiwara K, Naito K, Kurokawa Y, Ichikawa T, "Kidney injury induced by lipid peroxide produced by vitamin E deficiency and GSH depletion in rats," *J Nutr Sci Vitaminol* (Tokyo) 1991 Feb; 37(1):99-107.

[43] Tabary O, Escotte S, Couetil JP, Hubert D, Dusser D, Puchelle E, Jacquot J, "Genistein inhibits constitutive and inducible NFkappaB activation and decreases IL-8 production by human cystic fibrosis bronchial gland cells," *Am J Pathol* 1999 Aug;155(2):473-481.

[44] Wong CH et al., "Cough Induced by Low pH," *Respiratory Medicine.* 93(1):58-61, 1999 January.

[45] Jurima-Romet M and PN Shek, "Lung Uptake of Liposome-entrapped Glutathione After Intratracheal Administration," *J. Pharm. Pharmacol.* 43:6-10, 1991.

[46] Boxer LA, Oliver JM, Speilberg SP, Allen JM, Schulman JD, "Protection of Granulocytes by Vitamin E in Glutathione Synthetase Deficiency," *New Engl J Med* 1979 Oct 25;301(17): 901-905.

[47] Rahman Q, Abidi P, Afaq F, Schiffmann D, Mossman BT, Kamp DW, Athar M, "Glutathione redox system in oxidative lung injury," *Crit Rev Toxicol* 1999 Nov; 29(6):543-568.

[48] Smith LJ, Anderson J, "Oxygen-induced lung damage. Relationship to lung mitochondrial glutathione levels," *Am Rev Respir Dis* 1992 Dec;146(6):1452-1457.

[49] Abidi P, Afaq F, Arif JM, Lohani M, Rahman Q, "Chrysolite-mediated imbalance in the glutathione redox system in the development of pilmonary injury," *Toxicol Lett* 1999 May 20;106(1):31-39.

[50] Thanislass J, Raveendran M, Devaraj H, "Buthionine sulfoximine-induced glutathione depletion. Its effect on antioxidants, lipid peroxidation and calcium homeostasis in the lung," *Biochem Pharmacol* 1995 Jul 17; 50(2):229-234.

[51] Forman HJ, Gao L, Broughman J, Iwamoto T, Venglarik CJ, Tomich JM, "Glutathione Transpoet and Impaired Antioxidant Function in Cystic Fibrosis," *symposium session S16.4 presented at the Fourteenth Annual North American Cystic Fibrosis Conference,* Baltimore, Maryland, November 9-12, 2000.

[52] Lauterburg BH, and ME Velez, "Glutathione deficiency in alcoholics: risk factor for paracetamol hepatotoxicity," *Gut* 29(9):1153-1157, 1988 Sep.

[53] Fernandez-Checa JC et al., "Mitochondrial glutathione depletion in alcoholic liver disease," *Alcohol* 10(6):469-475.

[54] Purucker E et al., "Glutathione status in liver and plasma during development of biliary cirrhosis after bile duct ligation," *Res Exp Med* (Berlin) 198(4):167-174, 1998 Dec.

[55] Loguercio C et al., "Effect of liver cirrhosis and age on the glutathione concentration in the plasma, erythrocytes, and gastric mucosa of man," *Free Radic Biol Med* 20(3):483-488, 1996.

[56] Barbaro G, Di Lorenzo G, Soldini M, Bellomo G, Belloni G, Grisorio B, Barbarini G, "Vagal system impairment in human immunodeficiency virus-positive patients with

chronic hepatitis C: does hepatic glutathione deficiency have a pathogenic role?," *Sand J Gastroenterol* 1997 Dec; 32(12):1261-1256.

[57] Nath RG, Ocando JE, Richie JP Jr, Chung FL, "Effect of glutathione depletion on exocyclic adduct levels in the liver DNA of F344 rats," *Chem Res Toxicol* 1997 Nov;10(11):1250-1253.

[58] Sokol RJ, Taylor SF, Devereaux MW, Khandwala R, Sondheimer NJ, Shikes RH, Mierau G, "Hepatic oxidant injury and glutathione depletion during total parenteral nutrition in weanling rats," *Am J Physiol* 1996 Apr;270(4 Pt 1):G691-700.

[59] Ankrah NA, Dunyo SK, Nyarko AK, Appiah-Opong R, Ofsuhene M, "Biliary excretion in persons with low blood glutathione," *East Afr Med J* 1998 Apr;75(4):204-207.

[60] Wang X, Kanel GC, DeLeve LD, "Support of sinusoidal endothelial cell glutathione prevents hepatic veno-occlusive disease in the rat," *Hepatology* 2000 Feb;31(2):428-434.

[61] Bouchard G, Yousef IM, Barriault C, Tuchweber B, "Role of glutathione and oxidative stress in phalloidin-induced cholestasis," *J Heptaol* 2000 Apr; 32(4):550-560.

[62] Kobayashi T, Robinson MK, Robinson V, DeRosa E, Wilmore DW, Jacobs DO, "Glutathione depletion alters hepatocellular high-energy phosphate metabolism," *J Surg Res* 1993 Mar;54(3):189-195.

[63] Demols A, Van Laethem JL, Quertinmont E, Legros F, Louis H, LeMoine O, Deviere J, "N-acetylcysteine decreases severity of acute pancreatitits in mice," *Pancreas* 2000 Mar; 20(2):161-169.

[64] Gomez-Cambronero L, Camps B,de La Asuncion JG, Cerda M, Pellin A, Pallardo FV, Calvete J, Sweiry JH, Mann GE, Vina J, Sastre J, "Pentoxifylline ameliorates cerulein-induced pancreatitits in rats: role of glutathione and nitric oxide," *J Pharmacol Exp Ther* 2000 May 1;293(2):670-676.

[65] Wallig MA, *"Xenobiotic metabolism, oxidant stress and chronic pancreatitis: focus on glutathione,"* Digestion 1998;59 Suppl 4:13-24.

[66] Paulusma CC, van Geer MA, Evers R, Heijn M, Ottenhoff R, Borst P, Oude Elferink RP, "Canalicular multispecific organic anion transporter/multidrug resistance protein 2 mediates low-affinity transport of reduced glutathione," *Biochem J* 1999 Mar 1;338(Pt 2):393-401.

[67] Ho E, Chen G, Bray TM, "Supplementation of N-acetylcysteine inhibits NFkappaB activation and protects against alloxan-induced diabetes in CD-1 mice," *FASEB J* 1999 Oct; 13(13):1845-1854.

[68] Vijayalingam S, Parthiban A, Shanmugasundaram KR, Mohan V, "Abnormal antioxidant status in impaired glucose tolerance and non-insulin-dependent diabetes mellitus," *Diabet Med* 1996 Aug; 13(8):715-719.

[69] Papadopoulos MC, Koumenis IL, Dugan LL, Giffard RG, "Vulnerability to glucose deprivation injury correlates with glutathione levels in astrocytes," *Brain Res* 1997 Feb 14;748(1-2):151-156.

[70] Ciuchi E, Odetti P, Prando R, "The effect of acute glutathione treatment on sorbitol level in erythrocytes from diabetic patients," *Diabetes Metb* 1997 Feb;23(1):58-60.

[71] Ankrah NA, Appiah-Opong R, "Toxicity of low levels of methylglyoxal: depletion of blood glutathione and adverse effect on glucose tolerance in mice," *Toxicol Lett* 1999 Sep 20;109(1-2):61-67.

[72] Domninguez C, Ruiz E, Gussinye M, Carrascosa A, "Oxidative stress at onset and in early stages of type 1 diabetes in children and adolescents," *Diabetes Care* 1998 Oct;21(10):1736-1742.

[73] Paolisso G et al., "Plasma GSH/GSSG affects glucose homeostasis in healthy subjects and non-insulin dependent diabetics," *Am J Physiol* 262(3 Pt. 1): E435-40, 1992 Sep.

[74] Agha AM, El-Khatib AS, Al-Zuhair H, "Modulation of oxidant status by meloxicam in experimentally induced arthritis," *Pharmacol Res* 1999 Oct;40(4):385-392.

[75] Raya A, Gallego J, Bosch-Morell F, Roma J, Romero FJ, "Phenytoin-induced glutathione depletion in rat peripheral nerve," *Free Radic Biol Med* 1995 Nov;19(5):665-567.

[76] Lee KJ, Andrejuk T, Dziuban SW Jr, Goldfarb RD, "Deleterious effects of buthionine sulfoximine on cardiac function during continuous endotoxemia," *Proc Soc Exp Biol Med* 1995 Jun;209(2):178-184.

[77] Ardite E, Sanas M, Panes J, Romero FJ, Pique JM, Fernandez-Checa JC, "Replenishment of glutathione levels improves mucosal function in experimental acute colitis," *Lab Invest* 2000 May;80(5):735-744.

[78] Goldin E, Ardite E, Elizalde JI, Odriozola A, Panes J, Pique JM, Fernanadez-Checa JC, "Gastric mucosal damage in experimental diabetes in rats: role of endogenous glutathione," *Gastroenterology* 1997 Mar;112(3):855-863.

[79] Yoshikawa T, Minamiyama Y, Ichikawa H, Takahashi S, Naito Y, Kondo M, "Role of lipid peroxidation and antioxidants in gastric mucosal injury induced by hypoxanthine-xanthine oxidase system in rats," *Free Radic Biol Med* 1997;23(2):243-250.

[80] Sido B, Hack V, Hochlehnert A, Lipps H, Herfarth C, Droge W, "Impairment of intestinal glutathione synthesis in patients with inflammatory bowel disease," *Gut* 1998 Apr;42(4):485-492.

[81] Miralles-Barrachina O, Savoye G, Belmonte-Zalar L, Hochain P, Ducrotte P, Hecketsweiler B, Lerebours E, Dechelotte P, "Low levels of glutathione in endoscopic biopsies of patients with Crohn's colitis: the role of malnutrition," *Clin Nutr* 1999 Oct;18(5):313-317.

[82] Bengmark S and Heppsson B, "Gastrointestinal surface protection and mucosa reconditioning," *J. Parenter Enteral Nutr* 19(5):410-5, 1995 Sep-Oct.

[83] Tolosa de Talamini N, Marchionatti A, Baudino V, Alisio A, "Glutathione plays a role in the chick intestinal calcium absorption," *Comp Biochem Physiol A Physiol* 1996 Oct;115(2):127-132.

[84] Ushmorov A, Hack V, Droge W, "Differential reconstitution of mitochondrial respiratory chain activity and plasma redox state by cysteine and ornithine in a model of cancer cachexia," *Cancer Res* 1999 Jul 15;59(14):3527-3534.

[85] Liberman MW, Wiseman AL, Shi ZZ, Carter BZ, Barrios R, Ou CN, Chevez-Barrios P, Wang Y, Habib GM, Goodman JC, Huang SL, Lebovitz RM, Matzuk MM, "Growth retardation and cysteine deficiency in gamma-glutamyl transpeptidase-deficient mice," *Proc Natl Acad Sci USA* 1996 Jul 23;93(15):7923-7926.

[86] Droge W, "Cysteine and glutathione in catabolic conditions and immunological dysfunction," *Curr Opin Clin Nutr Metab Care*, 1999 May;2(3):227-233.

[87] Golden MH, "Oedematous malnutrition," *Br Med Bull* 1998;54(2):433-444.

[88] Scholz RW et al., "Mechanism of Interaction of Vitamin E and Glutathione in the Protection against Lipid Peroxidation," *Annals of the New York Academy of Sciences*, 570:514-517, 1989.

[89] Higuchi, Y, Matsukawa S, "Glutathione depletion induces giant DNA and high-molecular-weight DNA fragmentation associated with apoptosis through lipid peroxidation and protein kinase C activation in C6 glioma cells," *Arch Biochem Biphys* 1999 Mar; 1;363(1):33-42

[90] Scholz RW, Reddy PV, Wynn MK, Graham KS, Liken AD, Gumpricht E, Reddy CC, "Glutathione-dependent factors and inhibition of rat liver microsomal lipid peroxidation," *Free Radic Biol Med* 1997; 23(5):815-28

[91] Thanislass J, Raveendran M, Devaraj H, "Buthionine sulfoximine-induced glutathione depletion. Its effect on antioxidants, lipid peroxidation and calcium homeostasis in the lung," *Biochem Pharmacol* 1995 Jul 17; 50(2):229-34

[92] Hagiwara K, Naito K, Kurokawa Y, Ichikawa T, "Kidney injury induced by lipid peroxide produced by vitamin E deficiency and GSH depletion in rats," *J Nutr Sci Vitaminol* (Tokyo) 1991 Feb; 37(1):99-107

[93] Angelini P, Cirelli F, Quarticelli A, Chicco D, Vendemiale G, Altomare E, "Administration of glutatione and lipid peroxidation induced during fasting," *Boll Soc Ital Biol Sper* 1990 Nov; 66(11):1097-1104

[94] Rosenblat M, Aviram M, "Macrophage glutathione content and glutathione peroxidase activity are inversely related to cell-mediated oxidation of LDL: in vitro and in vivo studies," *Free Radic Biol Med* 1998 Jan 15;24(2):305-317.

[95] Freedman SD, Katz MH, Parker EM, Laposata M, Urman MY, Alvarez JG, "A membrane lipid imbalance plays a role in the phenotypic expression of cystic fibrosis in cftr (-/-) mice," *Proc Natl Acad Sci* USA 1999 Nov 23; 96(24):13995-4000.

[96] Chen Q, Galleano M, Cederbaum AI, "Cytotoxicity and apoptosis produced by arachidonic acid in Hep G2 cells overexpressing human cytochrome P4502E1," *J Biol Chem* 1997 Jun 6;272(23):14532-14541.

[97] Montuschi P, Karitonov SA, Ciabattoni G, Corradi M, van Rensen L, Geddes DM, Hodson ME, Barnes PJ, "Exhaled 8-isoprostane as a new non-invasive biomarker of oxidative stress in cystic fibrosis," *Thorax*, 2000, 55(3):205-209.

[98] Buhl R et al, "Oxidant-Protease Interaction in the Lung: Prospects for Antioxidant Therapy," *Chest*, 110(6): 267S-272S, 1996 December supplement.

[99] Gillissen A, Birrer P, McElvaney NG, Buhl R, Vogelmeier C, Hoyt RF Jr, Hubbard RC, Crystal RG, "Recombinant secretory leukoprotease inhibitor augments gluathione levels in lung epithelial lining fluid," *J Appl Physiol* 1993 Aug;75(2):825-32

[100] Vogelmeier C, Biedermann T, Maier K, Mazur G, Behr J, Krombach F, Buhl R, "Comparative loss of activity of recombinant sefretory leukoprotease inhibitor and alpha 1-protease inhibitor caused by different forms of oxidative streaa," *Eur Respir J* 1997 Sep;10(9):2114-9

[101] Barbero, GJ, "Therapeutic Approaches to Cystic Fibrosis," *Bulletin of the World Health Organization*, 72(3): 341-352, 1994.

[102] Brenneisen P. Briviba K, Wlaschek M, Wenk J, Scharffetter-Kochanel K, "Hydrogen peroxide (H2O2) increases the steady-state mRNA levels of collagenase/MMP-1 in human dermal fibroblasts," *Free Radic Biol Med* 1997;22(3):515-524.

[103] Jain A et al., "Ascorbic acid prevents oxidative stress in glutathione deficient mice: effects on lung type 2 cell lamellar bodies, lung surfactant, and skeletal muscle," *Proc. Natl. Acad. Sci.* USA 89(11):5093-7, 1992 June.

[104] Jain A, Mehta T, Auld PA, Rodrigues J, Ward RF, Schwartz MK, Martensson J, "Glutathione metabolism in newborns: evidence for glutathione deficiency in plasma, bronchoalveolar lavage fluid, and lymphocytes in prematures," *Pediatr Pulmonol* 1995 Sep;20(3):160-156.

[105] Madesh M, Benard O, Balasubramanian KA, "Glutathione modulates lipid composition of human colon derived HT-29 cells," *Int J Biochem Cell Biol* 1998 Dec;30(12):1345-1352.

[106] Boda D, Nemeth I, Pinter S, "Surface tension, glutathione contenet and redox ratio of the tracheal aspirate fluid of premature infants with IRDS," *Biol Neonate* 1998 Oct;74(4):281-288.

[107] Supinski G, "Free radical induced respiratory muscle dysfunction," *Mol Cell Biochem* 1998 Feb;179(1-2):99-110.

[108] Bounous G, Molson J, "Competition for glutathione precursors between the immune system and the skeletal muscle: pathogenesis of chronic fatigue syndrome," *Med Hypotheses* 1999 Oct;53(4):347-349.

[109] Shaheen SO, Sterne JA, Songhurst CE, Burney PG, "Frequent paracetamol use and asthma in adults," *Thorax* 2000 Apr;55(4):266-270.

[110] Ogino T et al., "Neutrophil Antioxidant Capacity During the Respiratory Burst -- Loss of Glutathione Induced by Chloramines," *Free Radical Biology and Medicine* 23(3): 445-452, 1997.

[111] Bilzer M and BH Lauterberg, "Gutathione metabolism in activated human neutrophils: stimulation of glutathione synthesis and consumption of glutathione by reactive oxygen species," *Eur. J. Clin. Investigation* 21(3): 316-322, 1991 June.

[112] Remiao F, Carmo H, Carvalho FD, Bastos ML, "Inhibition of glutathione reductase by isoproterenol oxidation products," *J Enzyme Inhib* 2000;15(1):47-61.

[113] Barker JE, Heales SJ, Cassidy A, Bolanos JP, Land JM, Clark JB, *"Depletion of brain glutathione results in a decrease of glutathione reductase activity; an enzyme susceptible to oxidative damage,"* Brain Res 1996 Apr 15;16(1-2):118-122.

[114] van Klaveren RJ, Hoet PH, Pype JL, Demedis M, Nemery B, "Increase in gamma-glutamyltransferase by glutathione depletion in rat type II pneumocytes," *Free Radic Biol Med* 1997;22(3):525-534.

[115] Li XY, Donaldson K, Rahman I, MacNee W, "An investigation of the role of glutathione in increased epithelial permeability induced by cigarette smoke in vivo and in vitro," *Am J Respir Crit Care Med* 1994 Jun;149(6):1518-1525.

[116] Kokura S, Wolf RE, Yoshikawa T, Granger DN, AW TY, "Molecular mechanisms of neutrophil-endothelial cell adhesion induced by redox imbalance," *Cric Res* 1999 Mar 19;84(5):516-524.

[117] Freeman ML, Huntley SA, Meredith MJ, Senisterra GA, Lepock J, "Destabilization and denaturation of cellular protein by glutathione depletion," *Cell Stress Chaperones* 1997 Sep;2(3):191-198.

[118] Calabreses V, Testa G, Ravagna A, Bates TE, Guiffrida Stella AM, "HSP70 induction in the brain following ethanol administration in the rat: regulation by glutathione redox state," *Biochem Biophys Res Commun* 2000 Mar 16;269(2):397-400.

[119] Liu H, Lightfoot R, Stevens JL, "Activation of heat shock factor by alkylating agents is triggered by glutathione depletion and oxidation of protein thiols," *J Biol Chem* 1996 Mar 1;271(9):4805-4812.

[120] Wilhelm D, Bender K, Knebel A, Angel P, "The level of intracellular glutathione is a key regulator for the induction of stress-activated signal transduction pathways including Jun N-terminal protein kinases and p38 kinase by alkylating agents," *Mol Cell Biol* 1997 Aug ; 17(8):4792-4800

[121] Kirlin WG, Cai J, Thompson SA, Diaz D, Kavanagh TJ, Jones DP, "Glutathione redox potential in response to differentiation and enzyme inducers," *Free Radic Biol Med* 1999 Dec;27(11-12):1208-18

[122] Lertratanangkoon K, Savaraj N, Scimeca JM, Thomas ML, "Glutathione depletion-induced thymidylate insufficiency for DNA repair synthesis," *Biochem Biophys Res Commun* 1997 May 19;234(2):470-475.

[123] Asensi M, Garcia-Espana A, Pallardo FV, Vina J, Esrrela JM, "Effect of nonprotein thiols on protein synthesis in isolated rat hepatocytes," *Experientia* 1996 Feb 15;52(2):111-114.

[124] Fussell JC, Kelly FJ, "Effects of deamethasone on lung protein turnover," *Biochem J* 273(Pt 1):93-7. 1991 Jan 1.

[125] Murthy MR, "Protein synthesis in growing-rat tissues. II. Polyribosome cocentration of brain and liver as a function of age," *Biochim Biophys Acta* 119(3):599-613, 1966 Jun 22.

[126] Thanislass J, Raveendran M, Sivasithamparam N, Devaraj H, "Effect of chronic glutathione deficiency on rat lung mitochondrial function," *Pulm Pharmacol* 1996 Apr;9(2):119-122.

[127] Rojas E, Valverde M, Kala SV, Kala G, Lieberman MW, "Accumulation of DNA damage in the organs of mice deficient in gamma-glutamyltranspeptidase," *Mutat Res* 2000 Feb 14;447(2):305-316.

[128] Gilmont RR, Dardano A, Young M, Engle JS, Adamson BS, Smith DJ Jr, Rees RS, "Effects of glutathione depletion on oxidant-induced endothelial cell injury," *J Surg Res* 1998 Nov;80(1):62-68.

[129] Fiorentini, C, Falzano L, Rivabene R, Fabbri A, Malorni W, "N-acetylcysteine protects epithelial cells against the antioxidant imbalance due to Clostridium difficile toxins," *FEBS Lett* 1999 Jun 18;453(1-2):124-128.

[130] Kamei H, "Cystine starvation induces reversible large-body formation from nuclear bodies in T24 cells," *Exp Cell Res* 1997 Nov 25;237(1):207-216.

[131] Zuelke KA, Jones DP, Perreault SD, "Glutathione oxidation is associated with altered microtubule function and disrupted fertilization in mature hamster oocytes," *Biol Reprod* 1997 Dec;57(6):1413-1439.

[132] Jain A, Martensson J, Mehta T, Krauss AN, Auld PM, Meister A, "Ascorbic acid prevents oxidative stress in glutathione-deficient mice: Effects on lung type 2 lamellar bodies, lung surfactant, and skeletal muscle," *Proc Natl Acad Sc USA*, 1992 June :89: 5093-5097.

[133] Moss M, Guidot DM, Wong-Lambertina M, Ten Hoor T, Perez RL, Brown LA, "The effects of chronic alcohol abuse on pulmonary glutathione homeostasis," *Am J Respir Crit Care Med* 2000 Feb 1;161(2 Pt 1):414-419

[134] Kitamura, S, "The 74th annual meeting president lecture: Pathogenesis and therapy of acute lung injury," *Kekkaku* 1999 Sep; 74(9):693-697.

[135] Rahman I, Skwarska E, Henry M, Davis M, O'Connor CM, FitzGerald MX, Greening A, MacNee, W, "Systemic and pulmonary oxidative stress in idiopathic pulmonary fibrosis," *Free Rad Biol Med* 1999 Jul;27(1-2):60-8

[136] Behr J, Degenkolb B, Maier K, Braun B, Beinert T, Krombach F, Vogelmeier C, Fruhmann G, "Increased oxidation of extracellular glutathione by bronchoalveolar inflammatory cells in diffuse fibrosing alveolitis," *Eur Respir J* 1995 Aug; 8(8):1286-1292.

[137] Staal FJT, Ela SW, Roederer M, Anderson MT, Herzenberg LA, "Glutathione deficiency and human immunodeficiency virus infection," *Lancet* 1992; 339:909-912.

[138] Pacht ER, Diaz P, Clanton T, Hart J, Gadek JE, "Alveolar glutathione fluid decreases in asymptomatic HIV-seropositive subjects over time," *Chest* 1997 Sep;112(3):785-788.

[139] Smith CV, Jones DP, Guenther TM, Lash, LH, Lauterberg BH, "Compartmentation of Glutathione: Implications for the Study of Toxicity and Disease," *Toxic and Appl Pharmacol* 140, 1-12, 1996.

[140] Houtmeyers E, Gosselink R, Gayan-Ramirez G, Decramer M, "Regulation of mucociliary clearance in health and disease," Eur Respir J 1999 May; 13(5):1177-1188.

[141] King M, Rubin BK, "Mucus-controlling agents: past and present," *Respir Care Clin N Am* 1999 Dec; 5(4):575-94

[142] Houtmeyers E, Gosselink R, Gayan-Ramirez G, Decramer M, "Effects of drugs on mucus clearance," *Eur Respir* J 1999 Aug;14(2):452-67

[143] Connolly MA, "Mucolytics and the critically ill patient: help or hindrance?" *AACN Clin Issues* 1995 May; 6(2):307-15

[144] Clarke SW, "Rationale of airway clearance," *Eur Respir J Suppl* 1989 Jul; 7:599s-603s.

[145] Jiang N, Dreher KL, Dye JA, Li Y, Richards JH, Martin LD, Adler KB, "Residual oil fly ash induces cytotoxicity and mucin secretion by guinea pig tracheal epithelial cells via an oxidant-mediated mechanism," *Toxicol Appl Pharmacol* 2000 Mar 15;163(3):221-230.

[146] Li JD, Feng W, Gallup M, Kim JH, Gum J, Kim Y, Basbaum C, "Activation of NF-kappaB via a Src-dependent Ras-MAPK-pp90rsk pathway is required for Pseudomonas aerugionosa-induced mucin overproduction in epithelial cells," *Proc Natl Acad Sci USA*, 1998, 95(10):5718-5723.

[147] Peterson JD, Herzenberg LA, Vasquez K, Waltenbaugh C, "Glutathione levels in antigen-presenting cells modulate Th1 versus Th2 response patterns," *PNAS* 1998 March 17;95(6):3071-3076.

[148] Galietta LJV, Folli C, Marchetti C, Romano L, Carpani D, Conese M, Zegarra-Moran O, "Modification of transepithelial ion transport in human cultured bronchial epithelial cells by interferon-gamma," *Am J Physiol - Lung Cell Mol Physiol* 2000 Jun;278(6):L1186-1194.

[149] Kelley TJ, Drumm ML, "Inducible nitric oxide synthase expression is reduced in cystic fibrosis murine and human airway epithelial cell lines," *J Clin Invest*, 1998 Sep;102(6):1200-1207.

[150] Mayer B, Pfeiffer S, Schrammel A, Koesling D, Schmidt K, Brunner F, "A new pathway of nitric oxide cylclic GMP signalling involving s-nitrosoglutathione," *J Biol Chem* 1998 Feb 6;273(6):3264-3270.

[151] Fischer B, Voynow J, "Neutrophil elastase induces MUC5AC messenger RNA expression by an oxidant-dependent mechanism," *Chest* 2000 May;117(5 Suppl 1):317S-320S.

[152] Cho S, Urata Y, Ilada T, Goto S, Yamaguchi M, Sumikawa K, Kondo T, "Glutathione downregulates the Phosphorylation of I kappa-B: Autoloop Regulation of the NF-kappa B-Mediated Expression of NF-kappa B Subunits by TNF-alpha in Mouse Vascular Endothelial Cells," *Biochemical and Biophysical Research Communications* 253(1):104-108, 1998.

[153] Droge W et al., "Modulation of Lymphocyte Functions and Immune Responses by Cysteine and Cysteine Derivatives," *The American Journal of Medicine* 91(3C): 140-143, 1991 September 30.

[154] Sen CK, Khanna S, Reznick AZ, Roy S, Packer L, "Glutathione regulation of tumor necrosis factor-alpha-induced NF-kappa B activation in skeletal muscle-derived L6 cells," *Biochem Biophys Res Commun* 1997 Aug 28;237(3):645-9

[155] Desai A, Huang X, Warren JS, "Intracellular glutathione redox status modulates MCP-1 expression in pulmonary granulomatous vasculitis," *Lab Invest* 1999 Jul;79(7):837-47

[156] Luo Y, Hattori A, Munoz J, Qin ZH, Roth GS, "Intrastriatal dopamine injection induces apoptosis through oxidation-involved activation of transcription factors AP-1 and NF-kappaB in rats," *Mol Pharmacol* 1999 Aug;56(2):254-64

[157] Haddad JJ, Olver RE, Land SC, "Antioxidant/pro-oxidant equilibrium regulates HIF-1alpha and NF-kappaB redox sensitivity: evidence for inhibition by glutathione oxidation in alveolar epithelial cells," *J Biol Chem* 2000 May 4

[158] Tanaka C, Kamata H, Takeshita H, Yagisawa H, Hirata H, "Redox regulation of lipopolysaccharide (LPS)-induced interleukin-8 (IL-8) gene expression mediated by NF kappa B and AP-1 in human astrocytoma U373 cells," *Biochem Biophys Res Commun* 1997 Mar 17;232(2):568-73

[159] Rahman I, MacNee W, "Regulation of redox glutathione levels and gene transcription in lung inflammation: therapeutic approaches," *Free Radic Biol Med* 28(9):1405-20, 2000 May 1

[160] Christman JW, Sadikot RT, Blackwell TS, "The role of nuclear factor-kappa B in pulmonary diseases," Chest, 2000, 117(5):1482-1487.

[161] Roederer M, Staal FJ, Osada H, Herzenberg LA, Herzenberg LA, "CD4 and CD8 T cells with high intracellular glutathione levels are selectively lost as the HIV infection progresses," *Int Immunol,* 1991 Sep; 3(9):933-7

[162] Garaci E, Palamara AT, Cirolo MR, D'Agostini C, del-Latif MS, Aquaro S, Lafavia E, Rotilio G, "Intracellular GSH content and HIV replication in human macrophages," *J Leukoc Biol,* 1997 Jul;62(1):54-9

[163] Palamara AT, Perno CF, Aquaro S, Bue MC, Dini L, Garaci E, "Glutathione inhibits HIV replication by acting at the late stages of the virus life cycle," *AIDS Res Hum Retroviruses*, 1996 Nov 1;12(16):1537-1541.

[164] Gosset P. Wallaert B, Tonnel AB, Fourneau C, "Thiol regulation of the production of TNF-alpha, IL-6 and IL-8 by human alveolar macrophages," *Eur Respir J* 1999 Jul;14(1):98-105

[165] Hashimoto S, Gon Y, Matsumoto K, Takeshita I, Asai Y, Asai Y, Machino T, Horie T, "Regulation by intracellular glutathione of TNF-alpha-induced p38 MAP kinase

activation and RANTES production by human pulmonary vascular endothelial cells," *Allergy* 2000 May;55(5):463-9

[166] Yamauchi N, Watanabe N, Kuriyama H, Neda H, Maeda M, Himeno T, Tsuji Y, Niitsu Y, "Suppressive effects of intracellular glutathione on hydroxyl radical production induced by tumor necrosis factor," *Int J Cancer* 1990 Nov 15;46(5):884-888.

[167] Peristeris P, Clark BD, Gatti S, Faggioani R, Mantovani A, Mengozzi M, Orencole SF, Sironi M, Ghezzi P, "N-acetylcysteine and glutathione as inhibitors of tumor necrosis factor production," *Cell Immunol* 1992 Apr;140(2):390-399.

[168] Rovin BH, Dickerson JA, Tan LC, Fassler J, "Modulation of IL-1-induced chemokine expression in human mesangial cells through alterations in redox status," *Cytokine* 1997 Mar;9(3):178-186.

[169] Pena LR et al., "Treatment with glutathione precursor decreases cytokine activity," *J. Parenter. Enteral. Nutr.* 23(1):1-6, 1999 January-February.

[170] Saccani A, Saccani S, Orlando S, Sironi M, Bernasconi S, Ghezzi P, Mantovani A, Sica A, "Redox regulation of chemokine receptor expression," *Proc Natl Acad Sci USA*, 2000 Mar 14;97(6):2761-2766.

[171] Morita A, Grewe M, Grether-Beck S, Olaizola-Horn S, Krutmann J, "Induction of proinflammatory cytokines in human epidermal carcinoma cells by in vitro ultraviolet A1 irradiation," *Photochem Photobiol* 1997 Apr;65(4):630-535

[172] Lombard-Gillooly K, Hubbard AK, "Modulation of silica-induced lung injury by reducing lung non-protein sulfhydryls with buthionine sulfoximine," *Toxicol Lett* 1993 Mar;66(3):305-15

[173] Cuzzocrea S, Constantino G, Zingarelli B, Mazzon E, Macali A, Caputi AP, "The protective role of endogenous gluathione in carrageenan-induced pleurisy in the rat," *Eur J Pharmacol* 1999 May 14;372(2):187-97.

[174] Liu B, Hannun YA, "Inhibition of neutral magnesium-dependent sphingomyelinase by glutathione," *J Biol Chem* 1997 Jun 27;272(26):16281-15287.

[175] Watson RW, Rotstein OD, Nathens AB, Dackiw AP, Marshall JC, "Thiol-mediated redox regulation of neutrophil apoptosis," *Surgery* 1996 Aug;120(2):150-157.

[176] Nakatani T, Tawaramoto M, Opare Kennedy D, Kojima A, Matsui-Yuasa I, "Apoptosis induced by chelation of intracellular zinc is associated with depletion of cellular reduced glutathione level in rat hepatocytes," *Chem Biol Interact* 2000 Mar 15;125(3):151-63

[177] Coppola S, Ghibelli L, "GSH extrusion and the mitochondrial pathway of apoptotic signalling," *Biochem Soc Trans* 2000 Feb;28(2):56-61

[178] Colell A, Garcia-Ruiz C, Miranda M, Ardite E, Mari M, Morales A, Corrales F, Kaplowitz N, Fernandez-Checa JC, "Selective glutathione depletion of mitochondria by ethanol sensitizes hepatocytes to tumor necrosis factor," *Gastroenterology* 1998 Dec;115(6):1541-51

[179] Nicole A, Santiard-Baron D, Ceballos-Picot I, "Direct evidence for glutathione as mediator of apoptosis in neuronal cells," *Biomed Pharmacother* 1998;52(9):349-55

[180] Rosenfeld ME, "Inflammation, lipids, and free radicals: lessons learned from te atherogenic process," *Semin Reprod Endrocrinol* 1998;16(4):249-61

[181] Hardwick SJ, Carpenter KL, Allen EA, Mitchinson MJ, "Glutathione (GSH) and the toxicity of oxidised low-density lipoprotein to human monocyte-macrophages," *Free Radic Res* 1999 Jan;30(1):11-9

[182] Aoshiba K, Yasui S, Nishimura K, Nagai A, "Thiol depletion induces apoptosis in cultured lung fibroblasts," *Am J Respir Cell Mol Biol* 1999 Jul;21(1):54-64

[183] Vahrmeijer AL, van Dierendonck JH, Schutrups J, van de Velde CJ, Mulder GJ, "Effect of glutathione depletion on inhibition of cell cycle progression and induction of apoptosis by mephalan (L-phenylalanine mustard) in human colorectal cancer cells," *Biochem Pharmacol* 1999 Aug 15;58(4):655-64

[184] Yang CF, Shen HM, Ong, CN, "Ebselen induces apoptosis in HepG(2) cells through rapid depletion of intracellular thiols," *Arch Biochem Biophys* 2000 Feb 15;374(2):142-52

[185] Li Y, Maher P, Schubert D, "A role for 12-lipoxygenase in nerve cell death caused by glutathione depletion," *Neuron* 1997 Aug;19(2):453-63.

[186] Iwata S et al., "Adult T cell leukemia (ATL)-derived factor/human thioredoxin prevents apoptosis of lymphoid cells induced by L-cystine and glutathione depletion: possible involvement of thiol-mediated redox regulation in apoptosis caused by pro-oxidant state," *J. Immunol.* 158(7):3108-17, 1997 April.

[187] Wedner HJ et al., "Inhibition of human polymorphonuclear leukocyte function by 2-cyclohexene-1-one: A role for glutathione in cell activation," *J. Clin. Invest.* 68(2):535-43, 1981 August

[188] Aziz AS et al., "Effects of selenium on polymorphonuclear leukocyte function in goats," *Am. J. Vet. Res.*, 45(9):1715-8, 1984 September.

[189] Voetman AA, Loos JA, Roos, D, "Changes in the Levels of Glutathione in Phagocytosing Human Neutrophils," *Blood* 1980 May;55(5):741-747.

[190] Tirouvanziam R, "CFTR, glutathione, and neutrophil function," 1999 Nov, http://63.193.197.190/Subsets/tirouv/index.htm

[191] Atalay M, Marnila P, Lilius, EM, Hanninen O, Sen OK, "Glutathione-dependent modulation of exhausting exercise-induced changes in neutrophil function of rats," *Eur J Appl Physiol* 1996;74(4):342-7.

[192] ven der Meide PH, de Labie MC, Botman CA, van Bennekom WP, Olsson T, Aten J, Weening JJ, "Mercuric chloride down-regulates T cell interferon-gamma production in brown Norway but not in Lewis rats; role of glutathione, *Eur J Immunol* 1993 Mar;23(3):675-81

[193] Smyth MJ, "Glutathione modulates activation-dependent proliferation of human peripheral blood lymphocyte populations without regulating their activated function," *J Immunol* 1991 Mar 15;146(6):1921-1927.

[194] Nathens AB, Rotstein OD, Dackiw AP, Gorczynski R, "The glutathione depleting agent diethylmaleate pronolong renal allograft survival," *J Surg Res* 1998 Jun;77(1):75-9

[195] Robinson MK, Rodrick ML, Jacobs DO, Rounds JD, Collins KH, Saporoschetz IB, Mannick JA, Wilmore DW, "Glutathione depletion in rats impairs T-cell and macrophage immune function," *Arch Surg* 1993 Jan;128(1):29-34

[196] Ginn-Pease ME, Whisler RL, "Optimal NF kappa B mediated transcriptional responses to Jurkat T cells exposed to oxidative stress are dependent on intracellular glutthione and costimulatory signals," *Biochem Biophys Res Commun* 1996 Sep 24;226(3):695-702

[197] Aukrust P. Svardal AM, Muller F, Lunden B, Nordoy I, Froland SS, "Markedly distrubed glutathione reodx status in CD45RA+CD4+ lymphocytes in human

immunodeficiency virus type 1 infection is associated with selective depletion of this lymphocyte subset," *Blood* 1996 Oct 1;88(7):2626-33

[198] Shenker BJ, Guo TL, O I, Shapiro IM, "Induction of apoptosis in human T-cells by methyl mercury: temporal relationship between mitochondiral dysfunction and loss of reductive reserve," *Toxicol Appl Pharmacol* 1999 May 15;157(1):23-35

[199] Herzenberg LA, De Rosa SC, Dubs JG, Roederer M, Anderson MT, Ela SW, Deresinski SC, Herzenberg LA, "Glutathione deficiency is asociated with impaired survival in HIV disease," *Proc Natl Acad Sci USA* 1997 Mar 4;94(5):1967-1972.

[200] Hamilos DL, Zelarney P, Mascari JJ, "Lymphocyte proliferation in glutathione-depleted lymphocytes: direct relationship between glutathione availability ant he proliferative response," *Immunopharmacology* 1989 Nov-Dec;18(3):223-35

[201] Gringhius SI, Leow A, Papendrecht-Van Der Voort EA, Remans PH, Breedveld FC, Verweij CL, "Displacement of linker for activation of T cells from the plasma membrane due to redox balance alterations results in hyporesponsiveness of synovial fluid T lymphocytes in rheumatoid arthritis," *J Immunol* 2000 Feb 15;164(4):2170-2179.

[202] Aidoo A, Lyn-Cook LE, Morris SM, Kodell RL, Casciano DA, "Comparative study of intracellular glutathione content in rat lymphocyte cultures treated with 2-mercaptoethanol and interleukin-2," *Cell Biol Toxicol* 1991 Jul;7(3):215-27

[203] Gmunder H, Roth S, Eck HP, Gallas H, Mihm S, Droge W, "Interleukin-2 mRNA expression, lymphokine production and DNA synthesis in glutathione-depleted rats," *Cell Immunol* 1990 Oct 15;130(2):520-8

[204] Ting CC, Wang J, Hargrove ME, "Reversal of multiple-site tumor cell-induced immunosuppression by specific cytokines and pharmacological agents," *Immunopharmacology* 1995 Aug;30(2):119-30

[205] Hyde H, Brothwick NJ, Janossy G, Salmon M, Akbar AN, "Upregulation of intracellular glutathione by fibroblast-derived factor(s): enhanced survival of activated T cells in the presence of low Bcl-2," *Blood* 1997 Apr 1;89(7):2453-2460.

[206] Messina JP, Lawrence DA, "Cell cycle progression of glutathione-depleted human peripheral blood mononuclear cells is inhibited at S phase," *J Immunol* 1989 Sep 15;143(6):1974-81.

[207] Fidelus RK and MF Tsan, "Glutathione and lymphocyte activation: a function of ageing and auto-immune disease," *Immunology* 61(4):503-8, 1987 August.

[208] Jeannin P, Delneste Y, Lecoanet-Henchoz S, Gauchat JF, Life P, Homes D, Bonnefoy JY, "Thiols decrease human interleukin (IL) 4 production and IL-4-induced immunoglobulin synthesis," *J Exp Med* 1995 Dec 1;182(6):1785-92

[209] Rigacci S, Iantomasi T, Marraccini P, Berti A, Vincenzini MT, Ramponi G, "Evidence for glutathione involvement in platelet-derived growth-factor-mediated signal," *Biochem J* 1997 Jun 15;324(Pt 3):791-6

[210] Romero DL, Mounho BJ, Lauer FT, Born JL, Burchiel SW, "Depletion of glutathione by benzo(a)pyrene metabolites, ionomycin, thatpsigargin, and phorbol myristate in human peripheral blood mononuclear cells," *Toxicol Appl Pharmacol* 1997 May;144(1):62-9

[211] Liang SM, Liang CM, Hargrove ME, Ting CC, "Regulation by glutathione of the effect of lymphokines on differentiation of primary activated lymphocytes. Influence of

glutathione on cytotoxic activity of CD3-AK-.," *J Immunol* 1991 Mar 15;146(6):1909-13

[212] Gmunder H, Droge W, "Differential effects of glutathione depletion on T cell subsets," *Cell Immunol* 1991 Nov;138(1):229-37

[213] Ting CC, Hargrove HE, Liang SM, Liang CM, Sharrow SO, "Dichotomy of glutathione regulation of the activation of resting and preactivated lymphocytes," *Cell Immunol* 1992 Jun;142(1):40-53

[214] Gmunder H, Eck HP, Benninghoff B, Roth S, Droge W, "Macrophages regulate intracellular glutathione levels of lymphocytes. Evidence for an immunoregulatroy role of cysteine," *Cell Immunol* 1990 Aug;129(1):32-46.

[215] Hargrove ME, Wang J, Ting CC, "Regulation by glutathione of the activation and differentiation of IL-4-dependent activated killer cells," *Cell Immunol* 1993 Jul;149(2):433-43

[216] Sprietsma JE, "Zinc-controlled Thl/Th2 switch significantly determines development of disease," *Med Hypotheses* 1997 Jul;49(1):1-14

[217] Spriestma JE, "Cysteine, glutathione (GSH) and zinc and copper ions together are effective, natral, intracellular inhibitors of (AIDS) viruses," *Med Hypotheses* 1999 Jun;52(6):529-38

[218] Spriestma JE, "Modern diets and diseases: NO-zinc balance. Under Thl, zinc and nitorgen monoxide (NO) collectively protect against viruses, AIDS, autoimmunity, diabetes, allergies, asthma, infectious diseases, atherosclerosis and cancer," *Med Hypotheses* 1999 Jul;53(1):6-16

[219] Moser C, Johansen HK, Song Z, Hougen HP, Rygaard J, Hoiby N, "Chronic Pseudomonas aeruginosa lung infection is more severe in Th2 responding BALB/c mice compared to Thl responding C3H/HeN mice," *APMIS* 1997 Nov;105(11):838-42

[220] Nishikawa M, Sato EF, Kashiba M, Kuroki T, Utsumi K, Inoue M, "Role of glutathione in nitric oxide-dependent regulation of energy metabolism in rat hepatoma cells," *Hepatology* 1998 Feb;27(2):422-426.

[221] Bolanos JP, Almeida A, Stewart V, Peuchen S, Land JM, Clark JB, Heales SJ, "Nitric oxide-mediated mitochondrial damage in the brain: mechanisms and implications for neurodegenerative diseases," *J Neurochem* 1997 Jun;68(6):2227-40.

[222] D'Emilia DM, Lipton SA, "Ratio of S-nitrosohomocyst(e)ine or other thiols determines neurotoxicity in rat cerebrocortical cultures," *Neuroscience Letters* 1999;265:103-106.

[223] Stefanelli C, Pignatti C, Tantani B, Stanic I, Bonavita F, Muscari C, Guarnieri C, Clo C, Caldarera CM, "Nitric oxide can function as either a killer molecule or an antiapoptotic effector in cardiomyocytes," *Biochim Biophys Acta* 1999 Jul 8;1450(3):406-13

[224] Rosenberg PA, Li Y, Ai S, Altiok N, Back SA, Volpe JJ, "Intracellular redox state determines whether nitric oxide is toxic or protective to rat oligodendrocytes in culture," *J Neurochem* 1999 Aug;73(2):476-84

[225] Chiueh CC, Rauhala P, "The redox pathway of S-nitrisoglutathione, glutathione and nitric oxide in cell to neuron communications," Free Radic Res 1999 Dec;31(6):641-50

[226] Boggs SE, McCormick TS, Lapetina EG, "Glutathione Levels Determine Apoptosis in Macrophages," *Biochem Biophys Res Commun* 1998 Jun 18;247(2):229-33

[227] Zhao ZH, Francis CE, Welch G, Loscalzo J, Ravid K, "Reduced glutathione prevents nitric oxide-induced apoptosis in vascular smooth muscle cells," *Biochimica er Biophysica Acta - Molecular Cell Research* 1997 Nov 27;1359(2):143-52

[228] Ju C, Yoon KN, Oh YK, Kim HC, Sin CY, Ryu JR, Ko KH, Kim WK, "Synergistic depletion of astrocytic glutathione by glucose deprivation and peroxynitrite: correlation with mitochondrial dysfunction and subsequent cell death," *J Neurochem* 2000 May;74(5):1989-98

[229] Callsen D, Brune B, "Role of mitogen-activated protein kinases in S-nitrosoglutathione-induced macrophage apoptosis," *Biochemistry* 1999 Feb 23;38(8):2279-86

[230] Lemaire G, Alvarez-Pachon FJ, Beuneu C, Lepoivre M, Petit JF, "Differential cytostatic effects of NO donors and NO producing cells," *Free Radic Biol Med* 1999 May;26(9-10):1274-83

[231] Romao PR, Fonseca SG, Hothersall JS, Noronha-Dutra AA, Ferreira SH, Cunha FQ, "Glutathione protects macrophages and Leishmania major against nitric oxide-mediated cytotoxicity," *Parasitology* 1999 Jun;118(Pt 6):559-66

[232] Aleryani S et al., "Superoxide-mediated decomposition of biological S-nitrosothiols," *J Biol Chem*, 273(11):601-5, 1998 March 13.

[233] Arnelle, DR and Stamler JS, "NO+, NO, and NO- donation by S-nitrosothiols: implications for regulation of physiological functions by S-nitrosylation and acceleration of disulfide formation," *Arch Biochem Biophys* 318(2):279-85, 1992 April 20.

[234] Jones KL, Bryan TW, Jinkins PA, Simpson KL, Grisham MB, Owens MW, Milligan SA, Markewitz BA, Robbins RA, "Superoxide released from neutrophils causes a reduction in nitric oxide gas," *AJP - Lung Cellular and Molecular Physiology* 1998 Dec;275(6):L1120-6

[235] Zavodnik IB, Lapshina EA, Rekawiecka K, Zavodnik LB, Barstosz G, Bryszewska M, "Membrane effects of nitrite-induced oxidation of human red blood cells," *Biochim Biophys Acta* 1999 Oct 15;1421(2):306-16

[236] Belvisi MG, Ward JK, Mitchell JA, Barnes PJ, "Nitric oxide as a neurotransmitter in human airways," *Arch Int Pharmacodyn Ther* 1995 Jan-Feb;329(1):97-110

[237] Gaston B et al., "Relaxation of Human Bronchial Smooth Muscle by S-Nitrosothiols in Vitro," *The Journal of pharmacology and experimental therapeutics*. 268(2): 978-984, 1994 February.

[238] Kamosinska B, Radomski MW, Duszyk M, Radomski A, Man SF, "Nitric oxide activates chloride currents in human lung epithelial cells," *Am J Physiol* 1997 Jun;272(6 PT 1):L1098-104

[239] Dong YJ, Chao AC, Kouyama K, Hsu YP, Bocian RC, Moss RB, Gardner P, "Activation of CFTR chloride current by nitric oxide in human T lymphocytes," *EMBO J* 1995 Jun 15;14(12):2700-2707.

[240] Gao L, Broughman JR, Iwamoto T, Tomich JM, Venglarik CJ, Forman HJ. "Synthetic chloride channel restorese glutathione secretion in cystic fibrosis airway epithelia." *Am. J. Physiol. Lung Cell Mol. Physiol* 2001 July; 28(1):L24-30.

[241] Buhl R, Vogelmeier C, Critenden M, Hubbard RC, Hoyt RF Jr., Wilson, EM, Cantin AM, Crystal RG, "Augmentation of the glutathione in the fluid lining the epithelium of the lower respiratory tract by directly administering glutathione," *Proc. Natl. Acad. Sci. USA*, 1990 June, 87:4063-67

[242] Buhl R, Holroyd K, Borok Z, Roum J, Bokser A, Grimes G, Czerski D, Cantin A, Crystal RG, "Reversal of the glutathione deficiency in the lower respiratory tract of

HIV-Seropositive individuals by glutathione aerosol therapy," *Clin. Res.*, 1990, 38(2): 596A

[243] Borok Z, Buhl R, Grimes GJ, Bokser AD, Hubbard RC, Holroyd KJ, Roum JH, Czerski DB, Cantin AM, Crystal RG, "Effect of Glutathione Aerosol on Oxidant-Antioxidant Imbalance in Idiopathic Pulmonary Fibrosis," *Lancet*, 1991 July 17, 338:215-6,

[244] Marrades RM, Roca J, Barbera JA, de Jover L, MacNee W, Rodriguez-Roisin R, "Nebulized Glutathione Induces Bronchoconstriction in Patients with Mild Asthma," *Am. J. Respir. Crit. Care Med.*, 1997, 156:425-30

[245] Bernorio S, Pecis M, Zucchi A, Guerra G, Migliorini V, Negri L, Corsano A, "Glutathione in Bronchial Hyperresponsiveness," *J. Aerosol Medicine* 9(2):207-213, 1996

[246] Testa B, Mesolella M, Testa D, Giuliano A, Costa G, Maione F, Iaccarino F, "Glutathione in the upper respiratory tract," *Ann Otol Rhinol Laryngol* 1995;104:117-9

[247] Roum JH, Borok Z, McElvaney NG, Grimes GJ, Bokser AD, Buhl R, Crystal RG, "Glutathione aerosol suppresses lung epithelial surface inflammatory cell-derived oxidants in cystic fibrosis," *J Appl Physiol* 1999 Jul;87(1):438-43

[248] Bagnato GF, Gulli S, DePasquale R, Giacobbe O, Spatari G, Purello D'Ambrosio F. "Effect of inhaled glutathione on airway response to 'fog' challenge in asthmatic patients." *Respiration* 1999 Nov-Dec; 66(6):518-521.

[249] Griese M, ramakers J, Krasselt A, Starosta V, Van Konigsbruggen S, Fischer R, Ratjen F, Mullinger B, Huber RM, Maier K, Rietschel E, Scheuch G. "Improvement of alveolar glutathione, lung function, but not oxidative stress in cystic fibrosis." *Am. J. Respir. Crit. Care Med*, 2004 Jan 15 (e published ahead of publication).

[250] Bishop C, Hudson VM, Hilton SC, Wilde CA, "A pilot study of the effect of inhaled buffered reduced glutathione on the clinical status of cystic fibrosis patients", *Chest*, in press.

[251] Snyder AH, McPherson ME, Hunt JF, Johnson M, Stumler JS, Gaston B. "Acute effects of aerosolized S-nitroglutathione in cystic fibrosis." *Am. J. Respir. Crit. Care Med*, 2002 April; 165(7):922-966.

[252] Sermet-Gaudelus I, Stoven V, Annereau JP, Witko-Sarsat V, Reinert P, Guyot M, Deschamps-Latscha B, Lallemand JY, Lenoir G. "Interest of colchicine for the treatment of cystic fibrosis patients. Preliminary report." *Mediators Inflamm.* 1999; *(1):13-5.

In: Progress in Cystic Fibrosis Research
Editor: Margaret A. Harrison, pp. 29-64
ISBN 1-59454-232-5

Chapter II

BILE ACID DYSFUNCTION IN THE CYSTIC FIBROSIS INTESTINE

Jacqueline Hardcastle[1,*] and Christopher J. Taylor[2]
[1]Department of Biomedical Science, University of Sheffield, Sheffield, UK
[2]Academic Unit of Child Health, University of Sheffield, Sheffield, UK

Abstract

Cystic fibrosis (CF) is characterised by defective epithelial transport. In the intestine this affects both absorption and secretion. Bile acids are released into the duodenum where they facilitate processing of dietary fat with subsequent reabsorption in the terminal ileum where 95% of bile salts are actively reabsorbed via the Na^+-dependent ileal bile acid transporter (IBAT). Bile acid dysfunction has been well described in CF suggesting that the handling of bile acids by the intestine is affected by the disease. Bile acid function in the CF intestine was therefore investigated using a transgenic mouse model in which the ΔF508 mutation, which is expressed in approximately 70% of CF chromosomes, was introduced into the CF gene.

Mucosal application of bile acids caused a biphasic increase in the short-circuit current (SCC) generated by ileal sheets from normal and wild-type mice. The initial phase was Na^+-dependent, but unaffected by the Cl^- channel blocker DPC, the NKCC inhibitor furosemide or the absence of Cl^-, suggesting that it reflected the activity of the IBAT. The second phase represented bile acid-induced secretion as it was Na^+-independent, but was inhibited by DPC, furosemide or absence of Cl^-. In more proximal regions of intestine and when applied serosally bile acids induced a monophasic secretory response. The secretory response involved the activation of mast cells that released secretory stimulants including histamine and 5-HT. In the case of taurocholic acid, but not ursodeoxycholic acid, a neural component was also present. In tissues from CF mice the secretory response to bile acids was absent in all regions of the intestine and the absorptive component in the ileum was reduced.

* Correspondence concerning this article should be addressed to Jacqueline Hardcastle, University of Sheffield, Sheffield, UK.

Absorption of taurocholic acid was measured directly in everted sacs of intestine. In ileal sacs from normal and wild-type mice active, Na^+-dependent bile acid uptake was demonstrated. In CF ileum taurocholic acid uptake was significantly lower, but this difference was not evident in brush-border membrane vesicles, suggesting that an intracellular component was required for this effect. In jejunum and mid-intestine taurocholic acid uptake was passive and there was no difference between wild-type and CF tissues.

These studies confirm that bile acid function in the intestine is disturbed in CF. The absence of bile acid-induced secretion in CF may contribute to the dehydration of the luminal contents that can lead to the development of obstructive symptoms such as meconium ileus. Impaired reuptake of bile acids by the terminal ileum could result in the excessive accumulation of these potentially toxic compounds in the intestinal lumen.

Abbreviations

ASBT	apical Na^+ bile salt transporter
cAMP	adenosine 3', 5'-cyclic monophosphate
CDCA	chenodeoxycholic acid
CA	cholic acid
CF	cystic fibrosis
CFTR	cystic fibrosis transmembrane conductance regulator
CMC	critical micellar concentration
DCA	deoxycholic acid
DRA	down-regulated in adenoma
GCA	glycocholic acid
cGMP	guanosine 3',5'-cyclic monophosphate
IBAT	ileal bile acid transporter
NHE	sodium/hydrogen exchanger
PD	potential difference
SCC	short-circuit current
SGLT	sodium/glucose transporter
TA	taurocholic acid
UDCA	ursodeoxycholic acid.

Introduction

Cystic fibrosis (CF) is a disease that affects the ability of epithelia to transport fluid and electrolytes from one side of the tissue to the other. The intestine is an organ that is lined with an epithelium whose cells, the enterocytes, possess a wide range of transport processes. It is therefore not surprising to find that patients with CF experience a range of intestinal symptoms, many of which can be attributed, at least in part, to disturbances in intestinal transport. Although the intestine is primarily concerned with the absorption of nutrients, electrolytes and fluid, it also has a secretory capacity that plays an important role in lubrication, providing Na^+ ions for Na^+-linked absorptive processes and washing immunoglubulins from the crypts. In CF secretion is impaired throughout the intestinal tract.

In vitro and *in vivo* studies have demonstrated that both the small (Taylor et al 1987, 1988; Berschneider et al 1987; Baxter et al 1989; O'Loughlin et al 1991) and large (Goldstein et al 1988, 1991; Hardcastle et al 1991; Mall et al 2000) intestine fail to respond to secretagogue challenge. In addition, there is evidence of enhanced Na^+ (Mall et al 1999) and Na^+-linked nutrient absorption (Baxter et al 1990) in CF. These transport changes will lead to excessive dehydration of the luminal contents and may contribute to the development of meconium ileus, observed in 10-20% of newborn CF children, and distal intestinal obstruction syndrome (meconium ileus equivalent) at later ages (Quinton 1999; Wyllie 1999).

In the intestine bile acids are secreted into the lumen of the duodenum where they contribute to the processing of dietary fat. They also activate secretory processes in the intestine (Binder 1980). Bile acids are conserved by active reabsorption via a Na^+-dependent mechanism localised to the enterocytes in the terminal ileum. They then enter the portal circulation and are returned to the liver for resecretion into the bile (Binder 1980). This enterohepatic circulation of bile acids is extremely efficient, with less than 10% escaping reabsorption and being lost in the faeces each day (Hofmann 1998). The first step in the uptake of bile acids involves a Na^+ gradient-driven cotransporter, the ileal bile acid transporter (IBAT), located on the luminal membranes of ileal enterocytes (Hofmann 1998). This operates in a similar fashion to the cotransporters responsible for Na^+-linked nutrient absorption whose activities are altered in CF. Thus two aspects of bile acid function in the intestine, their stimulation of secretion and their active reuptake by the terminal ileum, could be affected by the disease.

In 1989 the CF gene was identified (Rommens et al 1989) and was found to encode a 1480 amino acid product named the cystic fibrosis transmembrane conductance regulator (CFTR). CFTR is a 168-kDa integral membrane protein that is a member of the ATP binding cassette family. It consists of 6 pairs transmembrane domains, 2 cytoplasmic nucleotide-binding domains and a large cytoplasmic regulatory domain. More than 1200 mutations of the CF gene have now been identified, but the majority of patients in Europe (70-80%) have the ΔF508 mutation (Veeze 1992) in which phenyl alanine is deleted at position 508, part of the 2nd nucleotide binding domain. Loss of function in the ΔF508 form of CFTR is due to abnormal processing in the Golgi apparatus, leading to a failure of trafficking so that the protein never reaches its normal location at the cell membrane (Riordan 1993). Patients with this mutation suffer a severe phenotype and are typically pancreatic insufficient.

CFTR is localized to epithelial tissues where it has been found to function as a cAMP-regulated Cl^- channel (Riordan 1993), thus explaining why defects in its structure can lead to alterations in Cl^- transport. However, more recent studies have revealed that CFTR can also influence the behaviour of other transport proteins such as ENaC (the epithelial Na^+ channel), ORCC (the outwardly-rectifying Cl^- channel), aquaporins (see Greger et al 2001) and DRA (down-regulated in adenoma; Wheat el al 2000) the anion exchanger involved in intestinal electroneutral NaCl absorption.

Identification of the CF gene has led to the development of transgenic mouse models of the disease and many of these have been used to investigate the changes in intestinal function that occur in CF (Grubb & Gabriel 1997). The models fall into two categories: animals in which the CF gene has been disrupted so that no CFTR is produced (knockout mice), and animals in which specific mutations have been introduced into the CF gene. These include animals with the ΔF508 mutation such as the mice developed in Cambridge ($Cftr^{tm2Cam}$,

Colledge et al 1995) and Rotterdam (*Cftr*^{tm1Eur}, Van Doorninck et al 1995). Intestinal tissues from transgenic CF mice clearly exhibit the failure of secretion and enhanced Na^+ absorption that is observed in human CF intestine, but the enhanced glucose absorption reported in jejunal biopsies from CF patients (Baxter et al 1990) has not been replicated in mouse small intestine (Grubb & Gabriel 1997).

Bile Acid Dysfunction in CF Patients

The intrahepatic bile duct epithelium modulates both the fluidity and alkalinity of the primary hepatocellular bile. Fluids, amino acids, glucose and bile acids are reabsorbed, while water, electrolytes and immunoglobulin A are secreted. The transport function of the intrahepatic biliary epithelium is finely regulated by a number of gastrointestinal hormones, neuropeptides and neurotransmitters that promote either secretion or absorption (Strazzabosco et al 2000). CFTR the cystic fibrosis CF gene product, functions as a cAMP-regulated anion channel in the apical membrane of biliary epithelial cells, including gallbladder epithelial cells (Dray-Charier et al 1999; Chinet et al 1999). The loss of CFTR-mediated transepithelial Cl^- and HCO_3^- secretion, coupled to similar changes in the pancreatic duct epithelium, leads to viscid duodenal fluid with an abnormally low pH (Clarke et al 2000). This causes bile salt precipitation and impairs micellar formation.

Bile acid malabsorption is a constant finding in untreated CF. Bile acids are bound to the undigested protein fraction of the stool, making them unavailable for reabsorption. Faecal losses of bile acids range from 24 – 57 mg/kg/day. This leads to depletion of the bile acid pool in untreated patients. Duodenal bile shows decreased total bile salt concentrations with an increase in both the glycine/taurine ratio and dihydroxy bile salts. The latter produces toxic, hydrophobic bile acids that lower the critical micellar concentration (CMC) and further exacerbates malabsorption. In well nourished patients, however, control of steatorrhoea with pancreatic enzyme replacement normalises concentrations of bile acids in duodenal bile and results in normal to large pool sizes of bile acids (Strandvik et al 1996). Nevertheless, the bile acid distribution remains abnormal with higher percentages of cholic acid and lower percentages of chenodeoxycholic and deoxycholic acid.

Ursodeoxycholic acid, the 7-beta-epimer of chenodeoxycholic acid, has multiple hepatoprotective activities. Ursodeoxycholic acid modifies the bile acid pool, decreasing levels of endogenous, hydrophobic bile acids while increasing the proportion of non-toxic hydrophilic bile acids. Ursodeoxycholic acid also has a choleretic effect, increasing hepatocellular bile acid excretion, as well as cytoprotective, anti-apoptotic and immunomodulatory properties. It has been used for the treatment of cholestatic liver disease in doses of 13-20 mg/kg/day where it appears to improve serum liver chemistry and may delay disease progression (Paumgartner et al 2002). Ursodeoxycholic acid is widely used in CF to prevent the progression of liver disease. CF-associated liver disease affects up to 20% of patients, and is becoming more relevant clinically with increasing life expectancy. Hyperviscous bile accumulates in the biliary tree causing cholangiocyte and hepatocyte injury, stimulating focal fibrosis. Fibrosis is thought to lead on to cirrhosis over a period of years, a process that is usually asymptomatic (Diwaker et al 2001). Treatment with ursodeoxycholic acid with the aim of improving biliary secretion and reducing bile viscosity and correcting bile acid composition, is claimed to have beneficial effects on liver biochemistry, hepatic excretory function and liver histology (Colombo et al 1998). However, a Cochrane review of ursodeoxycholic acid in CF found its clinical effectiveness unproven (Cheng et al 2000).

Transport Processes in the Intestine

The secretory function of the intestine plays a vital role in maintaining the fluidity of the intestinal contents, facilitating the processes of digestion and absorption. Secretion of fluid and electrolytes involves changes in two transport processes: electrogenic Cl^- secretion is stimulated (see Barrett & Keely 2000) and electroneutral NaCl absorption is inhibited (Kunzelmann & Mall 2001).

Electrogenic Cl^- Secretion

The mechanism of electrogenic Cl^- secretion is illustrated in Figure 1A. Cl^- enters the enterocyte by means of the NKCC1 (Na^+, K^+, $2Cl^-$) cotransporter located at the basolateral membrane. This uses energy from the Na^+ gradient to accumulate Cl^- within the cell against its electrochemical potential. The Na^+ that enters the cell via the cotransporter is then extruded by the basolateral Na^+ pump, while K^+ leaves through basolateral K^+ channels. The cell is thus primed for secretion. When it is stimulated, Cl^- channels in the luminal membrane open, allowing the accumulated Cl^- to move into the lumen. The resulting increase in luminal negativity causes Na^+ to move into the lumen via the cation-selective paracellular pathway. The NaCl now present in the lumen creates an osmotic driving force for fluid secretion. As Cl^- exit from the cell is electrogenic it depolarises the luminal membrane, reducing the driving force for continued Cl^- efflux and so compromising the secretory process. To overcome this problem secretory stimulation also opens K^+ channels in the basolateral membrane. The resulting basolateral hyperpolarisation is transmitted via the low resistance paracellular pathway to the luminal side of the cell where it maintains the luminal membrane potential and hence allows continued Cl^- secretion. The process of Cl^- secretion is electrogenic. It generates an electrical current and this can be conveniently used to monitor its activity.

CFTR is expressed throughout the intestinal tract and is localised to the luminal membrane of the enterocyte (Crawford et al 1991; Strong et al 1994; O'Loughlin et al 1996; Ameen et al 2000) where it functions as the anion channel through which Cl^- leaves the cell during secretion. Mutations in the CF gene lead to defective CFTR so that the Cl^- exit process cannot operate normally and Cl^- secretion fails.

Electroneutral NaCl Absorption

The mechanism of electroneutral NaCl absorption is illustrated in Figure 1B. Na^+ and Cl^- enter the enterocyte from the intestinal lumen via two linked ion exchangers: a Na^+/H^+ exchanger (principally NHE3) and a Cl^-/HCO_3^- exchanger (DRA: down-regulated in adenoma). Na^+ is then actively extruded from the cell by the basolateral Na^+ pump, while Cl^-

leaves via a basolateral anion channel. As the stoichiometry of this process is 1:1 it is electrically silent.

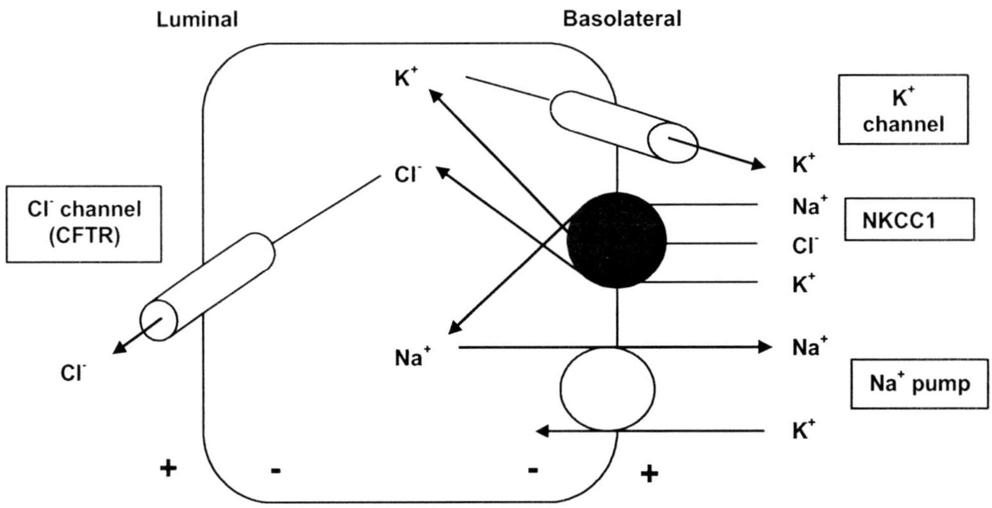

A. Electrogenic Cl⁻ secretion (stimulated)

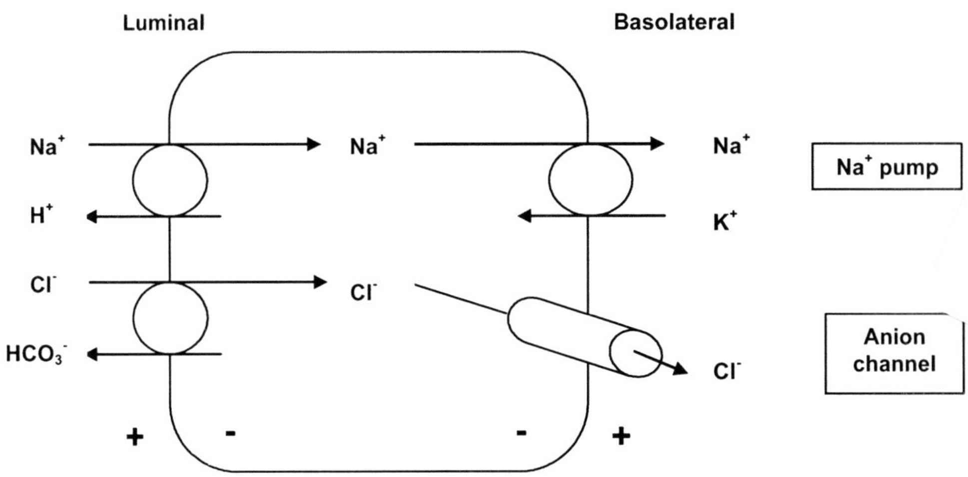

B. Electroneutral NaCl cotransport (inhibited)

Fig. 1. Mechanisms involved in the intestinal secretory response.

A wide range of agents, both endogenous and exogenous, can stimulate intestinal secretion. Their effects are mediated by increases in either cyclic nucleotides (cAMP and cGMP) or cytosolic Ca^{2+}. The defect in CF however, is downstream of intracellular signalling molecules and their production is unaffected by the disease (Hitchin et al 1990; Klaren et al 2001). Thus secretion fails no matter which intracellular signalling pathway is stimulated.

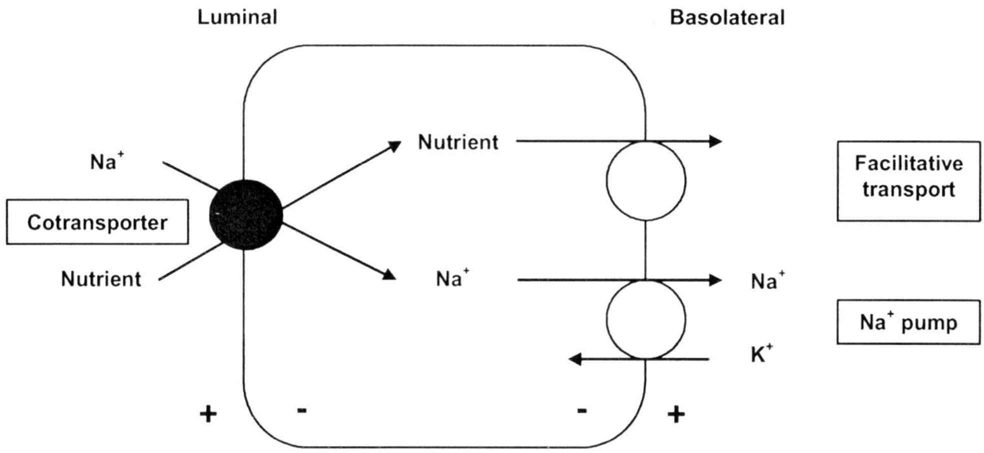

Fig. 2. Mechanism for the Na$^+$-dependent absorption of nutrients.

Na$^+$-Dependent Nutrient Absorption

A wide range of nutrients, including sugars, amino acids and bile acids, are actively absorbed by the small intestine in a process that is driven by the energy available from the inwardly-directed electrochemical gradient for Na$^+$ (Figure 2). A cotransporter, located at the luminal membrane, harnesses the energy from the Na$^+$ gradient, allowing the nutrient to be taken up by the enterocyte against its concentration gradient. The cotransporter possesses sites for both Na$^+$ and nutrient and when these are both occupied the inward movement of Na$^+$ down its gradient provides the energy for the active uptake of nutrient. In the case of bile acids the cotransporter involved is the IBAT, also known as the apical Na$^+$ bile salt transporter, ASBT (Meier & Stieger 2002). It is a protein of 348 amino acids and has 7, or possibly 9, transmembrane domains. It has a stoichiometry for Na$^+$:bile acid of 2:1, so functions electrogenically. Efflux of bile acid across the basolateral membrane is not well understood, but is believed to involve an anion exchange mechanism (Meier & Stieger 2002).

In the intestine bile acids not only stimulate secretion, but they are also actively absorbed. In view of the range of effects that CFTR is now known to exert on epithelial transport processes it is possible that bile acid function in the intestine is altered in CF. This has been explored using transgenic mouse models of the disease (Hardcastle et al 2001, 2001a, 2004).

Bile Acid-Induced Secretion in CF

Although the ability of bile acids to stimulate intestinal secretion has been known for many years (see Binder 1980), there are few reports of their effects in the mouse. Bile acids have been shown to induce secretion in the mouse colon (Gelbmann et al 1995), but the small intestine remained largely unstudied. Thus before investigating bile acid-induced secretion in transgenic CF mice it was necessary to characterise this process in normal (Swiss) mice (Hardcastle et al 2001, 2001a).

Methods Used to Investigate Bile Acid-Induced Secretion

Experiments were performed on intestinal tissues from mice killed by cervical dislocation in accordance with UK Home Office regulations and with local Ethics Committee approval. Male Swiss mice (age 12-13 weeks, body weight 20-30 g) together with two transgenic CF mouse models in which the ΔF508 mutation had been introduced into the CFTR gene were used. These were the $Cftr^{tm2Cam}$ (Colledge et al 1995) and the $Cftr^{tm1Eur}$ mouse model (Van Doorninck et al 1995). Animals used included mice homozygous for the ΔF508 mutation together with wild-type littermates.

As the secretory process is electrogenic its activity can be monitored by measuring transintestinal electrical activity. The potential difference (PD), short-circuit current (SCC) and tissue resistance were measured across paired sheets of mouse small intestine. Both intact and stripped (outer muscle layers and myenteric plexus removed) tissues were used. Jejunal tissues were taken from the region immediately distal to the ligament of Treitz, ileal tissues from the region just proximal to the caecum and mid-intestinal tissues were taken from the mid region. Each sheet was mounted in an Ussing chamber (Figure 3) with an aperture of 0.5 cm^2 and incubated at 37°C in Krebs bicarbonate saline gassed with 95% O_2/5% CO_2. The serosal fluid contained 10 mM glucose and the mucosal fluid 10 mM mannitol and each had a volume of 5 mL. The PD was measured using salt bridge electrodes connected via calomel half cells to a differential input electrometer with output to a two-channel chart recorder. Current was applied across the tissue via conductive plastic electrodes and tissue resistance determined from the PD change induced by a 50 μA current pulse, taking into account the fluid resistance. The SCC generated by the sheets was calculated from PD and resistance measurements using Ohm's law. Tissues were allowed to stabilise for 15 min after mounting and then readings of electrical activity were taken at 1 min intervals. Following 5 min basal readings bile acid was added to the mucosal or serosal fluid and readings were continued for a further 10 min.

In Cl^--free conditions all Cl^- in both mucosal and serosal solutions was replaced with gluconate. To test the Na^+-dependence of the taurocholic acid response the Na^+ concentration of the mucosal solution was reduced to 25 mM by replacing all the NaCl in the Krebs with isotonic mannitol. Inhibitors were added to test sheets as soon as the preparations were set up, with control sheets receiving an equivalent volume of vehicle. Vehicles used to prepare stock solutions were: furosemide, DMSO (dimethylsulphoxide); DPC (diphenylamine-2-carboxylic acid), ethanol; verapamil, methanol; capsaicin, 4% DMSO in saline; tetrodotoxin, 154 mM NaCl and in each case 25 μL was added to 5 mL bathing solution. Indomethacin was dissolved in 10% ethanol in 0.2% Na_2CO_3 and 100 μL was added to the serosal solution. All other drugs were dissolved in 154 mM NaCl and 100 μL was added 5 mL bathing solution. Taurocholic acid was dissolved in 154 mM NaCl, but all other bile acids were dissolved in ethanol. In each case 100μL stock solution was added to 5 mL bathing solution. Preliminary experiments indicated that the vehicles had no effect on basal electrical activity or on the responses to bile acids ($P>0.05$ in all cases). They also had no effect on the rise in SCC associated with Na^+-linked glucose absorption ($P>0.05$ in all cases).

The phenotype of the CF mice was confirmed by testing the intestinal response to secretagogue challenge. Acetylcholine (10^{-3}M) or 5-HT (10^{-4}M) was added to the serosal solution after 5 min basal readings, with glucose (10 mM) being added to the mucosal solution 5 min later to confirm tissue viability.

Results are expressed as mean values ± 1 s.e.m. of the number of observations indicated. Student's *t* test, paired or unpaired as appropriate, was used to assess significance. For multiple comparisons ANOVA, with post hoc analysis by Scheffé's method, was used.

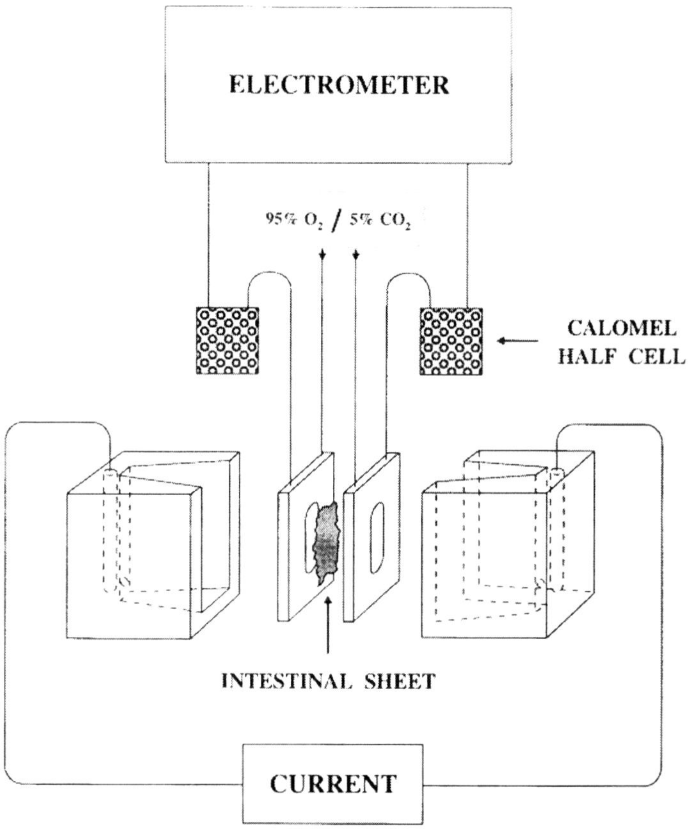

Fig. 3. Ussing chamber used to measure transintestinal electrical activity generated by intestinal sheets from the mouse.

Swiss Mice

Basal Electrical Activity in Intact and Stripped Sheets of Small Intestine

All regions of the intestine generated a basal PD and SCC with the serosal side being positive with respect to the mucosal side. In stripped ileal sheets basal PD, SCC and tissue resistance values were 2.0±0.1 mV, 63.2±2.4 μA cm^{-2} and 31.6±0.6 ohm cm^2 (n=92). Corresponding values were 0.8±0.1 mV, 30.9±2.2 μA cm^{-2} and 26.7±0.7 ohm cm^2 (n=83) in stripped mid-intestine and 1.7±0.1 mV, 61.7±4.3 μA cm^{-2} and 28.1±1.4 ohm cm^2 (n=23) in stripped jejunum.

Effects of Bile Acids on Transintestinal Electrical Activity

In the ileum luminal application of bile acids induced a biphasic increase in PD and SCC with intact and stripped sheets producing similar responses (Hardcastle et al 2001). There was an initial transient peak followed by a more gradual rise that reached a peak in approximately 2.5 min. This is illustrated by the effects of taurocholic acid (Figure 4).

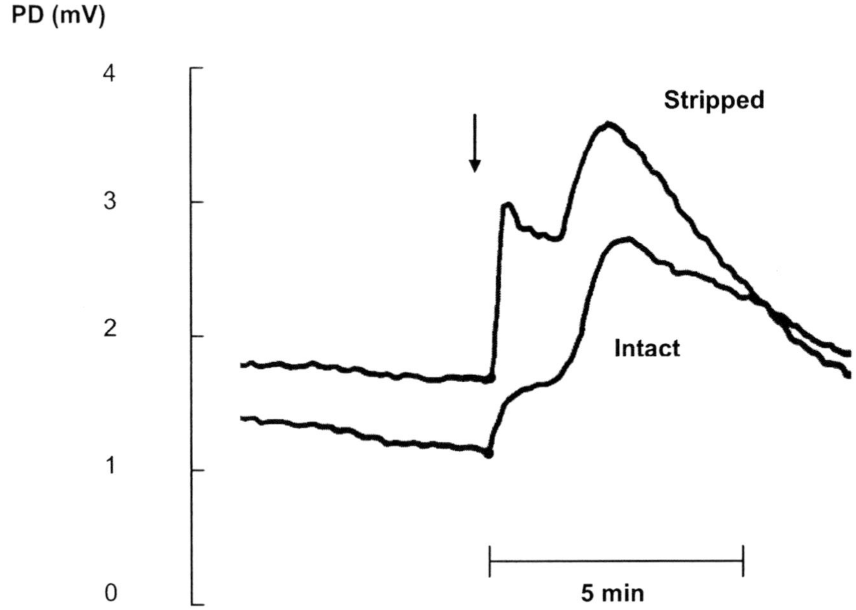

Fig. 4. Typical changes in the potential difference (PD) across intact and stripped sheets of ileum from Swiss mice induced by mucosal application of taurocholic acid (2.5 mM) added at the arrow.

The magnitude of the first phase was 45.8±2.2 μA cm^{-2} in stripped sheets and 34.5±5.1 μA cm^{-2} in intact sheets while that of the second phase was 97.0±10.4 μA cm^{-2} in stripped sheets and 101.8±17.4 μA cm^{-2} in intact sheets (n=7, P>0.05 in both cases). Serosal application of taurocholic acid (1 mM) to stripped sheets was without effect (1.6±2.0 μA cm^{-2}, n=4). The initial phase of the response to mucosal bile acid was decreased when the Na^+ concentration of the mucosal solution was reduced to 25 mM, but it was unaffected by conditions that inhibit intestinal secretion (absence of Cl^-, serosal furosemide, mucosal DPC; Figure 5A). In contrast, the second phase was unaffected by low mucosal Na^+, but it was reduced by conditions that inhibit the secretory response (Figure 5B). Moreover, the second phase of the response to 2.5 mM taurocholic acid was reduced by increasing the serosal K^+ concentration to 20 mM (control: 128.2±13.7 μA cm^{-2}; test: 57.3±9.1 μA cm^{-2}, n=7, P<0.01). Similar findings have been obtained with ursodeoxycholic acid (Hardcastle et al 2001a).

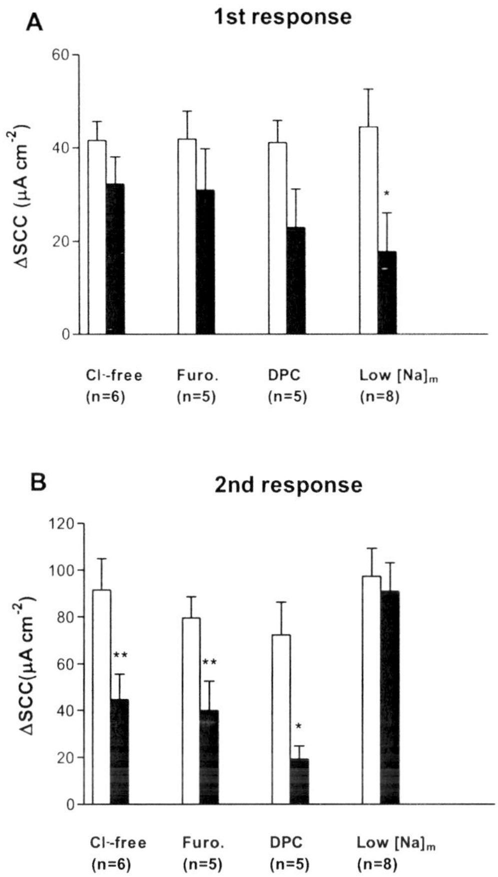

Fig. 5. Effect of taurocholic acid on stripped ileal sheets from Swiss mice. 2.5 mM taurocholic acid was added to the mucosal solution and the first (A) and second (B) peaks of the SCC response recorded. The effects of Cl^--free conditions, serosal furosemide (10^{-3}M), mucosal DPC (10^{-3}M) and low mucosal Na^+ concentration ($[Na^+]_m$ = 25mM) are shown. Values are mean ± 1 s.e.m. of the number of tissue pairs (n) indicated,with control values shown by the open bars and test values by solid bars. A paired *t* test was used to compare control (open bars) and test (solid bars) values. * $P<0.05$; ** $P<0.01$.

These observations suggest that the initial phase of the electrical response to taurocholic acid is associated with its active Na^+-dependent absorption. This is supported by the finding that lowering the mucosal Na^+ concentration to 25 mM reduced the rise in SCC induced by 10 mM mucosal glucose by 54.5±4.9% (n=8, $P<0.001$), but had no effect on the response to serosal application of the secretagogue acetylcholine (10^{-3}M, control: 210.2±21.7 μA cm^{-2}; test: 206.5±28.8 μA cm^{-2}, n=4, $P>0.05$). The first, absorptive, phase was observed in the ileum, but was absent in more proximial regions of intestine (Table 1) that lack the IBAT. The second phase represents bile acid-induced secretion and is present throughout the intestine (Table 1).

The magnitude of both the first and second ileal responses to taurocholic acid were concentration-dependent (Figures 6A and 6B) in stripped and intact sheets. For both the absorptive and secretory components a 50% maximum response was achieved at a concentration of approximately 0.5 mM.

Table 1. Comparison of the effects of bile acids on the SCC in stripped sheets of mouse small intestine.

		Mucosal		Serosal
	Bile acid	**M1 μA cm^{-2}**	**M2 μA cm^{-2}**	**S μA cm^{-2}**
Ileum	TA	35.0±5.1(6)	92.7±8.5(6)	1.6±2.0(4)
	UDCA	35.0±4.7(8)	49.2±5.8(8)	37.4±5.2(8)
	DCA	38.2±4.5(5)	7.2±6.4(5)	31.5±3.9(5)
	CDCA	28.8±5.6(6)	1.9±5.2(6)	27.9±2.0(5)
	GCA	25.1±3.3(5)	40.8±5.3(5)	7.2±3.1(5)
	CA	29.2±5.0(7)	12.3±3.3(7)	3.1±3.3(7)
Mid-intestine	TA	-	9.4±4.7(6)	3.6±1.2(6)
	UDCA	-	41.6±4.9(7)	45.0±6.3(7)
	DCA	-	-4.1±1.8(8)	63.8±7.7(4)
	CDCA	-	7.6±4.0(6)	62.0±5.3(6)
	GCA	-	10.5±4.5(6)	16.9±3.0(6)
	CA	-	7.8±3.4(6)	18.9±2.0(6)
Jejunum	TA	-	7.8±1.7(7)	96.7±20.1(8)
	UDCA	-	21.3±7.9(8)	12.1±2.8(8)
	DCA	-	-9.9±6.5(8)	54.6±7.9(8)
	CDCA	-	4.7±6.4(8)	48.8±5.9(8)
	GCA	-	0.2±0.8(4)	12.6±2.3(4)
	CA	-	11.5±4.4(7)	44.7±8.9(7)

1 mM taurocholic acid (TA), ursodeoxycholic acid (UDCA), deoxycholic acid (DCA), chenodeoxycholic acid (CDCA), glycocholic acid (GCA) or cholic acid (CA) was added to either the mucosal or serosal solution. M1 and M2 represent the first and second phases of the ileal response to mucosal application and S is the response to serosal application. Each value represents the mean ± 1 s.e.m. of the number of observations in parentheses.

The effects of other bile acids on the transintestinal electrical activity of the jejunum and mid-intestine, as well as the ileum, were also investigated. These included ursodeoxycholic, deoxycholic, chenodeoxycholic, glycocholic and cholic acids (Table 1). When applied mucosally, they all induced an initial increase in SCC in ileal sheets, indicating their ability to be actively absorbed by an electrogenic Na^+-dependent mechanism in this region of the intestine. However, only taurocholic, ursodeoxycholic and glycocholic acids caused a secondary increase. In contrast, serosal addition of taurocholic, glycocholic and cholic acids had little effect, but ursodeoxycholic, deoxycholic and chenodeoxycholic acids all increased the SCC. The response to serosal application of bile acids was monophasic and represented a secretory event as it was inhibited by absence of Cl^-, mucosal DPC or serosal furosemide, but unaffected by lowering the mucosal Na^+ concentration.

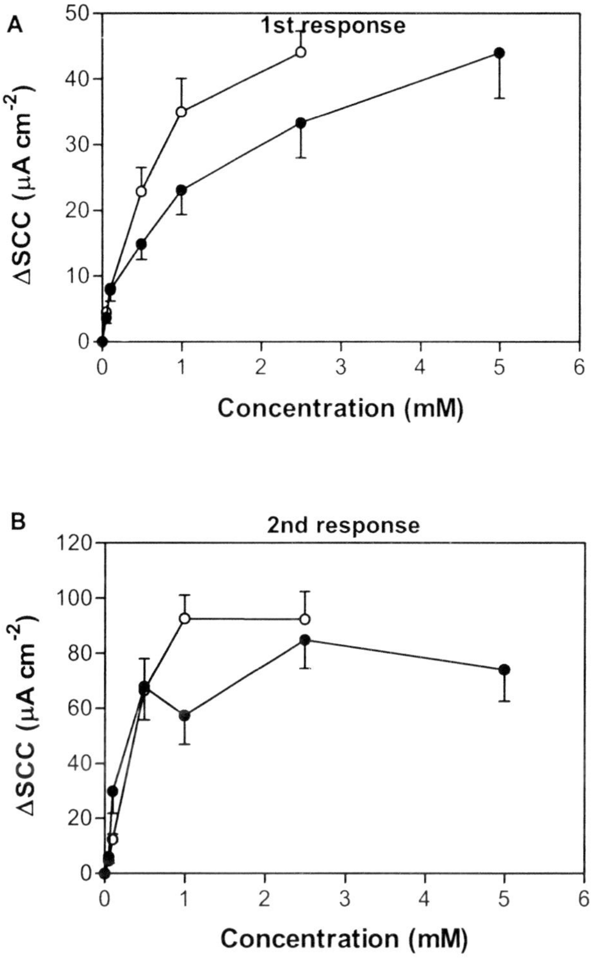

Fig. 6. Concentration-dependence of the first (A) and second (B) phases of taurocholic acid action in intact (●) and stripped (O) sheets of mouse ileum. Each point represents the mean ± 1 s.e.m. of 6-16 tissues.

In the mid-intestine and jejunum rises in SCC induced by bile acids were always monophasic and represented a stimulation of secretion (Hardcastle et al 2001a). Ursodeoxycholic acid was most effective in eliciting a response to mucosal application, with the other bile acids having little or no effect (Table 1). When added to the serosal side of the preparation ursodeoxycholic, deoxycholic, chenodeoxycholic, glycocholic and cholic acids all caused a rise in SCC. Serosal taurocholic acid was without effect in the mid-intestine, but caused a large response in the jejunum. There are, therefore, regional variations in the intestinal response to bile acids.

In jejunum and mid-intestine bile acid-induced secretion reached its maximum effect move quickly following serosal application, although in the ileum, mucosal application produced a more rapid response (Hardcastle et al 2001a).

The secretory component of the SCC response to taurocholic acid in the ileum was Ca^{2+}-dependent as it was reduced both by removal of serosal Ca^{2+} and by the addition of verapamil to the serosal solution (Figure 7). It is not clear however, whether this represented the involvement of Ca^{2+} at the level of the enterocyte. Neither removal of serosal Ca^{2+} nor the presence of verapamil affected the response to glucose ($P>0.05$ in both cases).

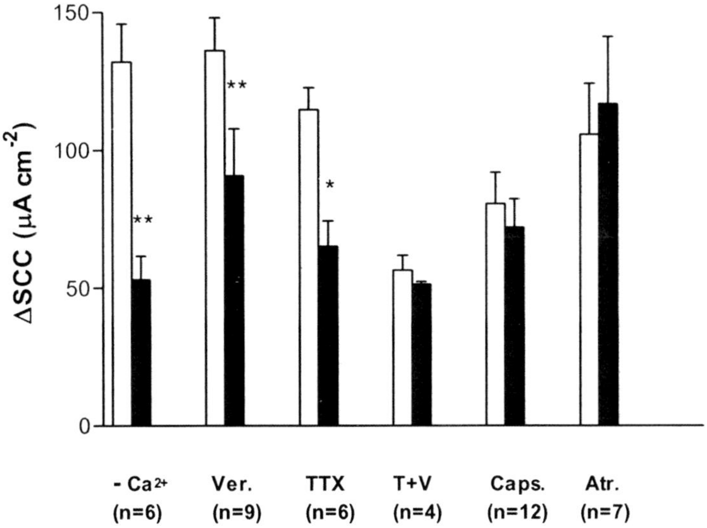

Fig. 7. Involvement of Ca^{2+} and neural mechanisms in the response of stripped sheets of mouse ileum to taurocholic acid. The effects of the absence of serosal Ca^{2+} ($-Ca^{2+}$) or the presence of serosal verapamil (Ver., 10^{-4}M), tetrodotoxin (TTX, 10^{-5} M), tetrodotoxin + verapamil (T+V), capsaicin (Caps., 10^{-6}M) or atropine (Atr., 10^{-5}M) on the SCC response to 2.5 mM mucosal taurocholic acid are shown. Each bar represents the mean ± 1 s.e.m. of the number of tissue pairs (n) indicated, with control values shown by the open bars and test values by the solid bars. A paired *t* test was used to assess significance. * $P<0.05$; ** $P<0.01$.

The possible involvement of neural pathways in taurocholic acid-induced ileal secretion was investigated by examining the effects of the neurotoxin, tetrodotoxin. Tetrodotoxin reduced the effect of taurocholic acid by 41.7±8.5% (n=6, $P<0.01$), indicating that neural mechanisms contribute to the response (Figure 7). In the presence of the neurotoxin verapamil caused no further inhibition, suggesting that the Ca^{2+}-dependence of taurocholic acid action represented an action on the neural pathways involved in the taurocholic acid response. There was no evidence for the involvement of capsaicin-sensitive afferent neurones as this agent did not inhibit the rise in SCC induced by taurocholic acid. Atropine did not inhibit the taurocholic acid response, although it reduced the effect of 10^{-3}M ACh by 85.4±3.6% (n=7, $P<0.001$), thus muscarinic cholinoreceptors make no contribution (Figure 7).

None of the experimental conditions designed to investigate the involvement of neural pathways inhibited the rise in SCC induced by glucose ($P>0.05$ in all cases).

The possibility that mast cells might contribute to bile acid-induced secretion was tested by examining the effects of mast cell stabilising agents and antagonists of mast cell degranulation products. Doxantrazole, which stabilises both mucosal and connective tissue-type mast cells (Pearce et al 1982), caused a significant inhibition of the secretory phase of the taurocholic acid-induced rise in SCC, whereas sodium chromoglycate, which acts only on connective tissue-type mast cells (Pearce et al 1982), did not (Figure 8).

Increased prostanoid production does not appear to contribute to taurocholic acid-induced ileal secretion as indomethacin did not reduce the SCC response. However, both the H_1 antagonist mepyramine and desensitisation to 5-HT (induced by prior exposure of the tissue to 10^{-4}M 5-HT) caused an inhibition (34.4±10.8%, n=6, $P<0.05$ and 41.4±5.1%, n=8, $P<0.05$ respectively, Figure 8), suggesting that histamine and 5-HT are involved in the secretory response to taurocholic acid. None of these treatments reduced the response to glucose ($P>0.05$ in all cases, n=4-6).

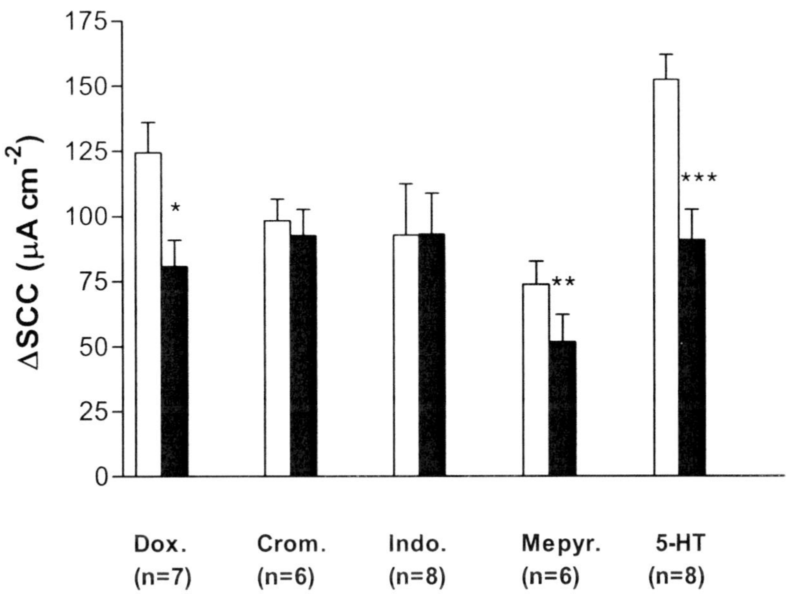

Fig. 8. Involvement of mast cell mediators in the response of stripped sheets of mouse ileum to taurocholic acid. The effects of mucosal + serosal doxantrazole (Dox., 10^{-3}M), mucosal + serosal sodium cromoglycate (Crom., 10^{-3}M), serosal indomethacin (Indo., 5×10^{-5} M), serosal mepyramine (Mepyr., 10^{-4}M), or desensitisation to 5-HT by prior exposure to 10^{-4}M serosal 5-HT on the SCC response to 2.5 mM mucosal taurocholic acid are shown. Each bar represents the mean ± 1 s.e.m. of the number of tissue pairs (n) indicated, with control values shown by the open bars and test values by the solid bars. A paired *t* test was used to assess significance. * $P<0.05$; ** $P<0.01$; *** $P<0.001$.

Ursodeoxycholic acid is a tertiary bile acid that is used therapeutically for its choleretic and cytoprotective effects in the treatment of primary biliary cirrhosis and gallstones (Hofmann 1998). It is also used to treat the hepatobiliary symptoms of CF (Cheng et al 1997). Like taurocholic acid, it causes a biphasic rise in ileal SCC with the first phase representing active Na^+-dependent uptake and the second phase bile acid-induced secretion. Its secretory effects are also Ca^{2+}-dependent and involve mast cell degranulation (Hardcastle et al 2001a). However, ursodeoxycholic acid differs from taurocholic acid in that there is no evidence for any neural involvement in its action, with tetrodotoxin failing to influence its effects (Hardcastle et al 2001a).

Transgenic CF mice

Basal Electrical Activity in CF Mice

Basal electrical activity was similar in intact ileal sheets from wild-type and CF (*Cftr*^{tm2Cam}) mice, with PD, SCC and tissue resistance values of 1.6±0.6 mV, 60.3±12.3 μA cm^{-2} and 23.8±3.6 ohm.cm^2 (n=5) in wild-type tissues and 1.4±0.3 mV, 46.8±10.9 μA cm^{-2}

and 30.0±0.3 ohm.cm^2 (n=5) in CF tissues (P>0.05 in all cases). The phenotype of the tissues was confirmed by testing their response to secretagogue challenge. Acetylcholine produced a very variable response in intact tissues from normal mice and in wild-type tissues 10^{-3}M acetylcholine increased the SCC by 25.0±14.3 μA cm^{-2} (n=5). Nevertheless this was significantly greater than the response observed in CF tissues (-9.3±5.9 μA cm^{-2}, n=5, P<0.05). The response to 5-HT was more consistent with 10^{-4}M 5-HT increasing the SCC by 75.2±20.2 μA cm^{-2} (n=5) in wild-type ilea and by 1.5±2.3 μA cm^{-2} (n=5, P<0.01) in CF ilea.

In stripped ileal sheets from CF (*Cftr*^{tm1Eur}) mice the basal PD, SCC and tissue resistance values were 1.3±0.3 mV, 53.9±9.4 μA cm^{-2} and 24.4±1.6 ohm.cm^2 (n=10) in wild-type tissues and 1.0±0.2 mV, 29.5±6.8 μA cm^{-2} and 35.9±2.1 ohm.cm^2 (n=8) in CF tissues. In this preparation the basal SCC was lower (P<0.05) and the tissue resistance was higher (P<0.001) in CF tissues. An increased tissue resistance has also been reported in human rectal biopsies (Mall et al 1999). The response to acetylcholine (10^{-3}M) in wild-type ilea was much larger (136.3±18.4 μA cm^{-2}, n=10) in stripped sheets than it was in intact sheets. Acetylcholine was added to the serosal side of the preparation and in intact preparations it had to penetrate a greater barrier to diffusion and was exposed to the high levels of cholinesterase present in the muscle layers and myenteric plexus (Ambache et al 1971). Both these factors would reduce the effective concentration of acetylcholine at its receptors on the basolateral membrane of the enterocyte. As in intact tissues, acetylcholine had very little effect in stripped ileal sheets from CF mice (11.3±1.6 μA cm^{-2}, n=8, P<0.001), confirming the phenotype of the tissues tested.

Effects of Bile Acids on Transintestinal Electrical Activity in CF Mice

In intact tissues from wild-type CF (*Cftr*^{tm2Cam}) mice taurocholic acid (2.5 mM) caused a biphasic rise in SCC (Figure 9) similar to that observed in tissues from Swiss mice (Figure 4), the magnitude of the first and second phases being 13.1±1.7 and 32.0±6.2 μA cm^{-2} (n=5) respectively. In CF tissues only the first absorptive phase of the response was still present (Figure 9) and the second phase was completely absent. Stripped ileal sheets from *Cft*^{rtm1Eur} mice behaved similarly, with wild type tissues producing a biphasic response to 2.5 mM taurocholic acid, with first and second phases of 44.4±5.6 and 89.9±16.5 μA cm^{-2} (n=10) respectively. CF tissues, in contrast, only produced an initial response and the secretory component was totally absent.

The effects of ursodeoxycholic acid have also been tested in stripped ileal sheets from CF (*Cftr*^{tm2Cam}) mice (Hardcastle et al 2001a). As with taurocholic acid, the secretory phase of the SCC response is absent (wild-type: 43.2±4.7 μA cm^{-2} (n=4); CF: -5.2±3.3 μA cm^{-2} (n=13), P<0.001). The initial phase was still present however, and its absorptive basis was confirmed by finding that it was unaffected by furosemide, but inhibited by a low mucosal Na^+ concentration.

It is clear that bile acids are capable of increasing the transintestinal electrical activity throughout the small intestine. In the ileum bile acids induced a biphasic rise in PD and SCC, with the first phase representing Na^+-dependent bile acid absorption, mediated by the IBAT, and the second phase a stimulation of electrogenic Cl^- secretion. In more proximal regions of intestine however, only a secretory response was observed and this is consistent with the distribution of the IBAT whose location is confined to the ileum (Stelzner et al 2000; St-Pierre et al 2001). There was some variability in the actions of the bile acids. Except for taurocholic acid, all the bile acids tested induced a secretory response in each of the regions of small intestine, although the effective site of application varied, with no consistent pattern being observed. Taurocholic acid had no effect in the mid-intestine, regardless of its site of application, but it produced large secretory responses when added serosally to the jejunum or mucosally to the ileum.

A number of observations point towards a stimulation of electrogenic Cl^- secretion as the ionic basis of the second component of the SCC response in the ileum and the monophasic response in more proximal regions of the intestine. The magnitude of this phase was reduced in the absence of Cl^- in the bathing medium. It was also reduced by serosal furosemide, which inhibits the NKCC1 cotransporter responsible for the accumulation of Cl^- within the enterocyte (Heintze et al 1983), or mucosal DPC, which blocks the luminal Cl^- channels through which Cl^- leaves the cell (Sahi et al 1994). Increasing the serosal K^+ concentration reduces the basolateral hyperpolarisation that contributes to the maintenance of Cl^- secretion (Hardcastle & Hardcastle 1987) and this too led to a decrease in the second phase of the response. The secretory response to taurocholic acid was observed at concentrations in the same range as those reported to be present in the intestinal lumen (Northfield & McColl 1973), suggesting that it represents a normal aspect of gut function.

Bile acids are actively absorbed in the terminal ileum by a Na^+-dependent mechanism that also generates electrical activity (Hofmann 1998) and this was responsible for the initial phase of the SCC response to mucosal application of bile acids to this region of the intestine. Lowering the mucosal Na^+ concentration to 25 mM inhibited the first component of the SCC response to taurocholic acid by 60%, an effect comparable to the 55% reduction in the glucose-dependent rise in SCC, generated by a similar Na^+-dependent mechanism (Schultz & Zalusky 1964), that is observed in low Na^+ conditions.

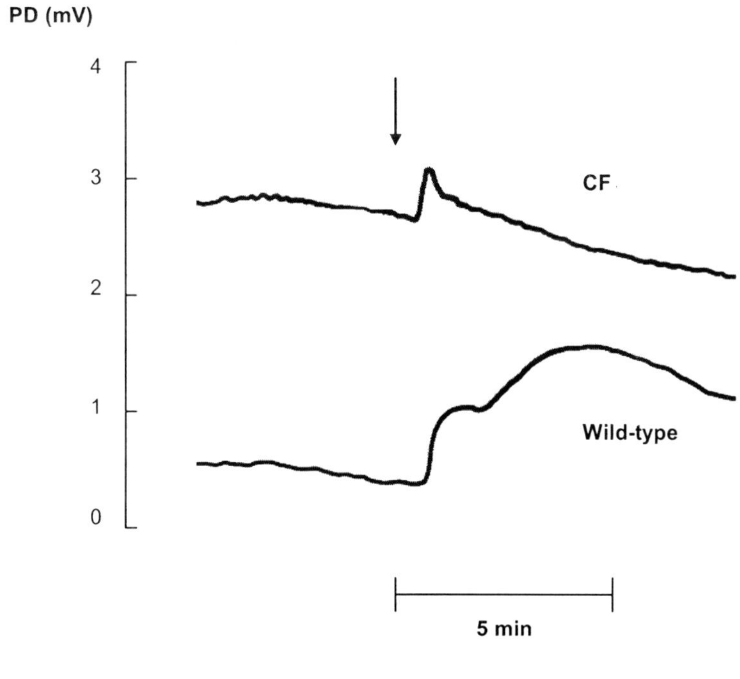

Fig. 9. Typical changes in the potential difference (PD) across intact sheets of ileum from transgenic CF mice ($Cftr^{tm2Cam}$) induced by mucosal application of taurocholic acid (2.5 mM) added at the arrow.

Activation of the enteric nervous system was responsible for at least part of the taurocholic acid-induced secretion as tetrodotoxin inhibited the SCC response of stripped ileal sheets to the bile acid by 42%. However, muscarinic cholinoreceptors were not involved. Neural mechanisms have also been shown to contribute to bile acid-induced secretion in rat small intestine, where the involvement of presynaptic cholinergic neurones and post-synaptic non-adrenergic, non-cholinergic neurones was demonstrated (Karlström et al 1981, 1983; Karlström 1986; Levin & Ayton 1995). In rat ileum it is the myenteric plexus that contributes to taurocholic acid-induced secretion as tetrodotoxin inhibits the response in intact tissues, but not in stripped preparations where the myenteric plexus is removed (Levin & Ayton 1995). In contrast, other components of the enteric nervous system must be involved in mouse ileum as tetrodotoxin was effective in stripped tissues. Activation of the enteric nervous system did not occur via stimulation of capsaicin-sensitive afferent neurones as pretreatment with capsaicin did not alter the response of mouse ileum to taurocholic acid. Similar observations have been made in the rat (Levin & Ayton 1995). In contrast, the secretory actions of ursodeoxycholic acid in stripped intestinal sheets do not seem to involve neural mechanisms, as tetrodotoxin had no inhibitory effects. However, the neurotoxin did inhibit ursodeoxycholic acid-induced secretion in intact intestinal sheets (Hardcastle et al 2001a), suggesting that in this preparation a neural pathway involving the myenteric plexus contributed to the response. This is similar to bile acid-induced secretion in rat ileum (Levin & Ayton 1995).

It is possible that bile acids could act on immune elements within the gut wall to release mediators that activate the enteric nerves, as an intimate relationship exists between the intestinal neural and immune systems (Cooke 1994). In mouse colon histamine and mast cells have been implicated in the response to bile acids (Gelbmann et al 1995) and in the mouse ileum there is evidence for the involvement of mucosal mast cells and their mediators in bile acid-induced secretion. Doxantrazole stabilises both mucosal and connective tissue-type mast cells (Pearce et al 1982) and it caused a significant inhibition of the secretory response to both taurocholic and ursodeoxycholic acids, whereas sodium cromoglycate, which acts only on connective tissue-type mast cells (Pearce et al 1982), was without effect. Mast cells have also been implicated in the secretory response of rat small intestine to antigen challenge (Crowe et al 1990) and a blunted response to bile acids has been observed in colonic tissues from mast cell-deficient mice (Gelbmann et al 1995). The mast cell mediators that contribute to bile acid-induced secretion include both histamine and 5-HT. The secretory response to bile acids was inhibited by mepyramine, an antagonist at the H_1 receptors that are responsible for histamine-mediated intestinal secretion (Hardcastle & Hardcastle 1987a). The secretory actions of 5-HT involve a number of different 5-HT receptor subtypes and sites of action (Hardcastle & Hardcastle 1997), with the result that no selective antagonist is capable of abolishing the response. However, desensitisation occurs following 5-HT challenge *in vitro* (Hardcastle et al 1994) and this provides an experimental approach to test the involvement of 5-HT in bile acid action. Both taurocholic acid and ursodeoxycholic acid were found to be less effective in eliciting a secretory response in ileal sheets that had been desensitised by prior exposure to 5-HT, implicating 5-HT involvement in their actions. 5-HT has also been shown to contribute to bile salt-induced secretion by rat jejunum *in vivo* (Timar Peregrin et al 1999). In contrast, there was no evidence for the involvement of prostanoids or substance P.

It appears that a number of mediators contribute to bile acid-induced secretion in mouse small intestine. Their release may involve Ca^{2+}-dependent mechanisms as the secretory response to bile acid stimulation was inhibited by lack of Ca^{2+} or the presence of the Ca^{2+}

channel blocker verapamil. Since verapamil caused no further inhibition in the presence of tetrodotoxin it is likely that it is the release of neurotransmitters that is Ca^{2+}-dependent rather than the action of the mediators on the transporting cells. In rat small intestine bile acid activation of the enteric nervous system occurs, at least in part, via the Ca^{2+}-dependent release of 5-HT from enterochromaffin cells (Timar Peregrin et al 1999) and it appears that a similar mechanism of action operates in mouse ileum. It is clear therefore, that indirect mechanisms contribute to the secretory response of mouse small intestine to bile acids. A similar conclusion has been reached with regard to the actions of deoxycholic acid in rat and rabbit colon where secretion was observed in intact mucosa, but not in isolated crypts (Mauricio et al 2000).

The secretory response of the jejunum and mid-intestine reached its maximum SCC value more rapidly when bile acids were added to the serosal compartment. This supports the concept that bile acids act subepithelially to exert their effects and is consistent with an action on mucosal mast cells. In the ileum the secretory response to bile acid stimulation is more rapid on mucosal application because there is an active mechanism for the reabsorption of bile acids in this region (Hofmann 1998) and this will accelerate the transport of bile acids from the lumen to their site of action.

Although indirect mechanisms contribute to the secretory response to taurocholic acid, a direct action on the transporting cell may also occur. Bile acids can induce secretion via a rise in cytosolic Ca^{2+} in T84 cells, a colonic cell line that exhibits many of the transport characteristics observed in normal enterocytes (Dharmsathaphorn et al 1989). They have also been shown to activate ion channels associated with the secretory process in T84 cells (Devor & Frizzell 1993), suggesting that the transporting cells themselves may possess the ability to respond to bile acid challenge.

The characteristics of the secretory response to bile acids were established in studies in Swiss mice and these laid the foundations for the investigation of bile acid-induced secretion in intestinal tissue from transgenic CF mice. Ileal tissues from wild-type mice exhibited taurocholic acid responses that were similar to those observed in Swiss mice, but there was a clear distinction between wild-type and CF mice. In intact ileal preparations from CF mice the secretory responses to acetylcholine and 5-HT were absent, mirroring the situation observed in intestinal tissues from human patients with CF (Taylor et al 1987, 1988), and indicating that the intestine from the ΔF508 CF mouse model exhibits the defective secretory response characteristic of the human disease. This failure of secretion arises as a result of defects in CFTR, the protein product of the CF gene, which acts as the channel that allows the exit of Cl^- during the secretory process. Thus any secretagogue, regardless of the intracellular signalling pathway that mediates its effects, is unable to activate the secretory process. Hence the generation of intracellular signalling molecules is normal in CF enterocytes (Hitchin et al 1990; Klaren et al 2001) and direct application of cAMP or A23187 (the Ca^{2+} ionophore that raises cytosolic Ca^{2+} levels) fails to activate secretion in CF tissues (Hardcastle et al 1990). The secretory component of the SCC responses to bile acids was also absent in CF ilea. Thus taurocholic acid did not elicit a secretory response in intact CF ilea while ursodeoxycholic acid failed to produce a secretory response in stripped ilea. It can therefore be concluded that bile acid-induced secretion is also abnormal in CF.

Bile acids induce secretion in the throughout the small intestine of normal mice and this response can involve both neural and immune elements within the gut wall. However, in CF intestine this response, like that to other secretagogues, is defective. The failure of normal bile acid-induced secretion may play a part in the excessive dehydration of the luminal contents that occurs in CF intestine and which contributes to the development of obstructive symptomatology such as meconium ileas.

Bile Acid Absorption in CF

In the intestine bile acids induce a secretory response that is absent in CF tissues. However, bile acids are also subject to an active reuptake mechanism in the terminal ileum. This process is mediated by the IBAT, a Na^+-dependent cotransporter that utilises the energy from the Na^+ gradient between the lumen and the intracellular fluid of the enterocyte to accumulate bile acids within the cell against their concentration gradient. Absorption mediated by other Na^+-dependent nutrient cotransporters is altered in CF (Frase et al 1985; Baxter et al 1990) and bile acid malabsorption has been reported in CF patients (Fondacaro et al 1982; O'Brien et al 1983), suggesting that the function of the IBAT may be disturbed in the disease. The terminal ileum is not easily accessible for study in human subjects, so the development of transgenic mouse models of CF has provided a valuable opportunity to examine the effects of the disease on the ileal mechanism for bile acid reabsorption in more detail (Hardcastle et al 2004).

Methods Used to Investigate Bile Acid Absorption

Experiments were performed on intestinal tissues from Swiss mice together with the $Cftr^{tm2Cam}$ and the $Cftr^{tm1Eur}$ transgenic mouse models. Animals used included mice homozygous for the ΔF508 mutation together with wild-type littermates.

As the Na^+-dependent mechanism for active bile acid uptake is electrogenic its activity can be monitored by measuring transintestinal electrical activity as described previously. In addition to these electrical measurements, taurocholic acid uptake was determined directly both in an intact tissue preparation, the everted sac, and an isolated membrane preparation, brush-border membrane vesicles (BBMVs).

Fluid and taurocholic acid uptakes were measured in everted sacs of small intestine. Jejunal sacs were taken from the region immediately distal to the ligament of Treitz, mid-intestinal sacs were taken from the mid region, while ileal sacs were taken from the region immediately proximal to the caecum. Each sac was approximately 5 cm long and was filled with 0.1-0.2 mL Krebs bicarbonate saline containing 10 mM glucose and incubated at 37°C for 30 min in 15 mL Krebs bicarbonate saline containing 10 mM mannitol, 1 mM taurocholic acid and 92.5 kBq/100 mL ^{3}H-taurocholic acid. During the incubation sacs were shaken at 80 oscillations per min. At the end of the incubation each sac was washed with 154 mM NaCl and gently blotted. It was then weighed and fluid uptake determined as the increase in weight of the filled sac during incubation. The serosal fluid was collected and the empty sac was deproteinised, homogenised and filtered. 100 μL samples of initial mucosal fluid, final mucosal fluid, final serosal fluid and gut homogenate were added to 3 mL Emulsifier Safe and counted in a liquid scintillation counter. Taurocholic acid uptake was determined as the amount taken up into the gut and serosal fluid. Fluid and taurocholic acid uptakes were related to the initial wet weight (iww) of the empty sac. The T/M ratio, the concentration of taurocholic acid in the tissue water compared with its concentration in the mucosal fluid at the end of the incubation, was used to determine whether active uptake (T/M ratio > 1) of the bile acid had occurred. The tissue water content was 80% initial wet weight (determined as 100 - dry weight x 100/wet weight) plus the volume of fluid taken up by the sac during incubation.

In low Na^+ conditions the Na^+ concentration of the mucosal solution was reduced to 25 mM by replacing all the NaCl in the Krebs with isotonic mannitol. The effects of glycocholic acid and ursodeoxycholic acid were tested by adding them to the mucosal fluid at the concentrations indicated. The ethanol vehicle used to dissolve the bile acids was present at a concentration of 0.67% (v/v) and this had no significant effect on either fluid or taurocholic acid uptake (P>0.05 in both cases).

Brush-border membrane vesicles (BBMVs) were isolated from the ileum of transgenic CF ($Cftr^{tm2Cam}$) mice using a magnesium precipitation technique as described in detail by Klaren et al (2000). The distal 8 cm of small intestine was removed, flushed with ice-cold saline (150 mM NaCl and 20 mM HEPES/Tris, pH 7.4), cut open lengthwise and the mucosa scraped off with a microscope slide. To ensure that sufficient BBMVs were prepared mucosae from 2 or 3 mice were pooled. The mucosae were homogenized in a 30 mL tissue grinder with a Teflon pestle in 15 mL ice-cold buffer (50 mM mannitol and 20 mM HEPES/Tris, pH 7.4). $MgCl_2$ was added to give a final concentration of 10 mM and the homogenate was stirred gently for 20 min. It was then centrifuged for 10 min in a cooled (to 4°C) rotor at 4725 g_{max} and the resultant supernatant was spun at 41400 g_{max} for 30 min. The pellet was resuspended in 1 mL buffer (300 mM mannitol, 0.1 mM $MgSO_4$, 20 mM HEPES/Tris, pH 7.4) by 25 passages through a 23-gauge needle. A further 15 mL buffer was added, the suspension was spun again at 4725 g_{max} for 15 min and the resultant supernatant spun at 41400 g_{max} for 30 min. The final pellet was resuspended in approximately 330 µL uptake buffer (200 mM mannitol, 0.1 mM $MgSO_4$, 20 mM HEPES/Tris, pH 7.4) to give a final concentration of approximately 1 mg protein mL^{-1}.

The protein content of the BBMV preparation was determined with a Coomassie Brilliant Blue reagent kit using BSA as a standard. Alkaline phosphatase (a marker enzyme for brush-border membranes) and Na^+, K^+-ATPase (a marker enzyme for basolateral membranes) activities were measured as described previously (Klaren et al, 2001). A 9.2±2.3-fold (n=6) enrichment of alkaline phosphatase activity occurred in the BBMV preparation (compared with the homogenate). This was significantly greater (P<0.01) than the change in Na^+, K^+-ATPase activity (2.6±0.4-fold, n=6).

Taurocholic acid uptake was measured in duplicate using a rapid filtration protocol. BBMVs were incubated at 20°C in a medium containing 100µM taurocholic acid, 843 kBq/mL ^{3}H-taurocholic acid, 100 mM Na-gluconate, 0.1 mM $MgSO_4$, 20 mM HEPES/Tris, pH 7.4 for periods between 10 and 900 sec. Uptake was terminated by adding an 18-fold surplus of ice-cold stop buffer (165 mM KCl, 100 µM taurocholic acid, 10 mM Tris, pH 7.4) and filtering immediately over a –80 kP_a vacuum using a cellulose nitrate membrane filter with a pore diameter of 0.45 µm. The filter was rapidly rinsed with 2 x 4 mL ice-cold stop buffer and transferred to a vial, 4.5 mL Emulsifier Safe was added and the filter allowed to dissolve. Vials were then counted in a liquid scintillation counter. Bile acid uptake was expressed as nmol taurocholic acid mg $protein^{-1}$.

Results are expressed as mean values ± 1 s.e.m. of the number of observations indicated. Student's *t* test, paired or unpaired as appropriate, was used to assess significance. For multiple comparisons ANOVA, with post hoc analysis by Scheffé's method, was used.

Effect of Taurocholic Acid on Transintestinal Electrical Activity in Swiss Mice

Addition of taurocholic acid to the mucosal solution caused a biphasic increase in PD and SCC (Figure 4) with intact and stripped sheets producing similar responses. Serosal application of taurocholic acid (1 mM) to stripped sheets was without effect (1.6 ± 2.0 μA cm^{-2}, n=4). The initial phase of the response to mucosal bile acid was decreased when the Na^+ concentration of the mucosal solution was reduced to 25 mM, but it was unaffected by conditions that inhibit intestinal secretion (absence of Cl^-, serosal furosemide, mucosal DPC; Figure 5A). In contrast, the second phase was unaffected by low mucosal Na^+, but it was reduced by conditions that inhibit the secretory response (Figure 5B). This suggests that the initial phase of the electrical response to taurocholic acid is associated with its active Na^+-dependent absorption, while the second phase represents bile acid-induced secretion.

The magnitude of the absorptive phase of the SCC response was related to the taurocholic acid concentration in both intact and stripped sheets (Figure 6). A Lineweaver Burke plot of the data provided apparent K_m and V_{max} values of 0.43 mM and 33.3 μA cm^{-2} in intact sheets and 0.50 mM and 50.0 μA cm^{-2} in stripped sheets. The presence of other actively transported bile acids in the mucosal solution inhibited the absorptive phase of the taurocholic acid-induced rise in SCC. In stripped ileal sheets ursodeoxycholic acid (1 mM) reduced the response to taurocholic acid (1 mM) from 18.5±3.3 to -5.1±1.8 μA cm^{-2} (n=7, $P<0.001$), while glycocholic acid (1 mM) reduced the response from 29.9±4.9 to 5.5±3.3 μA cm^{-2} (n=6, $P<0.01$).

Effect of Taurocholic Acid on Transintestinal Electrical Activity in CF Mice

The basal electrical activity was similar in intact ileal sheets from wild-type and CF mice (*Cftr*^{tm2Cam}), with PD, SCC and tissue resistance values of 1.6±0.6 mV, 60.3±12.3 μA cm^{-2} and 23.8±3.6 $ohm.cm^2$ (n=5) in wild-type tissues and 1.4±0.3 mV, 46.8±10.9 μA cm^{-2} and 30.0±0.3 $ohm.cm^2$ (n=5) in CF tissues ($P>0.05$ in all cases). The phenotype of the tissues was confirmed by testing their response to secretagogue challenge. Acetylcholine produced a very variable response in intact tissues from normal mice and in wild-type tissues 10^{-3}M acetylcholine increased the SCC by 25.0±14.3 μA cm^{-2} (n=5). Nevertheless this was significantly greater than the response observed in CF tissues (-9.3±5.9 μA cm^{-2} (n=5, $P<0.05$). The response to 5-HT was more consistent with 10^{-4}M 5-HT increasing the SCC by 75.2±20.2 μA cm^{-2} (n=5) in wild-type ilea and by 1.5±2.3 μA cm^{-2} (n=5, $P<0.01$) in CF ilea. In wild-type tissues taurocholic acid (2.5 mM) caused a biphasic rise in SCC (Figure 9) similar to that observed in tissues from Swiss mice, the magnitude of the first and second phases being 13.1±1.7 and 32.0±6.2 μA cm^{-2} (n=5) respectively. In CF tissues the first phase of the response was still present (Figure 9), although it was smaller (2.0±3.3 μA cm^{-2}, n=5, $P<0.05$) than that obtained in wild-type tissues. The second phase was completely absent.

In stripped ileal sheets from CF mice ($Cftr^{tm1Eur}$) the secretory component of the SCC response was again absent. The initial absorptive phase was present in both wild-type (44.4±5.6 μA cm^{-2}, n=10) and CF (40.5±6.0 μA cm^{-2}, n=8) tissues, and in this case there was no significant difference in values obtained from the two groups (P>0.05). The response to acetylcholine (10^{-3}M) confirmed the phenotype of the tissues tested, with wild-type tissues producing a response of 136.3±18.4 μA cm^{-2} (n=10) while in CF tissues the increase in SCC was only 11.3±1.6 μA cm^{-2} (n=8, P<0.001).

Fluid and Taurocholic Acid Uptake by Everted Sacs from Swiss Mice

In everted ileal sacs from Swiss mice fluid absorption was 0.58±0.07 ml/g iww/30 min and taurocholic acid uptake was 5.29±0.75 μmole/g iww/30 min (n=14). The T/M ratio was 2.39±0.24, indicating that taurocholic acid had been actively accumulated in the tissue. Taurocholic acid uptake was reduced when the mucosal Na^+ concentration was lowered (Figure 10). It was also inhibited in the presence of other actively absorbed bile acids (Figure 10). Fluid uptake was unaffected by any of these conditions (P>0.05 in all cases). The effect of ursodeoxycholic acid was concentration-dependent with 0.5, 1 and 2 mM reducing taurocholic acid uptake to 2.88±0.23 (n=5, P>0.05), 2.31±0.24 (n=6, P<0.05) and 1.15±0.12 (n=5, P<0.01) μmole/g iww/30 min respectively.

In everted sacs from more proximal regions of the mouse small intestine taurocholic acid uptake was much smaller, with no evidence of active absorption. In the jejunum fluid absorption was 0.30±0.03 ml/g iww/30 min, taurocholic acid uptake was 0.18±0.01 μmole/g iww/30 min and the T/M ratio was 0.16±0.01 (n=10), while in the mid-intestine equivalent values were 0.35±0.03 ml/g iww/30 min, 0.47±0.07 μmole/g iww/30 min and 0.31±0.04 (n=11) respectively.

Fluid and Taurocholic Acid Uptake by Everted Sacs from CF Mice ($Cftr^{tm2Cam}$)

In everted ileal sacs from wild-type mice fluid absorption, taurocholic acid uptake and the T/M ratio were similar to values obtained in ilea from Swiss mice (Figure 11, P>0.05 in all cases). In CF sacs however, taurocholic acid uptake and the T/M ratio were significantly reduced, although fluid uptake was similar (Figure 11).

In wild-type mice sacs from more proximal regions of the small intestine again exhibited much less taurocholic acid uptake with values for fluid transport, taurocholic acid uptake and the T/M ratio being 0.32±0.04 ml/g iww/30 min, 0.26±0.01 μmole/g iww/30 min and 0.22±0.01 (n=5) in the jejunum and 0.41±0.02 ml/g iww/30 min, 0.54±0.08 μmole/g iww/30 min and 0.30±0.04 (n=8) in the mid-intestine. In CF sacs equivalent values were 0.31±0.04 ml/g iww/30 min, 0.25±0.01 μmole/g iww/30 min and 0.22±0.01 (n=7) in the jejunum and 0.37±0.02 ml/g iww/30 min, 0.27±0.03 μmole/g iww/30 min and 0.23±0.02 (n=8) in the mid-intestine. In the jejunum there was no difference in taurocholic acid uptake between wild-type and CF tissues (P>0.05), but in the mid-intestine uptake of the bile acid was lower in CF sacs (P<0.01). This may be due to the presence of small amounts of the IBAT in more distal regions of sacs from the mid-intestine.

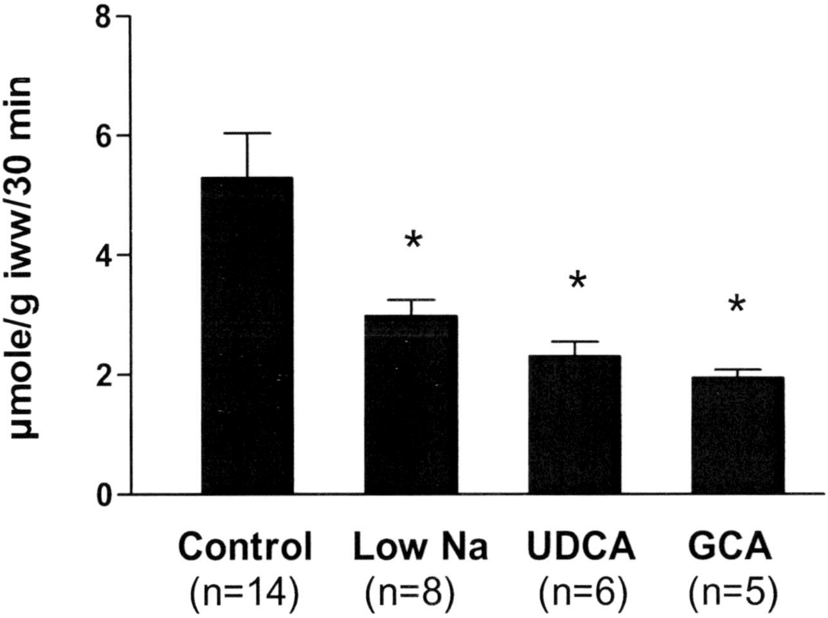

Fig. 10. Uptake of taurocholic acid by everted ileal sacs from Swiss mice. Sacs were incubated for 30 min in the presence of 1 mM taurocholic acid in the mucosal solution. In low Na^+ conditions the mucosal Na^+ concentration was reduced to 25 mM by replacement of NaCl with isotonic mannitol. The effects of 1 mM ursodeoxycholic acid (UDCA) or 1 mM glycocholic acid (GCA) in the mucosal solution were also tested. Each bar represents the mean ± 1 s.e.m. of the number of sacs (n) indicated and control and test data were compared using ANOVA. * P<0.05.

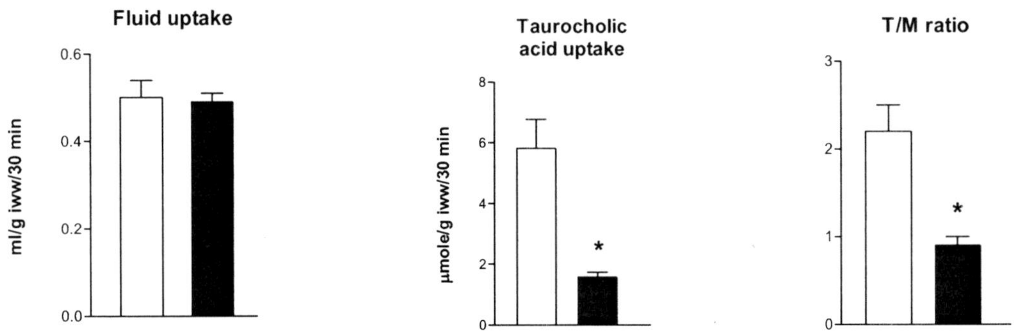

Fig. 11. Comparison of fluid and taurocholic acid uptake by everted ileal sacs from wild-type (open bars) and CF (solid bars) mice (*Cftr*^{tm2Cam}). Each bar represents the mean ± 1 s.e.m. of 8 sacs and an unpaired *t* test was used to compare control and test data. * *P*<0.05.

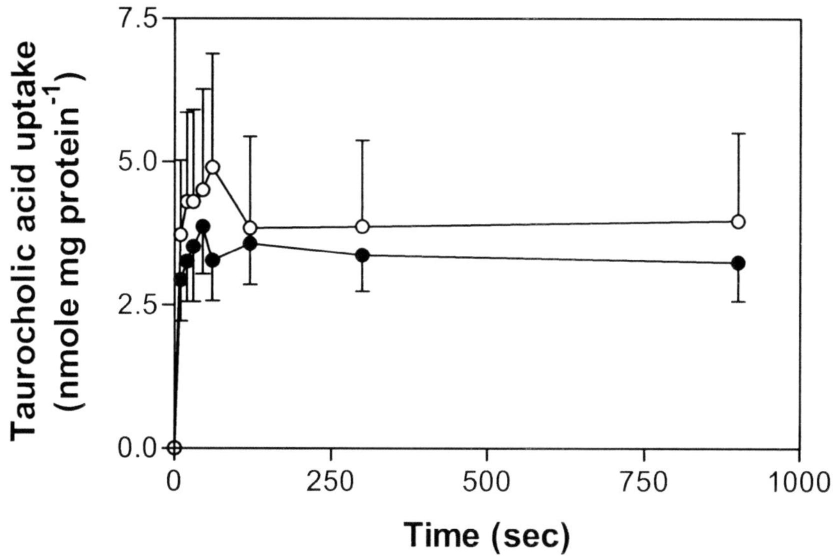

Fig. 12. Time course of taurocholic acid uptake by brush-border membrane vesicles from ilea of wild-type (○) and CF (●) mice (*Cftr*^{tm2Cam}). The taurocholic acid concentration was 100μM and uptake was measured in the presence of an inwardly-directed Na^+ gradient. Each point represents the mean ± 1 s.e.m. of 5 preparations.

Taurocholic acid uptake by brush-border membrane vesicles from wild-type and CF mice

In the presence of an inwardly-directed Na^+ gradient taurocholic acid uptake by BBMVs from both wild-type and CF ilea exhibited an overshoot (Figure 12). Peak uptake values were 4.90±1.99 (n=5) and 3.87±0.83 (n=5) nmole mg protein^{-1} (P>0.05) in vesicles from wild-type and CF ilea respectively. The times taken to achieve peak uptake were 46±7 and 37±5 sec (P>0.05).

Taurocholic acid uptake exhibited significant non-specific binding, indicated by the effects of increasing the extravesicular osmolarity (Hardcastle et al 2004). At conditions of infinite osmolarity a considerable uptake remained and this represented binding to the vesicle surface or incorporation into an osmotically-insensitive compartment rather than uptake into the intravesicular space. Similar observations have been reported for taurocholate uptake by human ileal BBMVs (Barnard & Ghishan 1987).

It is evident that a Na^+-dependent mechanism for the active reabsorption of bile acids exists in the terminal ileum of the mouse. In everted sacs taurocholic acid was accumulated within the tissue against its concentration gradient, leading to a T/M ratio significantly greater than unity and this process was inhibited when the Na^+ concentration of the mucosal solution was reduced. It was also inhibited by the presence of other actively transported bile acids that compete for the bile acid binding site on the IBAT. That both ursodeoxycholic acid and glycocholic acid can be actively absorbed by mouse ileum is demonstrated by their ability to elicit an absorptive component in their SCC response when applied to the luminal side of intestinal sheets. They also inhibited the initial phase of the SCC response of stripped ileal sheets to 1 mM taurocholic acid. The amount of taurocholic acid absorbed by mouse ileum is comparable to uptake of this bile acid by everted sacs of rat ileum (Caspary 1973) and by ileal biopsies from human patients (Ung et al 2002). In more proximal regions of the mouse small intestine taurocholic acid uptake was much smaller and there was no evidence for its active absorption. This is consistent with the known distribution of the IBAT whose expression is confined to the enterocytes of the terminal ileum (Binder 1980; Meier & Stieger 2002).

The activity of the IBAT could also be detected in both intact and stripped ileal sheets mounted in Ussing chambers. Mucosal application of taurocholic acid elicited a biphasic rise in SCC as has been noted previously (Hardcastle et al 2001). The first phase of this response was reduced by a low mucosal Na^+ concentration, but was unaffected by conditions that inhibit intestinal secretion. Thus removal of Cl^-, serosal furosemide (inhibits the Na^+, K^+, $2Cl^-$ cotransporter responsible for Cl^- accumulation within the enterocyte; Heintze et al 1983) or mucosal DPC (blocks luminal Cl^- channels; Sahi et al 1994) had no effect on the initial SCC response, although they did inhibit the second, secretory, phase. The magnitude of the initial SCC response was concentration-dependent and the apparent K_m, in the order of 0.5 mM, was very similar to that (0.3 mM) obtained by direct measurement of taurocholic acid uptake by everted sacs of rat ileum (Caspary 1973).

The possibility that bile acid absorption was disturbed in CF was examined using a transgenic mouse with the same genetic defect found in the majority of CF patients. In wild-type animals taurocholic acid uptake by everted ileal sacs was similar to that obtained in tissues from Swiss mice. In contrast, CF ilea exhibited a markedly reduced taurocholic acid uptake and a lower absorptive SCC response in intact ileal sheets, although in stripped sheets there was no significant difference between wild-type and CF tissues. The fact that the T/M ratio did not reach unity in CF sacs suggests that these tissues lack the capacity for active bile acid reabsorption. A similar conclusion was reached by Fondacaro et al (1982) in their study of taurocholic acid uptake by ileal biopsies from CF patients. Bile acid malabsorption has also been reported in a SeHCAT retention analysis of CF patients (O'Brien et al 1993), although an *in-vivo* perfusion study of human ileum failed to detect any difference in taurocholate and glycocholate uptake between control and CF subjects (Thompson & Davidson 1988). The only other study to use transgenic CF mice to investigate ileal bile acid reabsorption in CF found that, in contrast to the results presented here, taurocholic acid uptake was enhanced in an everted sleeve preparation of CF ileum (Stelzner et al 2001). However, this group used a knockout mouse in which no CFTR is produced while we have used mice with the ΔF508 mutation where aberrant CFTR is produced but, due to a trafficking defect, fails to reach its normal location at the luminal membrane of the enterocyte (Riordan 1993). In more proximal regions of the small intestine, where bile acid uptake is passive, taurocholic acid uptake was not reduced in CF tissues.

The reduction in taurocholic acid uptake observed in ilea from CF mice is in contrast to the enhanced absorption of sugars and amino acids reported in jejunal biopsies from CF patients (Baxter et al 1990), in spite of the fact that all the transport processes concerned are Na^+-dependent. Studies comparing the effects of glucose on the electrical activity of human and mouse jejunum in CF suggest that there may be a species difference in the way in which CF affects Na^+-dependent nutrient absorption. Glucose increases the SCC generated by the intestine as the process responsible for its active absorption is electrogenic. Thus the rise in SCC reflects the rate of active glucose absorption. In jejunal biopsies from control human patients mounted in modified Ussing chambers with an exposed tissue area of 3 mm^2 the basal PD, SCC and tissue resistance values were 1.7±0.1 mV, 58.7±3.8 $\mu A\ cm^{-2}$ and 30.9±2.0

ohm.cm^2 (n=53, mean age 5 years 3 months; range 2 days – 14 years 4 months). Equivalent values for CF patients homozygous for the ΔF508 mutation were 0.3±0.1 mV, 10.8±4.3 μA cm^{-2} and 28.3±2.5 ohm.cm^2 (n=15, mean age 4 years 5 months; range 2 months – 15 years 11 months). In the CF group the PD and SCC were significantly lower ($P<0.001$ in both cases), although tissue resistances were similar ($P>0.05$). A similar pattern was observed in stripped sheets of jejunum from wild-type and CF (*Cftr*^{tm1Eur}) mice (wild-type: PD = 1.5±0.2 mV, SCC = 57.9±8.6 μA cm^{-2}, tissue resistance = 27.4±2.7 ohm.cm^2, n=7; CF: PD = 0.1±0.2 mV ($P<0.001$), SCC = 10.8±4.3 μA cm^{-2} ($P<0.001$), tissue resistance = 30.4±0.9 ohm cm^2, ($P>0.05$), n=8). However, the effect of CF on the SCC response to glucose differed in human and mouse tissues. In human jejunal biopsies 10 mM glucose caused a greater increase in SCC in CF tissues (Baxter et al 1990), while in mouse jejunum the effect of 10 mM glucose was greater in wild-type tissues (Hardcastle et al 2004a). In both human and mouse jejunum the effect of acetylcholine (10^{-3}M) confirmed the phenotype (Figure 13).

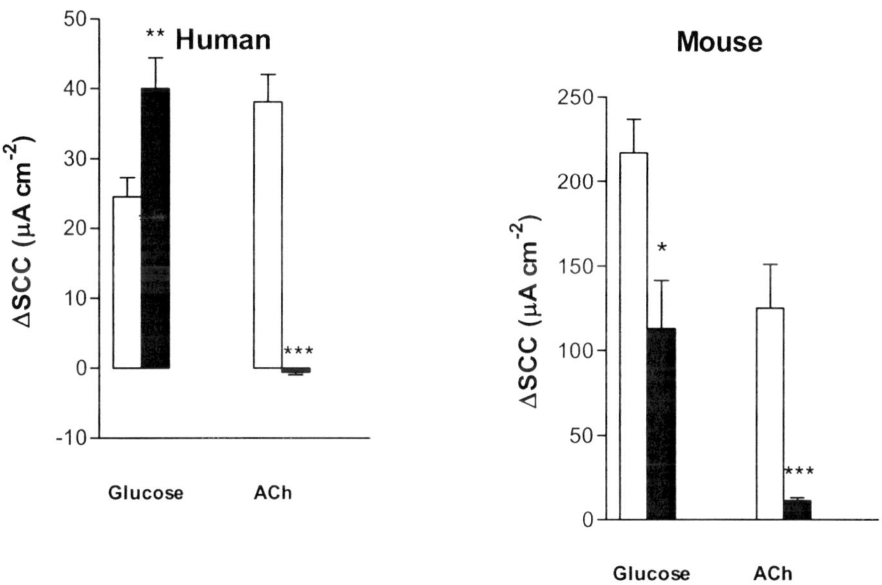

Fig. 13. Effect of glucose (10 mM) and acetylcholine (ACH, 10^{-3}M) on the SCC in human and mouse jejunum. Glucose was added to the mucosal solution and acetylcholine to the serosal solution of human jejunal biopsies from 53 control patients and 15 CF patients homozygous for the ΔF508 mutation, and stripped sheets of jejunum from 7 wild-type and 8 CF (*Cftr*^{tm1Eur}) mice. Each bar represents the mean ± 1 s.e.m., with control values shown by the open bars and CF values by the solid bars. * $P<0.05$; ** $P<0.01$; *** $P<0.001$.

The addition of a solute to the mucosal solution imposes an osmotic gradient across the intestine, leading to the development of an electrokinetic potential that reduces the SCC (Smyth & Wright 1966). Thus when glucose is added to the mucosal fluid the rise in SCC consists of two components: an increase due to active Na^+-dependent absorption and a decrease due to the osmotic effect. The magnitude of this osmotic effect can be assessed by determining the decrease in SCC that occurs when equimolar mannitol is added to the mucosal side of the tissue. In human jejunal biopsies the magnitude of this effect was larger in CF tissues (control: 3.5±0.9 μA cm^{-2}/10 mM (n=6); CF: 12.6±5.1 μA cm^{-2}/10 mM (n=3), P>0.05), while in mouse jejunum it was similar in wild-type (12.5±1.7 μA cm^{-2}/10 mM, n=7) and CF (11.7±1.1 μA cm^{-2}/10 mM, n=8, P>0.05) tissues. An increase in passive Cl^- absorption in CF has recently been reported in human jejunum *in-vivo* (Russo et al 2003) and it was suggested that this could result from an alteration in charged groups within the tight junctions. An increased net negative charge would explain both the reduced passive Cl^- permeability and an increased electrokinetic potential.

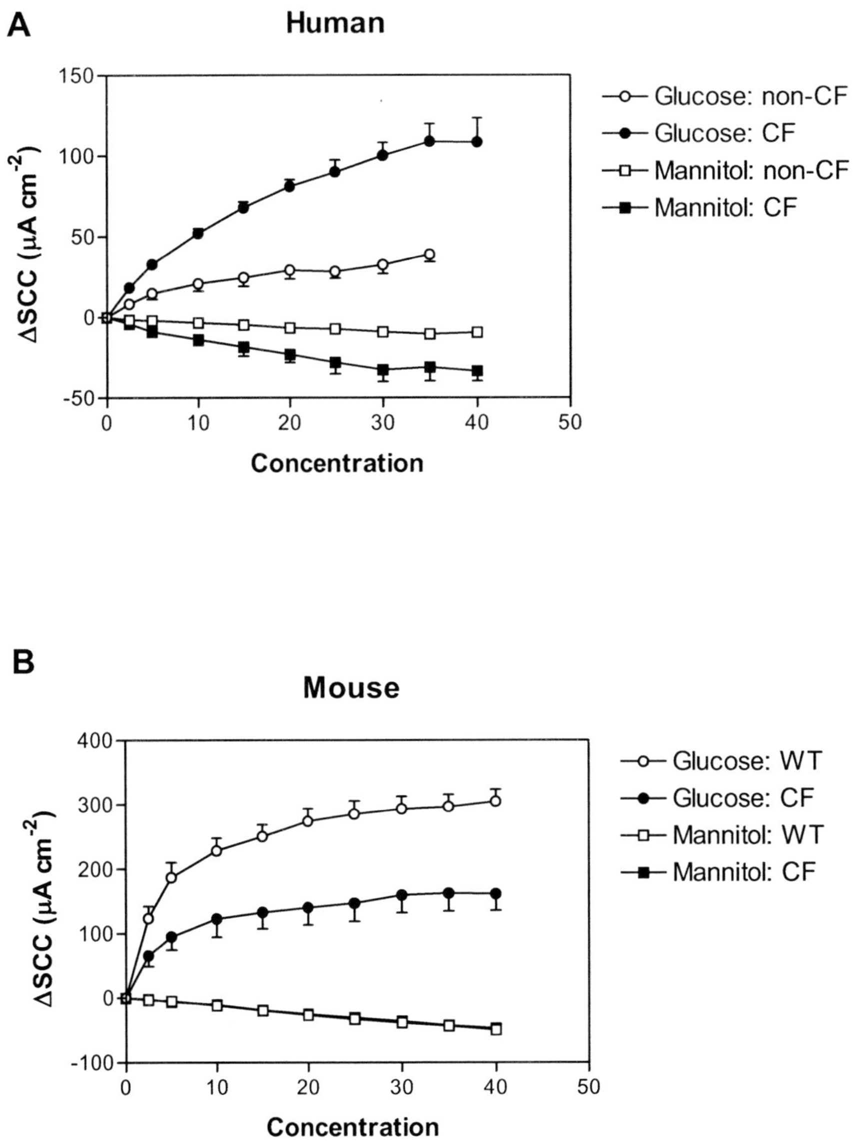

Fig. 14. Changes in SCC induced by glucose and mannitol in A: jejunal biopsies from patients with CF (n=6) and age-matched controls (n=5), and B: stripped sheets of jejunum from transgenic (*Cftr*^{tm1Eur}) wild-type (WT, n=7)) and CF (n=8) mice. Glucose or mannitol was added cumulatively to give the concentrations shown and each point represents the mean ± 1 s.e.m. of the number of observations indicated.

When the osmotic effect is taken into account the rise in SCC due to active Na^+-dependent glucose absorption can be determined. Glucose caused a concentration-dependent increase in SCC that exhibited saturation kinetics, while equimolar mannitol caused a decrease in SCC that was linearly related to its concentration (Figure 14).

By investigating the relationship between the rise in SCC and the glucose concentration the kinetics of the transport process can be determined. From the data in Figure 14 apparent K_m and V_{max} values were calculated (Table 2).

Table 2. Kinetics of the glucose-dependent rise in SCC in human and mouse jejunum. Each value represents the mean ± 1 s.e.m. of the number of observations indicated and an unpaired t test was used to assess the significance of the difference between control and CF tissues. ** *P*<0.01; * *P*<0.001.**

	Human		**Mouse**	
	Control (7)	**CF** (6)	**Wild-type** (7)	**CF** (8)
K_m (mM)	23.0±10.2	27.8±4.5	5.4±0.9	4.9±0.7
V_{max} (μA cm^{-2})	74.0±10.8	195.0±20.3***	342.2±23.5	190.4±20.3**

The apparent V_{max} value was substantially increased in CF tissues from human patients, but in mouse jejunum it was much lower in the CF group. Apparent K_m values were unchanged in both species. It is important to remember however, that the apparent K_m can be influenced by changes in the V_{max} as:

$$\text{apparent } K_m = \text{real } K_m + V_{max}\, d/D$$

where d is the thickness of the unstirred layer and D is the free diffusion coefficient of glucose (Levin 1979). An unchanged apparent K_m in the presence of an altered apparent V_{max} in stripped preparations suggests that the real K_m may have changed, reflecting an alteration in the affinity of the cotransporter for its substrate. *In vivo* perfusion studies have also demonstrated an enhanced intestinal absorption of glucose in CF patients, but this was attributed to reduced diffusion barriers (Frase et al 1985). In contrast, a recent *in vivo* perfusion study in human jejunum (Russo et al 2003) failed to detect any difference in glucose absorption between control and CF groups, but this technique does not distinguish between the active and passive components of glucose absorption. It is interesting to note that in this investigation the glucose-dependent PD (associated with active glucose absorption) was greater in CF patients. Previous measurements of the glucose-dependent SCC have not detected any significant difference between control and CF tissues (Taylor et al 1987, 1988; Berschneider et al 1988; O'Loughlin et al 1991), but in each of these reports the number of patients investigated was small. Alternatively, abnormal mucoid secretion in CF (Eggermont 1985) could alter both the thickness of the unstirred layer (d) or the free diffusion coefficient (D), but there is currently no information on this point. It is therefore impossible to draw any conclusions regarding the effect of CF on the affinity of the Na^+/glucose cotransporter. A decreased SCC response to glucose has not been observed previously in intestinal tissues from transgenic CF mice (Clarke et al 1992; Grubb 1995; Seidler et al 1997; Joo et al 1998). However, all these studies used knockout mice in which the CF gene was disrupted, whereas our experiments used mice homozygous for the ΔF508 mutation where aberrant CFTR is produced, but due to a trafficking defect, it is retained within the Golgi apparatus (Riordan 1993).

The different effects of CF on the glucose-dependent rise in SCC in human and mouse jejunum suggest that there may be a species variation in the actions of CFTR on other transport processes. It is known that SGLT1, the cotransporter responsible for active Na^+-dependent glucose uptake, is regulated by protein kinases and species differences have been reported for the actions of protein kinase C (Wright at el 1997). This kinase increases the activity of human SGLT1, but reduces that of rat and rabbit SGLT1 when the cotransporters are expressed in *Xenopus* oocytes. A similar process may be involved in regulating the IBAT. The fact that CFTR activates protein kinases (Riordan 1993), which could then have different effects in different species, suggests a mechanism by which this species variation could occur.

The reduced taurocholic acid absorption observed in CF intestine was not mirrored in an isolated brush-border membrane preparation where taurocholic acid uptake was similar in wild-type and CF vesicles. A limited study of taurocholic acid uptake by ileal BBMVs from two CF patients also concluded that bile acid uptake was not abnormal in the disease (de Rooij et al 1985). Similarly, in human jejunum there is no difference in glucose uptake by BBMVs (Beesley et al 1996), although control and CF jejunal biopsies exhibit an enhanced glucose-dependent rise in SCC, an index of active Na^+-dependent glucose absorption (Baxter et al 1990). Both CFTR (Ameen et al 2000; O'Loughlin et al 1996) and the IBAT (Stelzner et al 2000; St-Pierre et al 2001) are normally located at the luminal membrane of villous enterocytes, allowing possible interactions to occur. However, this may require the presence of intracellular components, such as ATP and protein kinase A that are required for CFTR activation (Riordan, 1993), that are absent in the vesicle preparation

Bile acid malabsorption is evident in intact ileal tissues from CF mice. Severe malabsorption can lead to decreased concentrations of bile acids in the intestinal lumen (Hofmann et al 1991) and this could exacerbate the maldigestion and malabsorption of fat that occurs in CF as a result of pancreatic exocrine insufficiency (Dodge 1986).

Conclusions

Studies of the effects of bile acids on intestinal transport processes in the mouse have demonstrated that these agents both induce secretion in all regions of the small intestine and that they are actively reabsorbed by a Na^+-dependent mechanism in the terminal ileum. The secretory response to bile acids involves both neural and immune processes, with histamine and 5-HT contributing to the effect. Electrogenic Cl^- secretion, together with an inhibition of electroneutral NaCl absorption, is the driving force for fluid secretion within the intestine. This process plays a vital role in the health of the gut by aiding lubrication, washing immunoglobulins from the crypts and providing Na^+ for Na^+-dependent nutrient absorption and the secretory actions of the bile acids will contribute to this aspect of gut function. In CF however, the ability of the intestine to secrete fluid and electrolytes is lost and this includes the secretory response to bile acids. As a result, the luminal contents will become increasingly viscous and this may contribute to the development of obstruction, a symptom associated with CF in both human and mouse intestine. It is clear that the active Na^+-dependent absorption of bile acids in the ileum is impaired in CF mice and this would explain reports of bile acid malabsorption in human patients. However, data with glucose indicate that extrapolating conclusions from mouse experiments to the human situation should only be undertaken with caution. In the case of active Na^+-dependent glucose absorption the effects of CF are quite different in human and mouse small intestine, with increased glucose absorption in human CF jejunum and a decrease in mouse CF jejunum. As the IBAT operates in a similar manner to SGLT1, the Na^+/glucose cotransporter, it is quite possible that the effects of CF on bile acid absorption may differ in human and mouse ileum and further human studies are required to resolve the situation. Thus although both human and mouse intestine exhibit the failure of secretion characteristic of CF, they differ in the way in which changes in absorption are expressed. Transgenic mouse models of CF do not, therefore, reflect faithfully all aspects of the human disease, so this chapter ends on a cautionary note.

Acknowlegements

We gratefully acknowledge financial support from the Sheffield Children's Hospital Children's Appeal.

We are grateful to the Journal of Pharmacy and Pharmacology for permission to use material from our papers published in that journal.

References

Ambache, N., Freeman, M. A., Hobbiger, F. (1971) Distribution of acetylcholinesterase and butyrylcholinesterase in the myenteric plexus and longitudinal muscle of guinea-pig intestine. *Biochem. Pharmacol.* 20: 1123-1132

Ameen, N., Alexis, J., Salas, P. (2000) Cellular localization of the cystic fibrosis transmembrane conductance regulator in mouse intestinal tract. *Histochem. Cell Biol.* 114: 60-75

Barnard, J. A., Ghishan, F. K. (1987) Taurocholate transport by human ileal brush border membrane vesicles. *Gastroenterology.* 93: 925-933

Barrett, K. E., Keely, S. J. (2000) Chloride secretion by the intestinal epithelium: molecular basis and regulatory aspects. *Ann. Rev. Physiol.* 62: 535-5572

Baxter, P. S., Goldhill, J., Hardcastle, J., Hardcastle, P. T., Taylor, C. J. (1990) Enhanced intestinal glucose and alanine transport in cystic fibrosis. *Gut* 31: 817-820

Baxter, P. S., Wilson, A. J., Read, N. W., Hardcastle, J., Hardcastle, P. T., Taylor, C. J. (1989) Abnormal jejunal potential difference in cystic fibrosis. *Lancet* no. 8636: 464-466

Beesley, A. H., Hardcastle, J., Hardcastle, P. T., Taylor, C. J. (1996) Sodium/glucose cotransporter activity in cystic fibrosis. *Arch. Dis. Child.* 75: 170

Berschneider, H. M., Knowles, M. R., Azizkhan, R. G., Boucher, R. C., Tobey, N. A., Orlando, R. C., Powell, D. W. (1988) Altered intestinal chloride transport in cystic fibrosis. *FASEB J.* 2: 2625-2629

Binder, H. J. (1980) Pathophysiology of bile acid- and fatty acid-induced diarrhea. In: Field, M., Fordtran, J. S., Schultz, S. G. (eds) *Secretory Diarrhea.* Waverley Press, Baltimore, pp 159-178

Caspary, W. F. (1973) Increase of active transport of conjugated bile salts in streptozotocin-diabetic rat small intestine. *Gut* 14: 949-999

Cheng, K., Ashby, D., Smyth, R. (2000) Ursodeoxycholic acid for cystic fibrosis-related liver disease. *Cochrane Database Syst. Rev.* 2: CD000222

Chinet, T., Fouassier, L., Dray-Charier, N., Imam-Ghali, M., Morel, H., Mergey, M., Dousset, B., Parc, R., Paul, A., Housset, C. (1999) Regulation of electrogenic anion secretion in normal and cystic fibrosis gallbladder mucosa. *Hepatology* 29: 5-13

Clarke, L. L., Grubb, B. R., Gabriel, S. E., Smithies, O. Koller, B. H., Boucher, R. C. (1992) Defective epithelial chloride transport in a gene-targeted mouse model of cystic fibrosis. *Science* 257: 1125-1128

Clarke, L. L., Harline, M. C., Gawenis, L. R., Walker, N. M., Turner, J. T., Weisman, G. A. (2000) Extracellular UTP stimulates electrogenic bicarbonate secretion across CFTR knockout gallbladder epithelium. *Am. J. Physiol.* 279: G132-G138

Colledge, W. H., Abella, B. S., Southern, K. W., Ratcliff, R., Jiang, C., Cheng, S. H., MacVinish, L. J., Anderson, J. R., Cuthbert, A. W., Evans, M. J. (1995) Generation and characterization of a ΔF508 cystic fibrosis mouse model. *Nature Gen.* 10: 445-452

Colombo, C., Battezzati, P. M., Strazzabosco, M., Podda, M. (1998) Liver and biliary problems in cystic fibrosis. *Semin. Liver Dis.* 18: 227-235

Cooke, H. J. (1994) Neuroimmune signaling in regulation of intestinal ion transport. *Am. J. Physiol.* 266: G167-G178

Crawford, I., Maloney, P. C., Zeitlin, P. L., Guggino, W. B., Hyde, S. C., Turley, H., Gatter, K. C., Harris, A., Higgins, C. F. (1991) Immunocytochemical localization of the cystic fibrosis gene product CFTR. *Proc. Natl. Acad. Sci.* 88: 9262-9266

Crowe, S. E., Sestini, P., Perdue, M. H. (1990) Allergic reactions of rat jejunal mucosa. Ion transport responses to luminal antigens and inflammatory mediators. *Gastroenterology* 99: 74-82

De Rooij, F. W. M., Van Den Berg, J. W. O., Sinaasappel, M., Bosman-Jacobs, E. P., Touw-Blommesteijn, A. C. (1985) Bile acid malabsorption in cystic fibrosis: membrane vesicles, a tool for revealing the role of the ileal brush border membrane. *Acta Ped. Scand.* Suppl 317: 28-30

Devor, D. C., Frizzell, R. A. (1993) Calcium-mediated agonists activate an inwardly rectified K^+ channel in colonic secretory cells. *Am. J. Physiol.* 265: C1271-C1280

Dharmsathaphorn, K., Huott, P. A., Vongkovit, P., Beuerlein, G., Pandol, S. J., Ammon, H. V. (1989) Cl^- secretion induced by bile salts. *J. Clin. Invest.* 84: 945-953

Diwakar, V., Pearson, L., Beath, S. (2001) Liver disease in children with cystic fibrosis. *Paediatr. Respir. Rev.* 2: 340-349.

Dodge, J. A. (1986) Gastrointestinal tract and nutrition in cystic fibrosis: pathophysiology. *J. Roy. Soc. Med.* 79 (suppl 12): 27-31

Dray-Charier, N., Paul, A., Scoazec, J. Y., Veissiere, D., Mergey, M., Capeau, J., Soubrane, O., Housset, C. (1999) Expression of delta F508 cystic fibrosis transmembrane conductance regulator protein and related chloride transport properties in the gallbladder epithelium from cystic fibrosis patients. *Hepatology* 29: 1624-1634

Eggermont, E. (1985) The role of the small intestine in cystic fibrosis patients. *Acta Paediatr. Scand.* 317 (suppl): 16-21

Fondacaro, J. D., Heubi, J. E., Kellogg, F. W. (1982) Intestinal bile acid malabsorption in cystic fibrosis: a primary mucosal cell defect. *Ped. Res.* 16: 494-498

Frase, L. L., Strickland, A. D., Kachel, G. W., Krejs, G. J. (1985) Enhanced glucose absorption in the jejunum of patients with cystic fibrosis. *Gastroenterology* 88: 478-484

Gelbmann, C. M., Schteingart, C. D., Thompson, S. M., Hofmann, A. F., Barrett, K. E. (1995). Mast cells and histamine contribute to bile acid-stimulated secretion in the mouse colon. *J. Clin. Invest.* 95: 2831-2839.

Goldstein, J. L., Nash, N. T., Al-Bazzaz, F., Layden, T. J., Rao, M. C. (1988) Rectum has abnormal ion transport but normal cAMP-binding proteins in cystic fibrosis. *Am. J. Physiol.* 254: C719-C724.

Goldstein, J. L., Shapiro, A. B., Rao, M. C., Layden, T. J. (1991) In vivo evidence of altered chloride, but not potassium secretion in cystic fibrosis rectal mucosa. *Gastroenterology* 101: 1012-1019

Greger, R., Schreiber, R., Mall, M., Wissner, A., Hopf, A., Briel, M., Bleich, M., Warth, R., Kunzelmann,K. (2001) Cystic fibrosis and CFTR. *Eur. J. Physiol.* 443 (suppl): 53-57

Grubb, B. R. (1995) Ion transport across the jejunum in normal and cystic fibrosis mice. *Am. J. Physiol.* 268: G505-G513

Grubb, B. R., Gabriel, S. E. (1997) Intestinal physiology and pathology in gene-targeted mouse models of cystic fibrosis. *Am. J. Physiol.* 273: G258-G266

Hardcastle, J., Hardcastle, P. T. (1987) Membrane permeability changes in intestinal secretion. *Med. Sci. Res.* 15: 471-473

Hardcastle, J., Hardcastle, P. T. (1987a) The secretory actions of histamine in rat small intestine. *J. Physiol.* 388: 521-532

Hardcastle, J., Hardcastle, P. T. (1997). Several receptor subtypes contribute to 5-hydroxytryptamine-induced secretion by rat ileum in-vitro. *J. Pharm. Pharmacol.* 49: 1114-1120

Hardcastle, J., Hardcastle, P. T., Carstairs, J. W. M., Franks, C. M. (1994). Is desensitization of intestinal 5-hydroxytryptamine receptors an in-vitro phenomenon? *J. Pharm. Pharmacol.* 46: 322-325

Hardcastle, J., Hardcastle, P. T., Chapman, J., Taylor, C. J. (2001) Taurocholic acid-induced secretion in normal and cystic fibrosis mouse ileum. *J. Pharm. Pharmacol.* 53: 711-719

Hardcastle, J., Hardcastle, P. T., Chapman, J., Taylor, C. J. (2001a) Ursodeoxycholic acid action on the transport function of the small intestine in normal and cystic fibrosis mice. *J. Pharm. Pharmacol.* 53: 1457-1467

Hardcastle, J., Hardcastle, P. T., Taylor, C. J., Goldhill, J. (1991) Failure of cholinergic stimulation to induce a secretory response from the rectal mucosa in cystic fibrosis. *Gut* 32: 1035-1039

Hardcastle, J., Harwood, M. D., Taylor, C. J. (2004) Absorption of taurocholic acid by the ileum of normal and transgenic ΔF508 cystic fibrosis mice. *J. Pharm. Pharmacol.* 54: 445-452.

Hardcastle, J., Harwood, M. D., Taylor, C. J. (2004a) Small intestinal glucose absorption in cystic fibrosis: a study in human and transgenic ΔF508 cystic fibrosis mouse tissues. *J. Pharm. Pharmacol.* 54: 329-338.

Heintze, K., Stewart, C. P., Frizzell, R. A. (1983) Sodium-dependent chloride secretion across rabbit descending colon. *Am. J. Physiol.* 244: G357-G365

Hitchin, B. W., Dobson, P. R. M., Brown, B. L., Hardcastle, J., Hardcastle, P. T., Taylor, C. J. (1990) Measurement of intracellular mediators in enterocytes isolated from jejunal biopsy specimens of control and cystic fibrosis patients. *Gut* 31: 893-899

Hofmann, A. F. (1998) Bile secretion and the enterohepatic circulation of bile acids. In: Feldman, M., Scharschmidt, B. F., Sleisenger, M. H. (eds) *Sleisenger & Fordtran's Gastrointestinal and Liver Disease*. 6th edn, W. B. Saunders Company, Philadelphia, pp 937-948

Hofmann, A. F., Schteingart, C. D., Lillienau, J. (1991) Biological and medical aspects of active ileal transport of bile-acids. *Ann. Med.* 23: 169-175

Joo, N. S., London, R. M., Kim, H. D., Forte, L. R., Clarke, L. L. (1998) Regulation of intestinal Cl^- and HCO_3^- secretion by uroguanylin. *Am. J. Physiol.* 274: G633-G644

Karlström, L. (1986). Evidence of involvement of the enteric nervous system in the effects of sodium deoxycholate on small-intestinal transepithelial fluid transport and motility. *Scand. J. Gastroenterol.* 21: 321-330

Karlström, L., Cassuto, J., Jodal, M., Lundgren, O. (1981) The effect of hexamethonium on the secretion induced by sodium deoxycholate in the rat jejunum. *Experientia*, 37: 991-992

Karlström, L., Cassuto, J., Jodal, M., Lundgren, O. (1983) The importance of the enteric nervous system for the bile-salt-induced secretion in the small intestine of the rat. *Scand. J. Gastroenterol.* 18: 117-123

Klaren, P. H. M., Giesberts, A. N., Chapman, J., White, S. J., Taylor, C. J., Hardcastle, P. T., Hardcastle, J. (2000) Effect of loperamide on Na^+/D-glucose cotransporter activity in mouse small intestine. *J. Pharm. Pharmacol.* 52: 679-686

Klaren, P. H. M., Hardcastle, J., Evans, S., Colledge, W. H., Evans, M. J., Taylor, C. J., Hardcastle, P. T., White, S. J. (2001) Acetylcholine induces Ca^{2+} mobilization in isolated distal colonic crypts from normal and cystic fibrosis mice. *J. Pharm. Pharmacol.* 53: 371-377

Kunzelmann, K., Mall, M. (2001) Electrolyte transport in the mammalian colon: mechanisms and implications for disease. *Physiol. Rev.* 82: 245-289

Levin, R. J. (1979) Fundamental concepts of structure and function of the intestinal epithelium. In: Duthie, H. L., Wormsley, K. G. (eds) *Scientific Basis of Gastroenterology*. Churchill Livingstone, Edinburgh, pp 308-337

Levin, R.J., Ayton, B. R. (1995). Electrogenic ion secretion induced by taurocholic acid in rat ileum *in vitro* is partially mediated through a myenteric reflex pathway. *J. Physiol.* 482: 30P

Mall, M., Bleich, M., Kuehr, J., Brandis, M., Greger, R., Kunzelmann, K. (1999) CFTR-mediated inhibition of epithelial Na^+ conductance is defective in cystic fibrosis. *Am. J. Physiol.* 277: G709-G716

Mall, M., Wissner, A., Seydewitz, H. H., Kuehr, J., Brandis, M., Greger, R., Kunzelmann, K. (2000) Defective cholinergic Cl^- secretion and detection of K^+ secretion in rectal biopsies from cystic fibrosis patients. *Am. J. Physiol.* 278: G617-G624

Mauricio, A. C., Slawik, M., Heitzmann, D., von Hahn, T., Warth, R., Bleich, M., Greger, R. (2000) Deoxycholic acid (DOC) affects the transport properties of distal colon. *Pflügers Arch.* 439: 532-540

Meier, P. J., Stieger, B. (2002) Bile salt transporters. *Ann. Rev. Physiol.* 64: 635-661

Northfield, T.C., McColl, I. (1973) Postprandial concentrations of free and conjugated bile acids down the length of the normal human small intestine. *Gut* 14: 513-518

O'Brien, S., Mulcahy, H., Fenlon, H., O'Broin, A., Casey, M., Burke, A., FitzGerald, M. X., Hegarty, J. E. (1993) Intestinal bile acid malabsorption in cystic fibrosis. *Gut* 34: 1137-1141

O'Loughlin, E. V., Hunt, D. M., Gaskin, K. J., Stiel, D., Bruzuszcak, I. M., Martin, H. C. O., Bambach, C., Smith, R. (1991) Abnormal epithelial transport in cystic fibrosis jejunum. *Am. J. Physiol.* 260: G758-G763

O'Loughlin, E. V., Hunt, D. M., Bostrom, T. E., Hunter, D., Gaskin, K. J., Gyory, A., Cockayne, D. J. H. (1996) X-ray microanalysis of cell elements in normal and cystic fibrosis jejunum: evidence for chloride secretion in villi. *Gastroenterology* 110: 411-418

Paumgartner, G., Beuers, U. (2002) Ursodeoxycholic acid in cholestatic liver disease: mechanisms of action and therapeutic use revisited. *Hepatology* 36: 525-531

Pearce, F. L., Befus, A. D., Gauldie, J., Bienenstock, J. (1982) Mucosal mast cells. II. Effects of anti-allergic compounds on histamine secretion by isolated intestinal mast cells. *J. Immunol.* 128: 2481-2486

Quinton, P. M. (1999) Physiological basis of cystic fibrosis: a historical perspective. *Physiol. Rev.* 79 (suppl.): S3-S22

Riordan, J. R. (1993) The cystic fibrosis transmembrane conductance regulator. *Ann. Rev. Physiol.* 55: 609-630

Rommens, J. M., Iannuzzi, M. C., Kerem, B., Drumm, M. L., Melmer, G., Dean, M., Rozmahel, R., Cole, J. L., Kennedy, D., Hidaka, N., Zsiga, M., Buchwald, M., Riordan, J. R., Tsui, L., Collins, F. S. (1989) Identification of the cystic fibrosis gene: chromosome walking and jumping. *Science* 245: 1059-1065

Russo, M. A., Högenauer, C., Coates, S. W., Santa Ana, C. A., Porter, J. L., Rosenblatt, R. L., Emmett, M., Fordtran, J. S. (2003) Abnormal passive chloride absorption in cystic fibrosis functionally opposes the classic chloride secretory defect. *J. Clin. Invest.* 112: 118-125

Sahi, J., Goldstein, J. L., Layden, T. J., Rao, M. C. (1994) Cyclic AMP- and phorbol ester-regulated Cl^- permeabilities in primary cultures of human and rabbit colonocytes. *Am. J. Physiol.* 266: G846-G855

Schultz, S. G., Zalusky, R. (1964) Ion transport in isolated rabbit ileum. II. The interaction between active sodium and active sugar transport. *J. Gen. Physiol.* 47: 1043-1059

Seidler, U., Blumenstein, I., Kretz, A., Viellard-Baron, D., Rossmann, H., Colledge, W. H., Evans, M., Ratcliff, R., Gregor, M. (1997) A functional CFTR protein is required for mouse intestinal cAMP-, cGMP- and Ca^{2+}-dependent HCO_3^- secretion. *J. Physiol.* 505: 411-423

Smyth, D. H. & Wright, E. M. (1966) Streaming potentials in the rat small intestine. *J. Physiol.* 182: 591-602

St-Pierre, M. V., Kullak-Ublick, G. A., Hagenbuch, B., Meier, P. J. (2001) Transport of bile acids in hepatic and non-hepatic tissues. *J. Exp. Biol.* 204: 1673-1686

Stelzner, M., Hoagland, V., Somasundaram, S. (2000) Distribution of bile acid absorption and bile acid transporter gene message in the hamster ileum. *Eur. J. Physiol.* 440: 157-162

Stelzner, M., Somasundaram, S., Lee, S. P., Kuver, R. (2001) Ileal mucosal bile acid absorption is increased in Cftr knockout mice. *BMC Gastroenterol.* 1:10-16

Strandvik, B., Einarsson, K., Lindblad, A., Angelin, B. (1996) Bile acid kinetics and biliary lipid composition in cystic fibrosis. *J Hepatol.* 25: 43-48

Strazzabosco, M., Spirli, C., Okolicsanyi, L. (2000) Pathophysiology of the intrahepatic biliary epithelium. *J. Gastroenterol. Hepatol.* 2000 15: 244-253

Strong, T. V., Boehm, K., Collins, F. S. (1994) Localization of cystic fibrosis transmembrane conductance regulator mRNA in the human gastrointestinal tract by in situ hybridization. *J. Clin. Invest.* 93: 437-354

Taylor, C. J., Baxter, P. S., Hardcastle, J., Hardcastle, P. T. (1987) Absence of secretory response in jejunal biopsy samples from children with cystic fibrosis. *Lancet* II: 107-108

Taylor, C. J., Baxter, P. S., Hardcastle, J., Hardcastle, P. T. (1988) Failure to induce secretion in jejunal biopsy samples from children with cystic fibrosis. *Gut* 29: 957-962

Thompson, G. N., Davidson, G. P. (1988) *In vivo* bile acid uptake from terminal ileum in cystic fibrosis. *Ped. Res.* 23: 323-328

Timar Peregrin, A., Ahlman, H., Jodal, M., Lundgren, O. (1999) Involvement of serotonin and calcium channels in the intestinal fluid secretion evoked by bile salt and cholera toxin. *Br. J. Pharmacol.* 127: 887-894.

Ung, K.-A., Olofsson, G., Fae, A., Kilander, A., Ohlsson, C., Jonsson, O. (2002) *In vitro* determination of active bile acid absorption in small biopsy specimens obtained endoscopically or surgically from the human intestine. *Eur. J. Clin. Invest.* 32: 115-121

Van Doorninck, J. H.; French, P. J., Verbeek, E., Peters, R. H. P. C., Morreau, H., Bijman, J., Scholte, B. J. (1995) A mouse model for the cystic fibrosis ΔF508 mutation. *EMBO J.* 14: 4403-4411

Veeze, H. J. (1992) Cystic fibrosis: genetics and intestinal secretion. *Neth. J. Med.* 41: 115-118

Wheat, V. J., Shumaker, H., Burnham, C., Shull, G. E., Yankaskas, J. R., Soleimani, M. (2000) CFTR induces the expression of DRA along with Cl^-/HCO_3^- exchange activity in tracheal epithelial cells. *Am. J. Physiol.* 279: C62-C71

Wright, E. M., Hirsch, J. R., Loo, D. D. F., Zampighi, G. A. (1997) Regulation of Na^+/glucose cotransporters. *J. Exp. Biol.* 200: 287-293

Wyllie, R. (1999) Gastrointestinal manifestations of cystic fibrosis. *Clin. Pediatr.* 38: 735-738

In: Progress in Cystic Fibrosis Research
Editor: Margaret A. Harrison, pp. 65-77
ISBN 1-59454-232-5

Chapter III

Electrolite Depletion with Metabolic Alkalosis in Infants with Cystic Fibrosis

Stojka Fustik*
Department of Pediatrics, Clinical Center, Skopje, Republic of Macedonia

Abstract

Metabolic alkalosis in association with low serum electrolyte concentration (hyponatremia, hypochloremia, and hypokalemia) is well known complication of cystic fibrosis (CF) in infancy. Two distinct clinical presentations of this metabolic disorder in CF are recognized: an acute one, with hypotonic dehydration or even shock, due to excess salt loss during sweating (heat exhaustion or prostration); and a chronic one, with gradual development of electrolyte depletion, metabolic alkalosis, failure to thrive, wasted condition, without marked dehydration.

The records of 109 children diagnosed as having CF before the age of 12 months, in the period from 1990 to 2002, were reviewed to ascertain the prevalence of the electrolyte depletion with metabolic alkalosis as a major presenting manifestation of CF in our region and to define the possible risk factors for its occurrence. The clinical and laboratory profiles (blood pH, serum bicarbonate, sodium, chloride and potassium levels, and urine chloride concentration) at the time of admission, sweat chloride test values, genotypes and past clinical data of patients were evaluated. The results from the study suggest that electrolyte depletion with metabolic alkalosis is a relatively common manifestation of CF in infancy. The prevalence of this sweat-related metabolic disorder in infant CF population in our region was 18.34%. Although episodes of electrolyte depletion and metabolic alkalosis were more common in the summer and early autumn months, they were not always associated with hot and arid weather. Early infant age, breastfeeding, delayed CF diagnosis, heat exhaustion and the presence of severe CFTR mutations are predisposed factors for the development of metabolic alkalosis with hypoelectrolytemia. The possibility of CF should be seriously considered in any infant

* Correspondence concerning this article should be addressed to Dr. Stojka Fustik, Department of Pediatrics, Clinical Center, Vodnjanska 17, 1000-Skopje, Republic of Macedonia

presenting with this metabolic disorder. Serum electrolytes should be assessed regularly in infants with CF, especially during hot weather months and in CF infants with weight loss or anorexia.

Key words: cystic fibrosis, electrolyte depletion, metabolic alkalosis, cystic fibrosis transmembrane conductance regulator mutations.

Cystic fibrosis (CF) is a complex inherited disorder causing by mutations in the single gene, the Cystic Fibrosis Transmembrane Conductance Regulator (CFTR), located on chromosome 7. It is characterized by chronic supportive lung disease, pancreatic fibrosis that usually leads to exocrine pancreatic failure, high sweat electrolyte concentration, and reduced life expectancy.

In 1953, Di Sant'Agnese demonstrated that excessive salt loss occurs in the sweat of children with CF [1], a finding that led soon after to the measurement of sodium and chloride in sweat as the diagnostic standard test for the disease [2]. The salt transport abnormality was further defined by Quinton, who demonstrated that CF duct epithelium has a markedly more negative potential difference than normal tissue, related to attenuated chloride transport in sweat ducts [3,4]. With the discovery of the CF gene and its protein product, CFTR, known to form a cAMP-regulatable chloride channel in normal cells, it has become possible to demonstrate the conclusive evidence that defective cAMP-related chloride transport in sweat ductal cells is the basic CF defect in this tissue [5]. Natrium absorption is reduced in CF ducts. This is likely to represent a secondary abnormality related to the chloride impermeability, the more negative intraluminal potential difference in these ducts retaining natrium within the lumen [6].

The sweat glands of patients with CF secrete a relatively normal iso-osmotic primary sweat. In the sweat duct, however, dysfunctional CFTR results in excessive chloride and sodium losses in final sweat. Infants with CF have much higher rates of unstimulated sweating than normal infants even in the absence of high environmental or endogenous temperatures. The difference is accentuated during sleep, while the sweat rates of CF infants may be up to 10 times as great as in normal control subjects [7]. With profuse sweating in warm environments, an infant with CF may lose up to 80 mEq of sodium and chloride, and 40 mEq of potassium per day depending on the individual's body surface area and sweat rate [8].

Due to excess salt loss with sweating, infants with CF are phoned to develop episodes of hyponatremic/hypochloremic dehydration. The extracellular fluid volume contraction and salt depletion will lead to activation of renin-angiotensin system and secondary hyperaldosteronism. The resulting effect is the increased renal potassium and hydrogen (proton) losses for the exchange with sodium in the distal tubule. The consequence hypokalemic alkalosis is a metabolic mimickery of Bartter's syndrome; therefore the condition is sometimes referred to as pseudo-Bartter's syndrome in CF [9].

Since the first description of electrolyte depletion with hyponatremic dehydration and heat prostration as a manifestation seen in CF, in 1951 [10], a number isolated reports of children with CF who have acute or chronic electrolyte depletion with metabolic alkalosis have been reported [8,11-21]. However, the important of this metabolic disorder as a major presenting manifestation of CF in the diagnosis of the disease is not well established. This is especially essential in the regions without neonatal screening program for CF, because early diagnosis and early appropriate treatment improve the clinical outcome of CF patients [22].

The aims of this study were to estimate the prevalence of metabolic alkalosis with hypoelectrolitemia in infants diagnosed as having CF; to find out the role of the possible risk factors for developing of this metabolic disorder in CF; and to define the importance of the manifestation as a form of presentation of CF in the diagnosis of CF.

Methods

The records of all children diagnosed as having CF before the age of 12 months in the period from January 1990 to December 2002 were reviewed, to find out the prevalence of metabolic alkalosis with hypoelectrolytemia as a presenting manifestation of CF in our region. Between 1990 and 2002, 109 newly diagnosed CF patients, each less than 12 months of age, were treated at Department of Pediatrics, Clinical Center, Skopje (Republic of Macedonia). Metabolic alkalosis with hypoelectrolytemia was identified in 20 infants with CF. In 18 of these infants diagnoses of CF had not been previously established.

Primary metabolic alkalosis was defined as an elevation of blood pH to greater than 7.45 and/or excess alkali in the serum (bicarbonate > 28 mmol/L), in the absence of respiratory insufficiency. Patients with combined metabolic alkalosis and respiratory acidosis were not included in the group of CF patients with primary metabolic abnormalities. Electrolyte depletion was considered as a decreased of serum sodium < 130 mmol/L, chloride < 90 mmol/L, and potassium < 3.5 mmol/L levels. Urine chloride concentration was measured before therapy in majority of patients with metabolic alkalosis and hypoelectrolytemia. Low urine chloride (< 10 mmol/l) characterizes alkalosis in which chloride depletion predominates.

Plasma and urine electrolyte concentrations were determined by flame photometry or autoanalyzer. Acid-base parameters were measured in arterialized capillary blood in the Astrup apparatus.

In addition to data of acid-base and electrolyte disequilibrium, the following information from medical history were collected: (1) age of patient; (2) season when the episode occurred; (3) dietary record of infant; (4) recent exposure to hot environment; (5) symptoms and signs predisposing to dyselectrolytemias such as fever, vomiting, diarrhea, or acute exacerbation of pulmonary disease; (6) physical findings suggested dehydration; (7) relative underweight, calculated on standard growth charts using body weight and length; and (8) past clinical data (respiratory and gastrointestinal manifestations). The sweat chloride test values (pilocarpine iontophoresis sweat test) were evaluated in 20 patients with electrolyte and acid-base abnormalities and in remained 89 CF infants with normal electrolyte and acid-base equilibrium. Furthermore, the patients with electrolyte depletion and metabolic alkalosis were analyzed with respect to genotype data to find out the influence of the CFTR mutations on developing of this sweat-related metabolic disorder.

The data were analyzed by Excel Ver. 9.0 (Microsoft LTD, Chicago, IL, USA). All values were expressed as mean (M) ± standard deviation (SD) and ranges. Statistical analysis was performed by analysis of variance. P-value less than 0.05 was considered significant.

Results

From the all study 109 infants with CF treated at the Department of Pediatrics, Clinical Center, Skopje, 20 infants, 13 boys and 7 girls, had manifestations of electrolyte depletion with metabolic alkalosis. The prevalence of metabolic alkalosis with hypoelectrolytemia in infant CF population in our region was 18.3%. Biochemical features in blood (blood pH, serum bicarbonate, sodium, chloride, and potassium levels.) and urine (chloride concentration) of CF patients presenting with electrolyte depletion and metabolic alkalosis are given in Table 1. Results are expressed as mean value (M), standard deviation (SD), minimum (Min) and maximum (Max). The metabolic disturbances were severe in most of the affected infants. In all CF patients with primary metabolic abnormalities urine chloride concentration was below 10 mmol/L, and sometimes even nil, indicated the presence of metabolic alkalosis with predominated chloride depletion.

The medium age of the CF patients with manifested electrolyte depletion and metabolic alkalosis was 3.1 months, and the age ranged from 2 to 8 months. With except of one patient who was 8 months old, all other CF patients with the presenting metabolic abnormalities were less than 6 months of age.

The episodes of metabolic alkalosis with hypoelectrolytemia took place in all seasons of the year, although more common during the summer and early autumn months (Figure 1). The hot clime during summer months, heated rooms, overclothing and bundling of infants during winter months were reasons for heat prostration and excess sweating.

All infants with metabolic alkalosis and hypoelectrolytemia were breastfed. Eighteen of them were on exclusive breast-milk feeding and two infants were on combined breast-milk feeding and formula-milk feeding. This finding suggested that low salt contained human milk is insufficient to compensate the increased electrolyte losses through the skin in CF infants during the high environmental temperature and profuse sweating.

Most of the children with metabolic alkalosis and hypoelectrolytemia were the first admitted patients without previous diagnosis of CF. Only two children had already been diagnosed by quantitative pilocarpine iontophoresis sweat test (sweat chloride concentration > 60 mmol/L) and genetic analysis as having CF. In the majority of the cases the diagnosis of CF was made following the episode of metabolic alkalosis with hypoelectrolytemia.

Table 1. Biochemical features of CF patients presenting with electrolyte depletion and metabolic alkalosis

Parameters	M	SD	Min	Max
pH	7.56	0.04	7.46	7.67
Bicarbonate (mmol/L)	41.43	6.87	32.5	52.3
Sodium (mmol/L)	119.6	6.93	108	130
Chloride (mmol/L)	69.5	10.17	54	90
Potassium (mmol/L)	3.02	0.46	1.7	3.6
Urinary chloride (mmol/L)	3.33	2.35	0	8

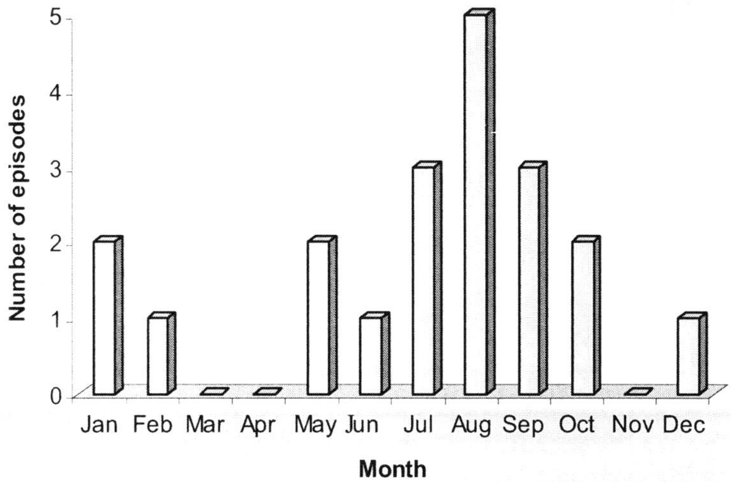

Figure 1. Seasonal occurrence of the episodes of electrolyte depletion with metabolic alkalosis

Clinical features related to episodes of electrolyte depletion with metabolic alkalosis are summarized in Table 2. Eleven patients had an acute presentation of the episode of metabolic alkalosis with hypoelectrolytemia. They had physical findings suggesting a state of mild to severe dehydration: body weight loss ranged from 5 to 13%. The percentage body weight loss at the time of admission was calculated from the difference between the weight on admission and that after correction of the electrolite depletion and metabolic alkalosis. The predominant clinical symptoms in patients with the acute episodes were vomiting, anorexia, nausea, fiver and excessive sweating, lasted for 1-3 days. These symptoms preceded the clinical presentation of the acute dehydration with electrolyte depletion and metabolic alkalosis.

Table 2. History and clinical findings in CF patients with acute (n=11) and chronic (n=9) electrolyte depletion and metabolic alkalosis

Symptoms	Acute Number	presentation %	Chronic Number	presentation %
Anorexia	9	81.8	9	100
Vomiting	11	100	7	77.8
Body weight loss	11	100	7	77.8
Diarrhea	4	36.4	1	11.1
Fever	6	54.5	0	0
Sweating	6	54.5	2	22.1
Cough	3	27.3	4	44.4
Dehydration	11	100	0	0
Lethargy	5	45.4	0	0
Cardio-vascular collapse/shock	4	36.4	0	0

In nine children with electrolyte depletion and metabolic alkalosis clinical signs of dehydration were not evident on admission, which indicated more chronic and gradual development of abnormally low serum electrolyte concentrations and metabolic alkalosis. All patients with chronic presentation of metabolic alkalosis with hypoelectrolytemia were wasted, prostrate and undernourished at admission. The majority of them had history of anorexia, poor intake, vomiting, failure to thrive or body weight loss. The symptoms often lasted for days and weeks. None of the infants with chronic electrolyte depletion and metabolic alkalosis were hyperpyrexic or in shock.

The nutritional status of the CF patients with primary metabolic abnormalities was assessment after correction of the electrolite depletion and metabolic alkalosis, when infants rapidly gained weight. The growth of patients was calculated on standard growth charts for age and gender using body weight and length. Index weight for length percentiles was used to expressed the relative undernourished (underweight) of the CF patients. The analysis of weight percentiles (W%), length percentiles (L%), and weight for length percentiles (W/L%) distribution of the patients with manifested electrolite depletion and metabolic alkalosis is given in Table 3. The proportion of CF patients who had body weight below 3th percentile, as the cut off point to identify malnutrition according to World Health Organisation [22] was 40% and the proportion of the patients who had weight for length percentiles below 3th percentile was 25%. The majority of infants with the presenting acid-base and electrolyte disturbance were undernourished and had suboptimal growth.

All children with metabolic alkalosis and hypoelectrolytemia had history of some loose stools and failure to thrive satisfactorily, although the gastrointestinal symptoms were not always severe enough to suggest possibility of CF. The precedent episodes of vomiting had 18 (90%) of infants with manifested electrolite depletion and metabolic alkalosis. The vomiting acted as a precipitating event to aggravate the patients' general condition as well as the electrolyte and acid-base disturbance.

Eigft infants with metabolic alkalosis and hypoelectrolytemia had had previous history of respiratory symptoms: cough, noisy respirations, upper respiratory tract infections, recurrent bouts of mild bronchitis. Night infants developed respiratory illness after rehydration and electrolyte supplementation therapy.

The diagnosis of CF was made by positive sweat test. The sweat chloride test values were compared with sweat chloride test values of CF patients without manifested episodes of electrolite depletion and metabolic alkalosis. CF patients with manifested metabolic alkalosis and hypoelectrolytemia tended to have higher sweat chloride values (128±41mmol/L) in comparison with CF patients without this manifestation (109±48mmol/L), but the difference was not significant ($p>0.05$).

Concerning the molecular basis of CF in patients with metabolic alkalosis and hypoelectrolytemia, 11 patients (55%) were homozygous for the most frequent disease causing mutation ΔF508 (Table 4). The genotypes of the remained 9 patients were: ΔF508/G542X (n=4), ΔF508/N1303K (n=1), ΔF508/CFTRdel.21Kb (n=1), G542X/N1303K (n=1), ΔF508/unknown (n=1), and CFTRdel.21Kb/unknown (n=1). All patients with metabolic alkalosis and hypoelectrolytemia had severe mutations with regard to pancreatic exocrine function.

Table 3. Growth indices of CF patients with manifested electrolyte depletion and metabolic alkalosis: weight percentiles (W%), length percentiles (L%), and weight for length percentiles (W/L%)

Index	<3% Number %	3-10% Number %	10-25% Number %	25-50% Number %
W%	8 40	9 45	3 15	0 0
L%	1 5	9 45	7 35	3 15
W/L%	5 25	7 35	6 30	2 10

Table 4. Genotypes of CF patients with manifested metabolic alkalosis and hypoelectrolytemia

Genotype	Number of patients	%
ΔF508/ΔF508	11	55
ΔF508/G542X	4	20
ΔF508/N1303K	1	5
ΔF508/CFTRdel.21Kb	1	5
G542X/N1303K	1	5
ΔF508/unknown	1	5
CFTRdel.21Kb/unknown	1	5

Discussion

Metabolic alkalosis in association with low serum electrolyte concentration is unusual metabolic disturbance in infancy. Disorders associated with repeated vomiting, especially pyloric stenosis, are the more common causes of metabolic alkalosis. Other less common primary causes of metabolic alkalosis are: continuous gastric drainage without appropriate electrolyte replacement, chloride-losing diarrhea, potassium-losing nephropathy, Bartter's syndrome, the use of thiazide diuretics and cystic fibrosis [16].

Primary metabolic alkalosis is recognized by increases in both arterial blood PH (alkalemia) and plasma bicarbonate concentration. The increase in arterial blood PH promptly, normally depresses ventilation resulting in increased $PaCO_2$ and the buffering of the alkalemia. The absence of respiratory distress in primary metabolic alkalosis excluded compensatory metabolic alkalosis for a primary respiratory acidosis (mixed metabolic alkalosis with respiratory acidosis).

Concerning the underlying patophysiology of the primary metabolic alkalosis, the most common group is those due to chloride depletion (chloride responsive metabolic alkalosis).The other group is that due to potassium depletion, usually with mineralocorticoid excess (primary or secondary aldosteronism). Metabolic alkalosis due to both potassium and chloride depletion also may occur and is not so rare [24].

CF is an autosomal recessive disease affecting exocrine gland function throughout the body. Patients with CF usually present with respiratory and gastrointestinal manifestations. Rarely, patients with CF present with electrolyte depletion and metabolic alkalosis, mainly in the young infant age. Sporadically, the metabolic disturbance is reported in older CF patients [25]. Our study confirmed that metabolic alkalosis with hypoelectrolytemia is not rare clinical presentation of CF in infancy. The prevalence of this sweat-related metabolic disorder in infant CF population in our region was 18.3%. The episodes of electrolyte depletion with metabolic alkalosis occurred mainly in geographical regions with hot, dry climate, and especially during the summer months [14,18]. We did not find strictly association between the manifestation of the metabolic abnormalities in CF infants and the season. Although episodes of electrolyte depletion and metabolic alkalosis were more common in the summer and early autumn months, they also occurred in the winter and spring months. The habits to bundle young babes in some areas, or to overheat the rooms where babes live, as well as the fiver due to intercurrent infection were the reasons for heat exhaustion of CF infants in the colder months of the year.

The profuse sweating, without sufficient salt replacement may lead to hypochloraemic, hyponatraemic metabolic alkalosis in CF children. In warm environments, where sweat rates may reach 2L/h [26], people with CF may have massive sweat sodium chloride losses, leading to extracellular fluid volume contraction and secondary hyperaldosteronism. The hyperaldosteronism will lead to potassium wasting in both the sweat and the urine, resulting in hypokalemia. The stimulated aldosterone production increases potassium secretion in the final sweat. Aldosteron-mediated effects on sweat potassium are likely the result of both increased glandular and ductal secretion [27]. In addition, hyperaldosteronism cause enhanced potassium secretion in the collecting ducts.

Metabolic alkalosis has a generation and maintenace phase [24]. Skin losses of chloride may generate alkalosis in CF. The effect of this electrolyte losses is the activation of the renin-angiotensin system and stimulation of sodium-cation (hydrogen, potassium) exchange, with resulted alkalosis and potassium depletion. The increased rate of sodium-hydrogen (proton) ion exchange in the kidney tubule leads indirectly to bicarbonate reabsorption, and the increased rate of sodium-potassium ion exchange leads to potassium secretion [28]. Therefore, the normal homeostatic response with increased secretion of aldosteron in condition of low body sodium is responsible for accentuating of metabolic alkalosis and hypokalaemia. Furthermore, the potassium depletion increases metabolic alkalosis by a shift of protons (hydrogen ions) from the extracellular to the intracellular fluid.

The factors contributing to maintenance of metabolic alkalosis in CF patients are multiple [24,25]. Because chloride-depletion alkaloses are usually characterized by concurrent deficits of sodium, potassium, and fluid, as well as chloride, controversy has arisen regarding which of these deficits is responsible for the maintenance of the alkalosis. First, extracellular fluid volume contraction causes a decrease in glomerular filtration and therefore a decrease in the filtered load of bicarbonate. Volume contraction accompanying alkalosis augments fluid reabsorption in the proximal tubule, and, because bicarbonate is preferentially reabsorbed compared with chloride in this segment, alkalosis is maintained. Based on this hypothesis with extracellular fluid volume expansion, fluid reabsorption in the proximal tubule is depressed, delivering more bicarbonate and chloride to the distal nephron, which possesses substantial capacity to reabsorb chloride but a limited one for bicarbonate. As a result, chloride is retained, bicarbonate excreted, and alkalosis corrected.

Second, chloride depletion alone has been shown to maintain metabolic alkalosis by increased reabsorption of bicarbonate. It has been shown that during either expansion or contraction of extracellular fluid volume, alkalosis was not corrected without chloride replacement [29]. Even during sustained volume contraction, chloride promptly increased bicarbonaturia and progressively corrected the alkalosis Thus, based on this hypothesis, chloride is necessary and sufficient for the correction of chloride depletion alkalosis [24,30]. Volume depletion is a commonly associated but not a causative or essential factor for the maintenance of alkalosis. Chloride depletion appears to decrease glomerular filtration by tubuloglomerular feedback. Chloride depletion also increases renin secretion by a macula densa mechanism, resulting in increased aldosterone secretion that may be disproportionate to the magnitude of an accompanying hypokalemia and thereby augment potassium wasting. Although normal functioning of the proximal tubule is essential to permit appropriate bicarbonate reabsorption, the collecting duct appears to be the major nephron site for altered electrolyte and proton transport in both maintenance of and recovery from metabolic alkalosis. The major cell stimulated by chloride-depletion alkalosis is the type B intercalated cell in the cortical segment [31]. During maintenance, bicarbonate secretion dose not occur because insufficient chloride is available for bicarbonate exchange and bicarbonate reabsorption is maintained distally in the medullary segments. When chloride is administrated and luminal or cellular chloride concentration increases, bicarbonate is promptly excreted and alkalosis is corrected.

Third, hypokalemia can maintain (and maybe generate) metabolic alkalosis by enhancing renal proximal and distal proton secretion, and increasing renal ammonia production. When potassium depletion and mineralocorticoid excess occur together, prominent metabolic alkalosis is common. However, these effects would be mitigated by a secondary decrease in aldosterone and by the inhibitory effects of alkalosis on ammoniagenesis [32,33].

Some disorders, including pseudo-Bartter's syndrome in CF, may be characterized by both chloride and potassium depletion, which serve to intensify the alkalosis. They are usually associated with sodium losses and normotension or hypotension. Thus in patients with CF, sweat sodium chloride losses coupled with significant hypokalemia could result in severe alkalosis

The metabolic abnormalities in the so-called pseudo-Bartter's syndrome in CF can mimicking biochemical features of Bartter's syndrome and misdiagnose of Bartter's syndrome to be made [9,16]. Although the biochemical hallmark of both Bartter's and pseudo-Bartter's syndrome is abnormally low plasma electrolyte concentrations, there are important differences between the two diseases. In Bartter's syndrome, the sweat electrolyte profile is normal and the renal handling of electrolytes is defective. In CF sweat electrolyte losses is increased, and intensive electrolyte reabsorption occurs in the renal tubules. In all our CF infants presenting with electrolyte depletion and metabolic alkalosis, the initial diagnosis of Bartter's syndrome was excluded by hypochloruria. Determination of urinary chloride before therapy is especially useful to distinguish these two conditions. The diagnosis of CF was confirmed by positive sweat test. Excessive sodium and chloride losses in the sweat should be excluded before a diagnosis of Bartter's syndrome [9].

During a period of profuse sweating (high environmental temperatures, fiver, bundling), an infant with CF may lose more than 80 mEq of sodium, 100 mEq of chloride, and 40 mEq of potassium per day depending on the individual's body surface area and sweat rate [13].Without sufficient salt replacement the infant may become hypochloremic, hyponatremic, and alkalotic. Older CF children probably compensate for excess losses of sodium, chloride and potassium in sweat by increasing the rate of aldosterone secretion and the salt intake. However, low salt contained human milk is insufficient to compensate the increased electrolyte losses with sweating in CF infants in warm environments. All our CF patients with metabolic alkalosis and hypoelectrolytemia were breast-fed, and only two infants were on combined breast-milk feeding and formula-milk feeding. Beside climatic conditions in Balkan region (hot summers and cold winters) and baby care habits in some areas, the relative high prevalence of breastfeeding in our country may explain the high incidence of metabolic alkalosis with hypoelectrolytemia in infants with CF.

The apparently increasing reports of children with pseudo-Bartter's syndrome and CF were noted after the change to low solute formula-milks in the mid 1970s, following the recommended guidelines for restraining the use of salt in commercial infant food [34].These measures reduce sodium intake from 25 to 50 mEq per day to 12 to 15 mEq per day for formula-fed infants, and 5 to 10 mEq per day for breast-fed infants [35]. Although these feeding recommendations satisfy sodium requirements for growth of healthy infants, they do not supply the necessary salt to offset increased losses through sweat in infants with CF. Therefore, breast-fed infants are at greatest risk for developing electrolyte depletion and metabolic alkalosis. However, formula-fed infants may also develop electrolyte depletion and metabolic alkalosis, especially during periods of increased sweating and additional gastrointestinal losses.

The exposition of CF infants to higher environmental temperature, associated with a low dietary salt intake, may last for days. In those cases the abnormally low serum electrolyte concentration and metabolic alkalosis are developed gradually, and signs of dehydration are less expressive or even absent. In CF infants with more acute salt and fluid losses due to heat prostration, signs of dehydration are well recognized. Eleven of our patients with metabolic alkalosis and hypoelectrolytemia had distinctive manifestations of dehydration, suggestive for the more acute depletion of electrolytes in excess of fluid losses.

In all CF infants with acute or chronic fluid and electrolyte losses with sweating, the metabolic abnormalities and condition of patients were aggravated by acute intercurrent episodes of vomiting, diarrhea, or respiratory symptoms. The intercurrent illness acts as a precipitating event to deteriorate an underlying metabolic alkalosis and hypoelectrolytemia. Almost all CF infants with acid-base and electrolyte disturbance had episodes of vomiting before admission. Vomiting was most probably initiated by the hyponatremia, but it itself aggravated electrolyte losses and metabolic alkalosis. The predominant symptoms of salt depletion, often seen in our patients with metabolic alkalosis and hypoelectrolytemia, are anorexia, nausea, vomiting and body weight loss. Therefore, careful monitoring of serum electrolyte levels and acid-base parameters, when infants with CF experience anorexia or excessive gastrointestinal losses and weight loss is especially important, particularly during the periods of increased sweating.

The majority of infants with metabolic alkalosis and hypoelectrolytemia were first admitted patients without previous diagnosis of CF. Although they had failed to thrive satisfactory, their gastrointestinal and/or respiratory symptoms were not severe enough to suggest the possibility of CF before the episode of metabolic alkalosis with hypoelectrolytemia occurred. So, electrolyte depletion and metabolic alkalosis has been recognized as an initial manifestation of CF. All CF patients with sweat-related metabolic disturbance were pancreatic insufficient (faecal chymotrypsin concentration < 3 U/g).

We did not find a significant difference in sweat electrolyte values between CF infants with manifested metabolic alkalosis and hypoelectrolytemia and CF infants without that manifestation, even though the CF infants with manifested metabolic disturbance tended to have higher average sweat electrolyte concentration. Higher rate of sweating and above average electrolyte losses with sweat may be reason some CF individuals to be biochemically more vulnerable, and more disposed to develop episodes of metabolic alkalosis with hypoelectrolytemia. The predisposition may be determinated by the genotype. The dysfunctional CFTR in the sweat ducts of CF patients causes inappropriate sweat chloride and sodium losses, but also the dysfunctional CFTR in the renal tubular cells may contribute for precipitating of alkalosis [25].

All CF infants with presented episodes of metabolic alkalosis and hypoelectrolytemia had severe CFTR mutations, associated with pancreatic insufficiency and more severe clinical course of the disease. Biochemical abnormalities due to insufficient CFTR chloride canal function are more accented in CF patients with severe disease caused mutations.

The treatment of children presenting with acute or chronic episodes of electrolyte depletion and metabolic alkalosis was consisted of intravenous administration of both sodium and potassium chloride. Salt supplementation in the diet was recommended in all these patients, at list until they reached the age of 2 years. Since human milk is low in sodium (160 mg/L), breast-fed CF babies need supplementation, especially during fever or hot summer months. Generally, salt added to meals is sufficient for older CF children, but with vigorous exercise or prolonged exposure to heat, salt tablets may be necessary.

Conclusion

- Due to the increased losses of chloride and sodium in the sweat, young CF children are predisposed to develop episodes of acute or chronic hyponatremic/hypochloremic dehydration with hypokalemia and metabolic alkalosis when they sweat excessively, especially during the wormer months of the year.
- The results from this study indicate that early infant age, breastfeeding, delayed diagnosis, heat exhaustion, and the presence of CFTR mutations associated with a severe phenotype are predisposed factors for development of electrolyte depletion and metabolic alkalosis.
- This metabolic disorder is a relatively common presenting manifestation of CF in infancy and appears to be often initial presentation of CF.
- The diagnosis of CF should be seriously considered in any infant with metabolic alkalosis and hypoelectrolytemia, whether or not there are associated pulmonary and/or gastrointestinal symptoms typical for CF.
- In infants known to have CF, serum electrolytes and acid-base balance should be measured if the infant is experiencing weight loss or anorexia, particularly during periods of excessive sweating.
- All CF infants at risk for development episodes of electrolyte depletion and metabolic alkalosis should receive daily salt supplementation in their diet.

References

[1] di Sant'Agnese PA, Darling RE, Perera GA, Shea E. Abnormal electrolyte composition of sweat in cystic fibrosis of the pancreas: Clinical significance and relationship to the disease. *Pediatrics* 1953; 12:549-63.

[2] Gibson LE, Cooke RE. A test for concentration of electrolytes in sweat in cystic fibrosis of the pancreas - utilizing pilocarpine iontophoresis. *Pediatrics* 1959; 23:545-9.

[3] Quinton PM. Chloride impermeability in cystic fibrosis. *Nature* 1983; 301:421-2.

[4] Quinton PM, Bijman J. Higher bioelectric potentials due to decreased chloride absorption in sweat glands of patients with cystic fibrosis. *N Engl J Med* 1983; 308:1189-91.

[5] Kartner N, Augustinas O, Jensen TJ. Mislokalization of ΔF508 CFTR in cystic fibrosis sweat gland. *Nature Genet* 1992; 1:321-7.

[6] Alton EWFW, Smith SN. *Applied cell biology*. In: Cystic Fibrosis, 2nd edition. Ed. Hodson ME and Geddes DM, London, Arnold 2000; 61-81.

[7] Sibings MS, Barbero GJ. Studies in the physiology of sweating in cystic fibrosis. II. Elevated night sweating rates. *Arch Dis Child* 1961; 36:537-40.

[8] Avranitakis SN, Lobeck CC. Metabolic alkalosis and salt depletion in cystic fibrosis. *J Pediatr* 1973; 82:535-6.

[9] Davison AG, Snodgrass GJAI. Cystic fibrosis mimicking Bartter's syndrome. *Acta Paediatr Scand* 1983; 72: 781-3.

[10] Kessler WR, Anderson DH. Heat prostration in fibrocystic disease of the pancreas and other conditions. *Pediatrics* 1951; 8:648-56.

[11] Gottlieb RP. Metabolic alkalosis in cystic fibrosis. *J Pediatr* 1971; 79:930-6.

[12] Sheth KJ, Heimler R. Cystic fibrosis in an infant presenting with metabolic alkalosis. *Wis Med J* 1977; 76(suppl):47-9.

[13] Beckerman RC, Taussing LM. Hypoelectrolytemia and metabolic alkalosis in infants with cystic fibrosis. *Pediatrics* 1979; 63:580-3.

[14] Nussbaum E, Boat TF, Wood RE, Doershuk CD. Cystic fibrosis with acute hypoelectrolytemia and metabolic alkalosis in infancy. *Am J Dis Child* 1979; 133:965-6.

[15] Ruddy R, Anolik R, Scanlin TF. Hypoelectrolytemia as a presentation and complication of cystic fibrosis. *Clin Pediatr* 1981; 21:367-9.

[16] Kennedy JD, Dinwiddie R, Daman-Willems C, Dillon MJ, Matthew DJ. Pseudo-Bartter's syndrome in cystic fibrosis. *Arch Dis Child* 1990; 65: 786-7.

[17] Özccelik U, Göcmen A, Kiper N, Coskun T, Yilmaz E, Özgüc M. Sodium chloride deficiency in cystic fibrosis patients. *Eur J Pedatr* 1994; 153:829-31.

[18] Sojo A, Rodriguez-Soriano J, Vitoria JC, Vazquez C, Ariceta G, Villate A. Chloride deficiency as a presentation or complication of metabolic alkalosis. *Eur J Pediatr* 1994; 153: 825-8.

[19] Pedroli G, Liechti-Gallati S, Mauri S, Birrer P, Kraemer R, Foletti-Jaggi C. Chronic metabolic alkalosis: Not uncommon in young children with severe metabolic alkalosis. *Am J Nephrol* 1995; 15:245-50.

[20] Mauri S, Pedroli G, Rüdeberg A, Laux-End R, Monotti R, Bianchetti M. Acute metabolic alkalosis in cystic fibrosis: Prospective study and review of literature. *Miner Electrolyte Metab* 1997; 23:33-7.
[21] Fustik S, Pop-Jordanova N, Slaveska N, Koceva S, Efremov G. Metabolic alkalosis with hypoelectrolytemia in infants with cystic fibrosis. *Pediatr International* 2002; 44:289-92.
[22] WHO working group. Use and interpretation of anthropometric indicators of nutritional status. *Bull WHO* 1986; 64:929-41
[23] Waters DL, Wilcken B, Irwing L, Van Asperen P, Mellis C, Simpson JM, Brown J, Gaskin KJ. Clinical outcomes of newborn screening for cystic fibrosis. *Arch Dis Child Fetal Neonatal Ed* 1999; 80:F1-7.
[24] Galla JH. Metabolic alkalosis. *J Am Soc Nephrol* 2000; 11:1-12.
[25] Bates CM, Baum M, Quigley R. Cystic fibrosis presenting with hypokalemia and metabolic alkalosis in a previously healthy adolescent. *J Am Soc Nephrol* 1997; 8:352-6.
[26] Quinton PM. Physiology of sweat secretion. *Kidney Int* 1987; 32:S102-8.
[27] Sato K, Kang WH, Saga KT. Biology of sweat glands and their disorders. I. Normal sweat gland function. *J Am Acad Dermatol* 1989; 20:537-63.
[28] Simopoulos AP, Lapey A, Boat TF, di Sant'Agnese PA, Bartter FC. The renin-angiotensin-aldosterone system in patients with cystic fibrosis of the pancreas. *Pediatr Res* 1971; 5: 626-32.
[29] Galla JH, Bonduris DN, Luke RG. Effects of chloride and extracellular fluid volume on bicarbonat reabsorption along the nephron in metabolic alkalosis in the rat. *J Clin Invest* 1987; 80:41-50.
[30] Schwartz WB, Ypersele de Strihou C, Kassirer JP. Role of anions in metabolic alkalosis and potassium deficiency. *N Engl J Med* 1968; 279:630-9.
[31] Verlander JW, Madsen KM, Galla JH, Luke RG, Tisher CC. Response of intercalated cells to chloride depletion metabolic alkalosis. *Am J Physiol* 1991; 262:F309-19.
[32] Alpern RJ, Emmet M, Seldin DW. *Metabolic alkalosis*. In: The Kidney: Physiology and Patophysiology, 2nd edition. Ed. Seldin DW and Giebisch G, New York, Raven Press 1992; 2273-758.
[33] DuBose TD, Good DW. Effects of chronic chloride depletion alkalosis on proximal tubule transport and renal production of ammonium. *Am J Physiol* 1995; 269:F508-14.
[34] Committee on Nutrition, American Academy of Pediatrics. Salt intake and eating patterns of infants and children in relation to blood pressure. *Pediatrics* 1974; 53:115-9.
[35] Laughlin JJ, Brady MS, Eigen H. Changing feeding trends as a cause of electrolyte depletion in infants with cystic fibrosis. *Pediatrics* 1981; 68:203-7.

In: Progress in Cystic Fibrosis Research
Editor: Margaret A. Harrison, pp. 79-98
ISBN 1-59454-232-5

Chapter IV

Markers of Oxidative Damage and Antioxidant Status in Blood of Children with Cystic Fibrosis

Teresa Laskowska-Klita and Magdalena Chelchowska*
Department of Biochemistry and Diagnostics Laboratories, Research Institute of Mother and Child, Warsaw, Poland

Abstract

Cystic fibrosis (CF) is the most frequent genetic disease affecting Caucasian populations. In cystic fibrosis, as a result of chronic pulmonary infections and digestive malabsorption, an imbalance between the production of reactive oxygen species and their inactivation by protective systems is observed. This imbalance may cause impairment of cell metabolism and oxidative injury. The aim of this study was to examine whether the antioxidant status in cystic fibrosis patients with pancreatic insufficiency provided sufficient protection against oxidative damage to protein and lipids. We have found that in plasma the mean concentration of lipid peroxides (measured as malondialdehyde-MDA) as well as index of oxidative modification of protein (protein carbonyls) was higher by 23% ($p<0.001$) in cystic fibrosis patients ($n=57$) than in healthy children ($n=21$). This was accompanied by significantly lower total radical-trapping antioxidant parameters (TRAP) in CF group (629 μmol/l ± 133 μmol/l) than in control (735 μmol/l ± 110 μmol/l; $p<0.001$). Plasma concentrations of antioxidant vitamins E, A and β-carotene were all reduced in CF patients as compared to controls. This reduction was particularly pronounced for β-carotene (50%; $p<0.0001$). In CF patients, concentrations of α-tocopherol and retinol were 13,7 μmol/l and 1,2 μmol/l respectively, whereas in the control it was higher by 30% ($p<0.0001$). MDA and some antioxidants were measured also in erythrocytes. In CF children, an enhanced lipid peroxidation was observed. In that group, the concentration of vitamin E was one half (1,39 μmol/l) that found in healthy

* Correspondence concerning this article should be addressed to Teresa Laskowska-Klita & Magdalena Chełchowska, Department of Biochemistry and Diagnostics Laboratories, Research Institute of Mother and Child ul. Kasprzaka 17A 01-211 Warsaw, Poland E-mail: lipidy@imid.med.pl

children (2,95 μmol/l). In RBC, antioxidant enzymatic activities (superoxide dismutase-SOD, glutathione peroxidase-GPx, catalase) were studied. Among them, that of GPx showed the same level in both groups. In CF patients, the activity of catalase was lower by 23% ($p<0.001$) and that of SOD higher by 30% ($p<0.0001$), than in erythrocytes of the control group. The obtained results indicated that in CF patients oxidative stress caused oxidative modification of proteins and peroxidation of lipids accompanied by a lowering of antioxidant protection. We concluded that CF children with exocrine pancreatic insufficiency are susceptible to oxidative damage. Therefore it seems that an adequate and balanced diet is essential for achieving and maintaining normal antioxidant status.

Key words: cystic fibrosis, oxidative damage, antioxidant status, children

Introduction

Cystic fibrosis (CF) is the most common life-shortening autosomal recessively inherited disorder in populations of European origin, with an incidence of approximately 1 in 2,500 live births. CF is caused by a defect in a gene on a long arm of chromosome 7 encoding cystic fibrosis transmembrane conductance regulator (CFTR). The CFTR protein has been shown to function as a cAMP-regulated chloride channel in an apical membrane of epithelial cells including those of the respiratory and gastrointestinal tract, pancreatic biliary and sweat ducts. The abnormal CFTR protein enhancing sodium reabsorption into cells and blocking chloride conductance modifies mucus secretion. Desiccated mucus is more viscous and elastic which provides progressive obstruction and destruction of the affected organ. A major clinical manifestation observed in 85% – 95% of patients with cystic fibrosis is chronic bacterial (Staphylococcus aureus, Pseudomonas aeruginosa, Haemophilus influenzae) endobronchial infection and chronic predominantly neutrophilic inflammatory response combined with exocrine pancreatic insufficiency that results in malnutrition and fat malabsorption.

The precise mechanism by which bacterial colonization, recurrent infection, pulmonary destruction and respiratory failure is not yet fully understood. One possible mechanism is an increased level of oxidative stress resulting in oxidative damage of pulmonary tissue. In the presence of chronic lung inflammation, increased generation oxygen free radicals is assumed to occur [1].

Polymorphonuclear neutrophils and macrophages release superoxide anion radical, hydrogen peroxide, hydroxyl radical and also powerful oxidant hypochlorous acid. An overwhelming generation of highly reactive species may be harmful, especially when it exceeds the antioxidant capacity. Exocrine pancreatic insufficiency leads to severe deficiencies in fat-soluble antioxidants, such as vitamin E and carotenoids and as a result to impaired antioxidant protection. An oxidant-antioxidant imbalance is likely to result in oxygen free radicals induced tissue injury.

It is assumed that oxygen free radicals induced tissue injury mediated by an attack on unsaturated fatty acids of lipid structures, DNA as well as protein (especially enzymes).

The most frequently assessed aspect of such an attack is increased lipid peroxidation. Free radicals initiate hydrogen abstraction, molecular rearrangement of polyunsaturated fatty acids (PUFA) and chain reactions resulting in the formation of lipid hydro peroxides, cyclic peroxides and secondary aldehydes such as malondialdehyde (MDA). In CF patients, an elevated level of thiobarbituric acid reactive substances, which are formed from breakdown products during the oxidation of PUFA have been shown [2]. Such breakdown is associated with increased susceptibility of low-density lipoprotein (LDL) to oxidation.

The attack of free radicals on DNA has been shown to cause the formation of DNA-protein cross-links, strand breakage and an alteration of the purine and pirimidine bases. Products of lipid peroxidation may mediate an increase in the production of 8OHdG in DNA. It has been established that following an oxidative hydroxyl radical attack on DNA, guanine bases undergo 8-hydroxylation. The damage is then repaired by exonucleases, releasing water soluble 8OHdG, which is excreted in urine. According to Brown et al. [3], an increased concentration of 8OHdG can be observed in the urine of CF patients indicating oxidative damage to the DNA although this appears to be independent of the clinical status.

Oxidative damage to various amino acids residues as well as to peptide backbone can adversely affects protein activity, stability and function which leads to the accumulation of oxidatively modified molecules. Reactive oxygen species have been shown to convert some amino acids residues to carbonyl derivatives. Therefore, the level of carbonyl groups has been accepted as a marker of protein oxidative injury. Brown and Kelly [4] did not observe in plasma protein carbonyl content a significant differences between CF patients and healthy subjects. However, a much wider distribution of this marker may indicate that some CF patients are more susceptible to oxidative damage than others.

To prevent free radical induced damage, an oxidant-antioxidant balance is needed. However patients with CF, because of their CFTR dysfunction and malabsorption condition, are predisposed to have a low store of antioxidants. A variety of studies have shown that exogenous, both lipophilic (tocopherols, carotenoids) and water-soluble (ascorbate) and also endogenous enzymatic antioxidants (glutathione peroxidase, superoxide dismutase, catalase) as well as non-enzymatic ones (glutathione, urate, albumine, ferritin and ceruloplasmine) are depleted [5,6].

In cystic fibrosis as a result of depleted antioxidant protection the risk of oxidative injury of erythrocytes has been suggested [7]. Oxidative stress in red blood cells (RBC) can cause changes in hemoglobin as well as in the cell membrane. Spontaneous autooxidation of hemoglobin to methemoglobin and next to hemichromes is involved in Heinz body formation. Oxidative damage to the membrane is manifested usually as lipid peroxidation. Direct exposure of RBC to malondialdehyde resulted in a modification of membrane proteins. In red blood cells, high membrane content of unsaturated lipid, aerobic conditions and the presence of metal ion (Fe3+) facilitate free radical generation, peroxidative processes and are linked to unstability of membranes and impaired integrity of the cell. This is a rare occurrence except in cases where defects exist in the red cells antioxidant capacity. Several studies have demonstrated that erythrocytes of CF patients have shortened survival time and were susceptible in vitro to peroxide induced hemolysis but lipid peroxidation, vitamin E status and some enzymatic activities were not studied frequently [8,9].

The purpose of this study was to investigate whether in cystic fibrosis patients with exocrine pancreatic insufficiency, the antioxidant status provided sufficient protection against oxidative damage to protein and lipids.

Materials and Methods

Patients

Our study population consisted of 57 (32 males and 25 females) CF patients with exocrine pancreatic insufficiency under surveillance at the Department of Pediatrics at the Institute of Mother and Child in Warsaw. All patients (median age 7 years, range 1-18 years) have been diagnosed on the basis of clinical history. The diagnosis of CF had been confirmed by elevated sweat chloride concentration (>60 mEq/L) and δ508 mutation. The patients were maintained on their routine medication and were treated with supplemental pancreatic enzymes. In addition to their dietary intakes, they all received standard vitamin supplementation (vitamin A as retinol from 1,500 – 4,000 IU/day and vitamin E from 100 – 1000 mg/day).

The control group consisted of 21 subjects (10 males and 11 females, median age 8 years, range 1 - 18 years) without digestive and pulmonary disease. The studies were approved by the institutional review board. Informed consent was obtained from the parents of the examined children.

Materials

Fasting blood was obtained by venipuncture into glass and heparinized tubes. Serum and plasma were prepared by centrifugation of blood at 4000 rpm and were used for lipids, protein and MDA determinations. Residual plasma and serum were frozen at –70°C until vitamins, TRAP and carbonyl groups content were measured. In washed erythrocytes hemoglobin and MDA were measured immediately. Vitamin E and activities of glutathione peroxidase (GPx), superoxide dismutase (SOD) and catalase (CAT) were determined in RBC stored frozen after dilution in phosphate buffer (pH 7,0).

Methods

Malondialdehyde (MDA) in Plasma and Erythrocytes

Lipid peroxidation as MDA was measured as thiobarbituric acid (TBA)-reactive materials [10]. The samples of plasma (200 μl) and hemolysate (50 μl red blood cells and distilled water 1:9 v/v) were mixed with 1 ml TBA-TCA-HCl solution. TBA-TCA-HCl solution was prepared by dissolving 41,6 mg TBA in 10 ml TCA (16,8% w/v in 0,25 N HCl). After heating (15 min, 100°C) and centrifugation (10 min, 4000 x g) the absorbance at 535 nm vs 600 nm was measured. The MDA concentration was expressed in nmol/l plasma or nmol/g Hb.

Carbonyls Content in Plasma

Protein carbonyls content in plasma has been previously determined by Levine et al. [11]. A sample of plasma (100 μl) was diluted 2-fold in 5 mmol/l EDTA, pH 7.4. This sample was then divided into two separate aliquots, precipitated protein with 500 μl of 20% TCA and centrifuged at 13,000 × g for 3 min. Both supernatants were discarded; one pellet was redissolved in 2M HCl containing 0,1% DNP solution and the other, which acted as the blank, was run in parallel, in 2M HCl alone. The pellets were sonicated at 10 microns for 10 s to aid dissolution. The samples were then left to stand at room temperature for 1 hour (mixing every 15 min); at the end of this period 500 μl of 20% TCA was added to reprecipitate the protein. The mixture was centrifuged at 13,000 × g for 3 min. The pellets were washed 3 times with 1 ml of ethanol/ethyl acetate (1:1) to remove the free reagent, with the sample allowed to stand for 10 min before centrifugation and the supernatant discarded each time. The final pellet produced from the washings was redissolved in 1 ml of 6 mol/l guanidine-HCl by warming gently at 37° C for 15 min followed by sonication at 14 microns for 10 s. After a last spin at 13,000 × g for 3 min, the absorbance of each sample and its corresponding blank was read against a blank containing 6 mol/l guanidine-HCl using Beckman DU® 640 (USA) at a wavelength of 370 nm. The carbonyl content was calculated as μmol/g protein.

Total Protein in Serum

Total protein concentrations were determined by the biuret method with commercially available kits from Hoffman La-Roche (Switzerland) by Cobas Mira analyzer.

Total Radical-Trapping Antioxidant Parameter in Plasma

Total plasma antioxidant activity was measured according to Wayner et al. [12] using an oxygen electrode (model 5300 Biological Oxygen Monitor, Yellow Springs Instruments, OH, USA), with automatic data recording. TRAP was defined as moles of peroxyl radical trapped by 1 l of plasma. The determination is performed in two stages. The first stage represents the antioxidative activity of the plasma, which inhibits lipid peroxidation by 2,2-azo-bis(2-amidinopropane hydrochloride) (ABAP). For a period, limited oxygen utilization is observed. Subsequently, when antioxidative abilities of the plasma are depleted, oxygen utilization rapidly increases due to intensive lipid peroxidation. Then in the second stage of determination, a commercially available antioxidant, Trolox (6-hydroxy-2,5,7,8-tetramethylchroman-2-carboxylic acid), is added to the reaction. Trolox inhibits oxygen consumption until its antioxidative abilities become exhausted, which is followed by rapid oxygen utilization resulting from intensified lipid peroxidation. The TRAP value (in μmol/l of plasma) was calculated as follows:

$$\text{TRAP}\frac{2(\text{Trolox})\times(\text{T serum})\times(\text{V Trolx})}{2(\text{Trolox})\times(\text{T serum})\times(\text{V Trolox})}$$

Where V Trolox and V serum are the volumes of the Trolox and serum solutions, respectively; 2 is the coefficient resulting from the fact that each Trolox molecule traps two peroxyl radicals; Trolox = Trolox solution (0,4 mmol/l); T Trolox and T serum are the lengths of segments obtained that delineate a tangent to the curve, which represents depletion of oxygen content in the incubation mixture.

Vitamin A, E, Beta-Carotene in Plasma and Vitamin E in Erythrocytes

Vitamin A, E, beta-carotene in plasma and vitamin E in erythrocytes were determined by the high-pressure liquid chromatography method (HPLC), (Knauer, Germany) [13]. The samples were thawed and deproteinized with ethanol, after which hexane was added (1000 μl). After being mixed by vortex, the samples were centrifuged (5000 rpm) and the hexane phase was removed. The samples (100 μl) were injected into an HPLC column. Separation was accomplished on 4x25 mm Hypersil ODS column (Knauer, Germany), 5 μm. particle size using isocratic elution, 1,5 ml/min with a mobile phase of 95% heksane and 5% 1.4 dioxane. Quantitation of Vitamin E was with UV 290 nm, vitamin A with 320 nm and beta-carotene with UV 450 nm detection using a known amount of retinyl acetate as an internal standard and a standard curve containing known amounts of α-tocopherol and all trans retinol (Sigma-Aldrich, USA). The concentrations of vitamins were expressed in μmol/l.

Lipids and Lipoproteins in Serum

Total cholesterol (TC), HDL-cholesterol (HDL-C), LDL-cholesterol (LDL-C) and trigliceride (TG) concentrations were measured enzymatically by the Cobas Mira analyzer (Hoffman La-Roche, Switzerland) using available commercial kits from Bio-Merieux (France). For HDL determination, serum LDL and very-low-density lipoprotein (VLDL) fractions were precipitated with the phospho-tungstic acid-MgCl2 reagent. In the clear supernatant, HDL levels were measured. Serum LDL-cholesterol was determined in the precipitate obtained by reaction with amphipatic polymers. Control Serum N (Hoffman La-Roche) and Lyotrol "N" (Bio-Merieux) were the quality control. Levels of lipids were expressed in mg/dl and mmol/l.

Catalase in Erythrocytes (EC.1.11.1.6)

The activity of catalase was determined according to Beers and Sizer [14]. The method is based on monitoring the rate of decomposition of H2O2 at room temperature. The time of decrease of optical density at 240 nm was measured. A 10 μl volume of hemolysate (red blood cells and distilled water 1:30 v/v, equivalent to about 0,1 mg Hb) was used for each sample. Enzyme activity was calculated as U/gHb.

Superoxide Dismutase in Erythrocytes (EC. 1.15.1.1)

Superoxide dismutase activity was determined using a RANSOD kit (Randox Laboratories Ltd. GB) by the Cobas Mira analyzer (Hoffman La-Roche, Switzerland). This method employs xanthine and xanthine oxidase to generate superoxide radicals which react with 2-(4-iodophenyl)-3-(4-nitrophenol)-5-phenyltetrazolium chloride (INT) to form a red formazan dye. The superoxide dismutase activity was then measured by the degree of inhibition of this reaction. For determination a 50 μl of hemolysate (red blood cells and distilled water 1:200 v/v, equivalent to about 75 μg Hb) was used. Enzyme activity was calculated as U/gHb.

Glutathione Peroxidase in Erythrocytes (EC. 1.11.1.9)

Glutathione peroxidase activity was determined using a RANSEL kit (Randox Laboratories Ltd. GB) by Cobas Mira analyzer (Hoffman La-Roche, Switzerland). This method is based on coupled enzyme assay of Paglia and Valentine [15]. GPx catalyses the oxidation of glutathione by cumene hydroperoxide. In the presence GPx and NADPH, the oxidized glutathione is immediately converted into the reduced form with a concomitant oxidation of NADPH to NADP+. The decrease in absorbance at 340 nm was measured. First, washed erythrocytes were mixed with Drabkin reagent at a ratio of 1:1. Then, 30 μl of mixture (approximately 4.5 mg Hb) were used for determination of the enzyme's activity, which was expressed as U/gHb.

Hemoglobin in Erythrocytes

Hemoglobin determination was carried out by the hemoglobin cyanide method (kit, Technoplastyka, Poland).

Statistical Analysis

Data are presented as means ±SD (standard deviation). The differences were evaluated by ANOVA (STATISTICA 6.0, StatSoft, USA). The significance was set a $p<0.05$.

Results

In cystic fibrosis patients with pancreatic insufficiency, peroxidation was significantly elevated. Mean values were 2,98 ± 0,72 μmol/l and 2,27 ± 0,32 μmol/l respectively ($p<0.001$) (Table I). Concentration of MDA in plasma was distributed in a wider range in patients (1,23 – 4,77 μmol/l) than in the control group (1,43 – 2,80 μmol/l) (Figure 1). Among 57 patients in 32 subjects, the level of MDA exceeded the upper value found in the healthy group.

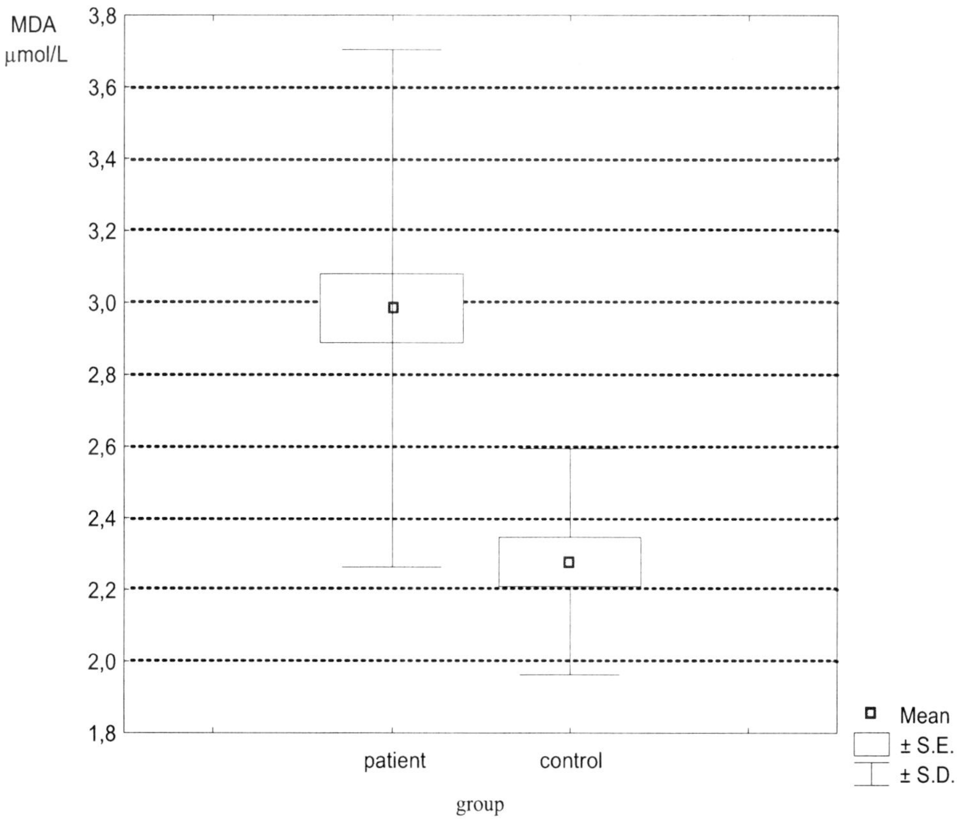

Figure 1. Concentration of MDA in plasma of cystic fibrosis patients and healthy children

As is shown in Table 1, plasma protein carbonyls content differed significantly between the two groups ($p<0.001$). In CF children, the mean value was 0,84 ± 0,37 µmol/g protein and was higher than in the control (0,64 ± 0,09 µmol/g protein). The range of protein carbonyl concentration was wider in patients (0,31 - 1,71 µmol/g protein) than in healthy children (0,45 - 0,76 µmol/g protein) (Figure 2). Protein carbonyls level in 63% of patients (36/57) exceeded mean values of control and in 53% (30/57) was above the highest concentration found in the healthy group.

Table 1. Concentration of malondialdehyde and protein carbonyls in plasma of cystic fibrosis patients and healthy children

Group	Malondialdehyde µmol/1	Protein carbonyls µmol/g protein
CF Patients	2,98 ± 0,72**	0,84 ± 0,37**
Control	2,27 ± 0,32	0,64 ± 0,09

Data are mean ± SD, statistically significance ** $p<0.001$

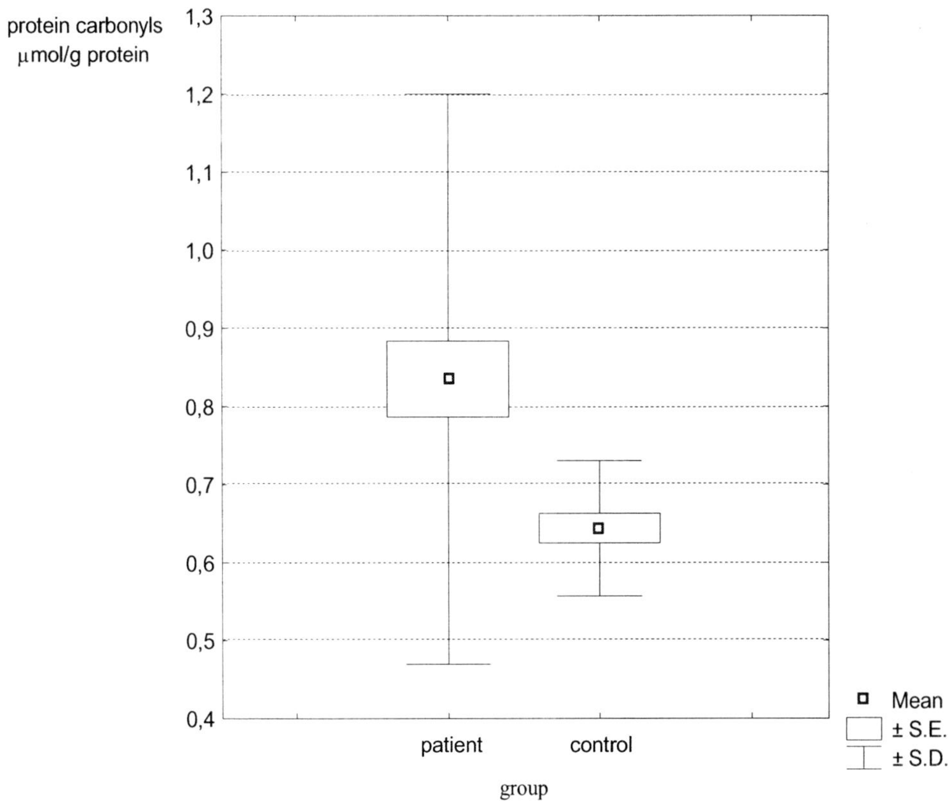

Figure 2. Concentration of protein carbonyls in plasma of cystic fibrosis patients and healthy children

Children with CF had reduced total radical trapping potential. Results presented in Figure 3 indicated that in patients mean concentration of TRAP amounted to 629 ± 132 µmol/l whereas in healthy subjects it was 735 ± 110 µmol/l ($p<0.001$).

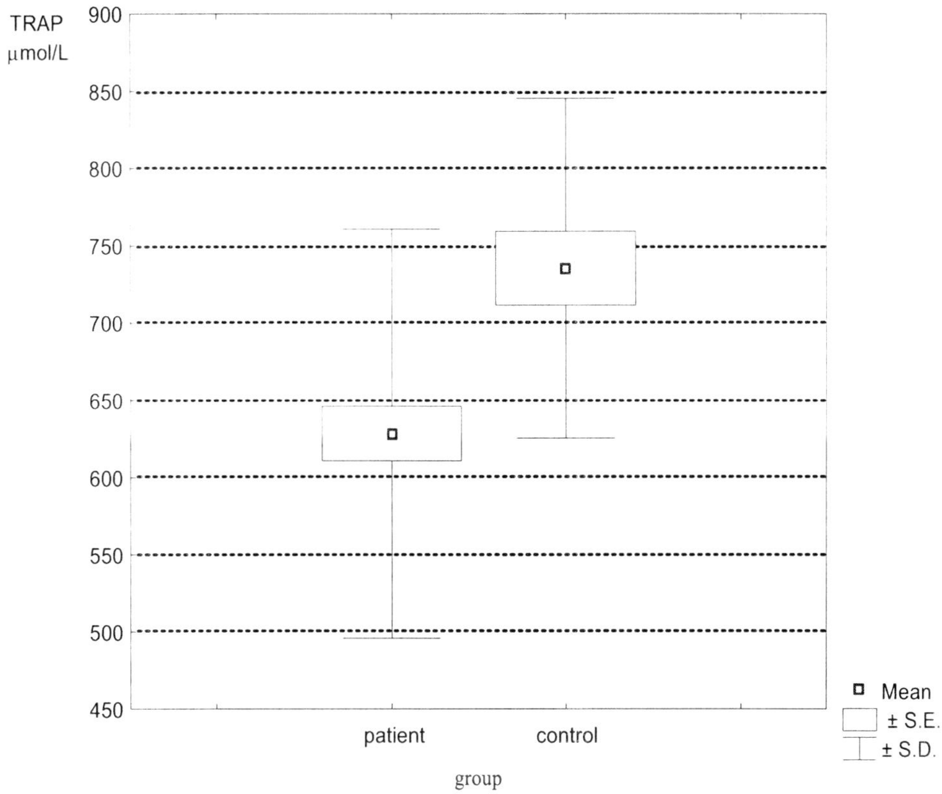

Figure 3. Concentration of TRAP in plasma of cystic fibrosis patients and healthy children

As is shown in Table 2, in the plasma of sick children, concentrations of total lipids, total cholesterol, cholesterol in HDL and LDL fractions were reduced respectively by 20% ($p<0.001$), 25% ($p<0.0001$), 38% ($p<0.0001$) and 16% ($p<0.05$) in comparison to the control.

Table 2. Serum lipids in cystic fibrosis patients and healthy children

Concentration		Group	
		CF Patients	Control
Total cholesterol	mmol/l	3,05 ± 0,75***	4,09 ± 0,48
	mg/dl	117,80 ± 29,15***	158,33 ± 18,53
HDL cholesterol mg/dl		33,26 ± 9,61***	53,33 ± 7,84
LDL cholesterol mg/dl		72,56 ± 20,36*	86,33 ± 15,95
Triglyceride	mmol/l	0,85 ± 0,23	0,79 ± 0,28
	mg/dl	74,70 ± 20,36	69,67 ± 24,06
LipidsTC + TG mmol/l		3,90 ± 0,80***	4,89 ± 0,61

Data are mean ± SD, statistically significance *$p<0.01$; *** $p<0.0001$

It was accompanied with severe deficiency of beta-carotene. In the plasma of CF patients, the mean value of β-carotene was 1,56 ± 0,38 μmol/l and was one half of that found in the control (3,12 ± 0,56 μmol/l; $p<0.0001$) (Figure 4). Ratios of beta-carotene to lipids and to total cholesterol in patients were lower than in the control by 36% and by 30% respectively (Table 3). Concentration of β-carotene below the lowest value of control was found in 55 children.

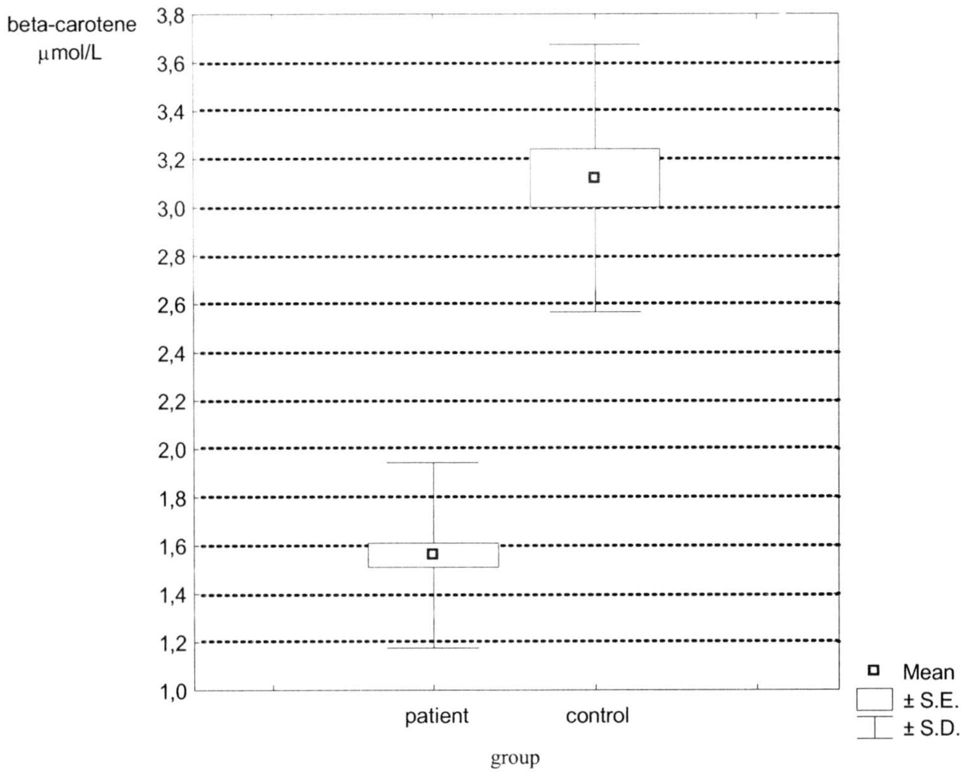

Figure 4.Concentration of beta-carotene in plasma of cystic fibrosis patients and healthy children

Table 3. Concentration of β-carotene in plasma of cystic fibrosis patients and healthy children

Group	β-carotene μmol/l	β-carotene/total cholesterol μmol/mmol	β-carotene/lipids μmol/mmol
CF Patients	1,56 ± 0,38***	0,54 ± 0,18***	0,42 ± 0,13***
Control	3,12 ± 0,58	0,78 ± 0,19	0,65 ± 0,16

Data are mean ± SD, statistically significance *** p<0.0001

CF children had also a concentration of vitamin A in the range of deficiency. The mean value of plasma retinol content in CF children amounted to 1,22 ± 0,45 μmol/l then was almost 30% lower in comparison to the control (1,69 ± 0,37 μmol/l). The differences were significant (p<0.0001) (Figure 5). However, ratios of vitamin A to lipids and to total cholesterol were the same in both studied groups (Table 4). A wide distribution of vitamin A was observed and in about 25% of patients, concentration of this vitamin was below the limit of healthy children.

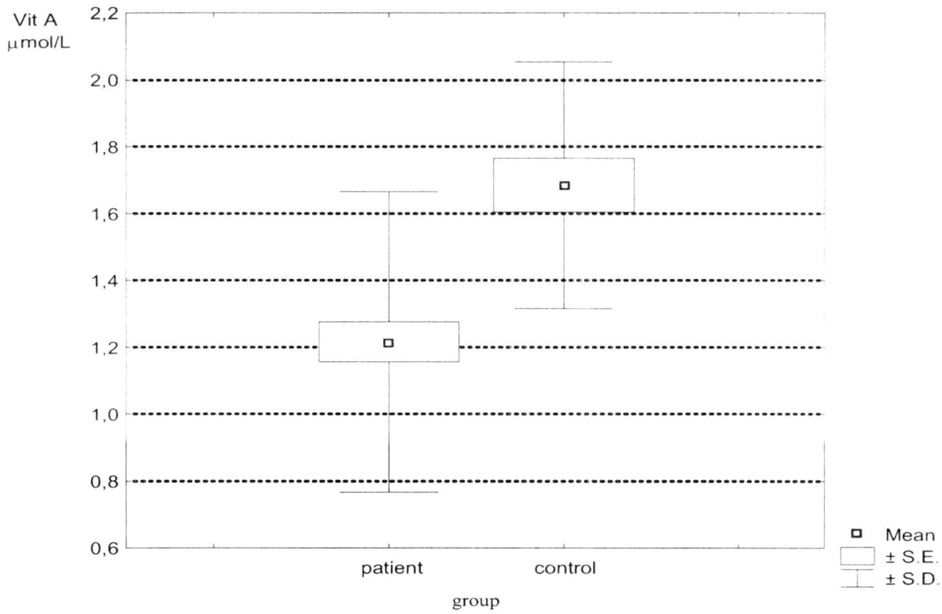

Figure 5. Concentration of vitamin A in plasma of cystic fibrosis patients and healthy children

Table 4. Concentration of vitamin A in plasma of cystic fibrosis patients and healthy children

Group	Vitamin A μmol/l	Vitamin A/total cholesterol μmol/mmol	Vitamin A/lipids μmol/mmol
CF Patients	1,22 ± 0,45***	0,42 ± 0,20	0,32 ± 0,14
Control	1,69 ± 0,37	0,42 ± 0,10	0,35 ± 0,09

Data are mean ± SD, statistically significance *** $p<0.0001$

The mean concentration of vitamin E (13,69 ± 4,90 μmol/l) in plasma of patients was 27% lower than that found in control ($p<0.0001$) (Figure 6). The ratio of vitamin E to total lipids was the same in patients and in the healthy group. However, the ratio of α-tocopherol to total cholesterol in subjects was reduced to 74% of the control (Table 5).

The deficiency of antioxidants in plasma seems to reflect an antioxidant defence system of red blood cells. In erythrocytes of CF children, the mean concentration of MDA was 128,73 ± 32,97 μmol/gHb whereas in the healthy group it was 113,77 ± 11,74 μmol/gHb. The difference was quite significant ($p<0.0001$). The range of MDA concentration was wide (60,86 – 216,80 μmol/gHb) and in 26/57 children was above the highest level of the control (Figure 7).

In erythrocytes, the mean values of α-tocopherol were 1,39 ± 0,42 μmol/l in patients and 2,95 ± 0,43 μmol/l in the control ($p<0.0001$) (Figure 8). Among 57 patients studied, in the erythrocytes of 53 children vitamin E concentrations were below these found in the healthy subjects.

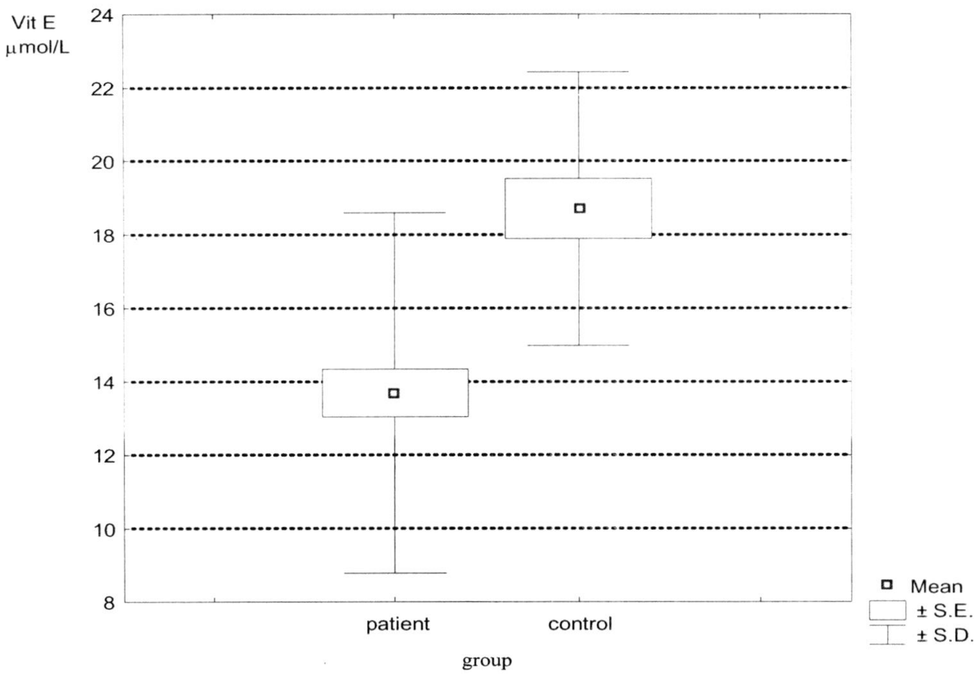

Figure 6. Concentration of vitamin E in plasma of cystic fibrosis patients and healthy children

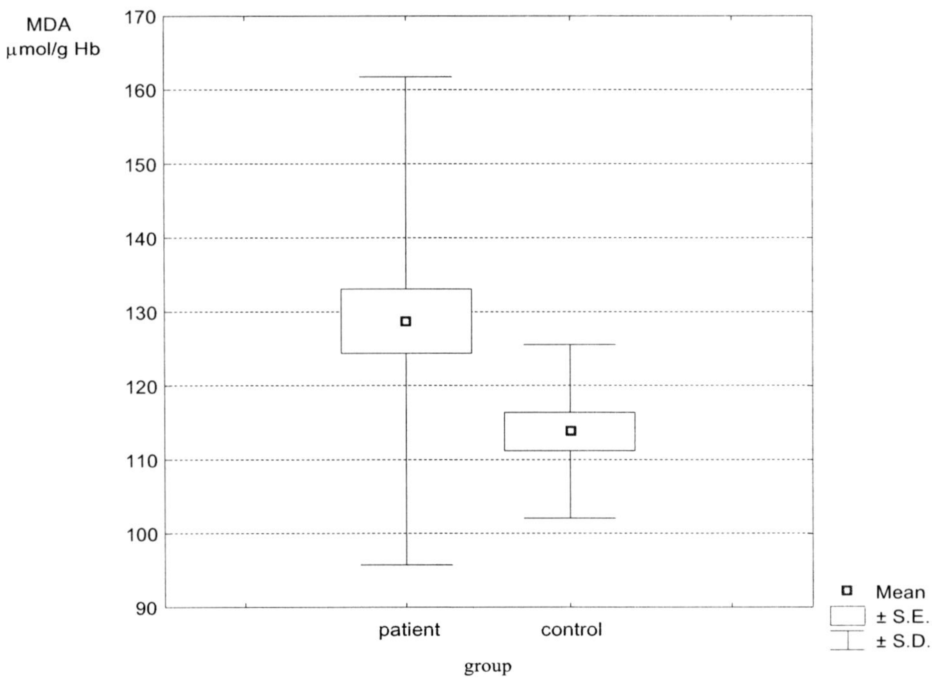

Figure 7. Concentration of MDA in red blood cells of cystic fibrosis patients and healthy children

Table 5. Concentration of vitamin E in plasma of cystic fibrosis patients and healthy children

Group	Vitamin E µmol/l	Vitamin E/total cholesterol µmol/mmol	Vitamin E/lipids µmol/mmol
CF Patients	13,69 ± 4,90***	3,90 ± 0,80	3,65 ± 1,54
Control	18,71 ± 3,73	4,64 ± 1,14	3,89 ± 0,98

Data are mean ± SD, statistically significance *** p<0.0001

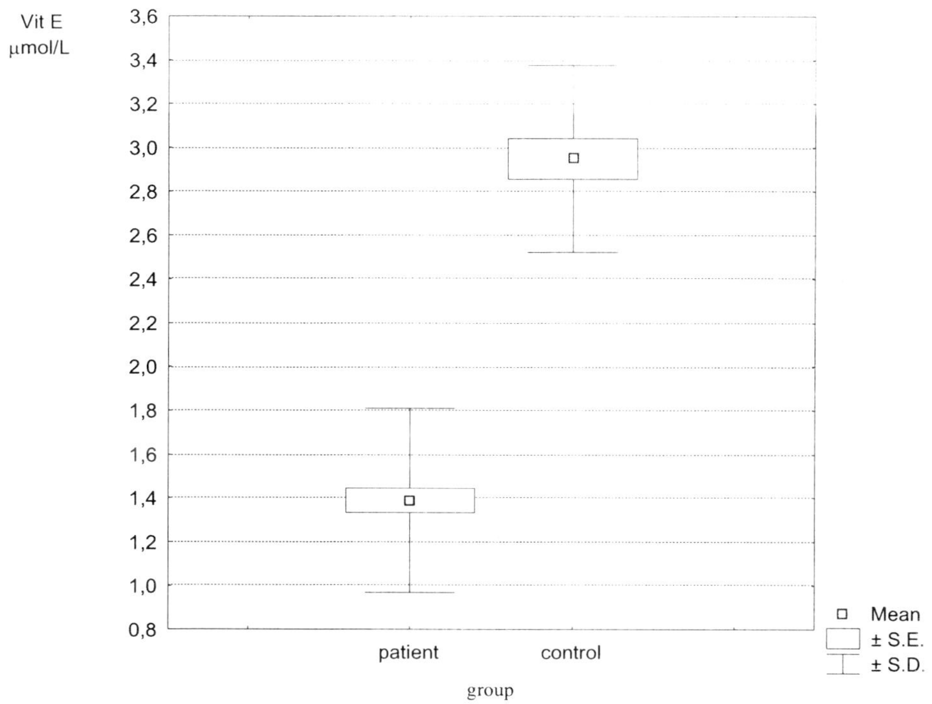

Figure 8. Concentration of vitamin E in red blood

Enzymatic antioxidant activities in erythrocytes of the CF group and of the control were different (Table 6). Activity of catalase was 23% lower (p<0.001) and superoxidase dismutase 30% higher (p<0.001) in patients than in healthy children. There was no significant difference in the activity of glutathione peroxidase in both studied groups.

Table 6. Activities of superoxidase dismutase, glutathione peroxidase and catalase in erythrocytes of cystic fibrosis patients and healthy children

Group	Superoxidase dismutase U/gHb	Glutathione peroxidase U/gHb	Catalase U/gHb
CF Patients	1450,17 ± 381,16***	30,30 ± 7,95	14,31 ± 5,64**
Control	1116,22 ± 168,99	31,12 ± 8,10	18,57 ± 3,65

Data are mean ± SD, statistically significance** p<0.001;***p<0.0001

Discussion

Digestive malabsorption in CF patients, especially those with exocrine pancreatic insufficiency, may lead to malnutrition and to amplification of oxidative conditions generated by chronic pulmonary infections. In patients, an imbalance between the production of reactive oxygen species and their inactivation by protective systems has been suggested [1].

It is currently believed that measurements of biomarkers of oxidative stress and antioxidant status may be useful in detecting those patients at risk at an early stage of imbalance and seems to be necessary for clinical management and therapeutic treatment of sick children.

Evidence of increased lipid peroxidation, the most frequently assessed aspect of oxidant-antioxidant imbalance, has been observed previously in CF patients. Portal et al. [16] reported higher lipid peroxidation in patients than in healthy children, regardless of whether it was determined by organic hydroperoxides or by MDA - secondary product of lipid peroxidation. Brown and Kelly [17] observed in CF subjects increased contents of both MDA and fatty acid hydroperoxides determined directly by the HPLC method. Benabdeslam et al. [2] found in CF patients an elevated index of lipid peroxidation by measuring in serum concentration not only of MDA but also of autoantibodies against oxidized low-density lipoproteins. We have previously shown that almost in 50% of the Polish CF population, plasma concentration of MDA exceeded the highest values found in the healthy children [18]. In current studies, we have confirmed these observations and have shown elevated (by 30%) mean values of MDA in patients than in the control.

Lipids are not a target for free radical attack in vivo only. In comparison, radical induced protein modifications have received less attention, although it is recognized that radical damage to proteins results in changes in their structure, stability and function. Oxidative attacks to various amino acid residues can lead to formation of carbonyl products. Brown and Kelly [4] have reported that concentrations of plasma carbonyl groups did not differ significantly between CF patients and healthy subjects. In our group of CF children, the increase of the concentration of protein carbonyl groups by 25% was significant and in the same range as reported by others in adult cystic fibrosis patients [19]. Distribution in values was wider in patients than in the control. The same was also observed by Brown and Kelly [4] and Range et al. [19] and might indicate different susceptibility of some subjects to oxidation of protein. In order to explain the relation of protein and lipid oxidation either to pancreatic insufficiency or to impairment of antioxidant capacity, more studies appear to be needed.

During the past few years, a deficiency of antioxidants in cystic fibrosis has been frequently reported. Using TRAP assay to investigate of total trapping antioxidant potency, several authors documented a significantly decreased ability of plasma to withstand oxidative stress. Mean values of TRAP decreased by about 16% in the plasma of CF patients in comparison to the control in not only in our study, but also in other previous studies by Langley et al. [20] and Lands et al. [6]. TRAP values appear to represent a mixed antioxidant response. Among individual plasma antioxidants contributed to TRAP, the most common in cystic fibrosis are deficiencies of β-carotene and α-tocopherol. The main carriers of carotenoids and vitamin E in the blood are low-density and high-density lipoprotein fractions and their concentration should be taken into account in assessment of lipophilic antioxidant status.

In cystic fibrosis pancreatic insufficiency, liver malfunction and impairment of resorption may have an important influence on the profile of lipid in blood. Severity of fat malabsorption could reflect the impairment in blood lipid level. Several studies reported those CF patients had low concentration of blood cholesterol associated presumably with a fall of cholesterol in the HDL and LDL fractions. The content of triglycerides in serum of patients and control subjects was not statistically different [21]. We also found in CF children significantly lower concentrations of total blood cholesterol and cholesterol in HDL and LDL lipoproteins and similar level of triglyceride as compared to the control.

Some authors suggest that ratios of lipophilic antioxidants to cholesterol or to total lipids rather than their concentrations in plasma might be the preferable index for characterizing the status in patients with disturbances in the lipid metabolism [16].

In CF patients, the status of vitamin A and E, when expressed on the basis of the concentrations of total cholesterol, were no different from those in control subjects. When those concentrations were not expressed as a ratio to cholesterol or lipids, the levels of β-carotene, retinol and α-tocopherol were drastically lower [16]. Our results showed that almost all CF patients with pancreatic insufficiency exhibited severe β-carotene deficiency expressed both as μmol/l and also on basis of cholesterol and lipids content. β-carotene as a metabolic precursor of retinol has contributed to the vitamin A status. The degree of β-carotene conversion into retinol is known to be regulated by dietary supplies and saturation of reserves of vitamin A. We have observed that the retinol status in CF children was not different from that in the control group when expressed as the ratio to cholesterol or lipids. Nevertheless, plasma concentrations of vitamin A remained lower in some subjects than in the control. The same was reported by Portal et al. [16] and Chase et al. [22]. Carotenoids as a single oxygen quencher and a chain-breaking antioxidant are complementary to peroxyl radical scavenging tocopherols and synergistically inhibited oxidative injury.

In CF patients, a deficiency of vitamin E has been frequently exhibited even early in the course of the disease [23]. Winklhofer et al. [21] have shown severe deficiency of plasma α-tocopherol in CF patients with exocrine pancreatic insufficiency. Their concentration of vitamin E did not exceed 35% of values found in the healthy group and correlated well with the cholesterol concentration. We also observed decreased plasma vitamin E content in CF subjects, but only by 30% in comparison to the control. The ratio of this vitamin to total lipid was the same, but to total cholesterol was lower in patients than in healthy children. According to James et al. [8], a ratio of α-tocopherol to cholesterol exceeding 4,8 μmol/mmol is necessary to protect against peroxidative damage sufficiently. In our CF children, the ratio of plasma α-tocopherol to cholesterol was 3,9 μmol/mmol (lower than the value needed).

Deficiencies of carotenoids and vitamin E in plasma could lead to impaired antioxidant protection and to increased sensitivity to oxidative stress under red blood cells as well. The level of MDA is not frequently determined in CF erythrocytes. Erythrocyte membranes, because of their high content of PUFA, are susceptible to peroxidation, especially under conditions of antioxidant imbalance. However, published data on lipid peroxidation in erythrocytes of CF patients is limited and somewhat contradictory.

Matkovics et al. [24], in 8 patients studied, observed significantly reduced levels of MDA in RBC. Gyurkovits et al. [25] found that reduced lipid peroxidation in erythrocytes was accompanied by an increase in antioxidant enzyme activities. Our CF group consisted of 57 patients with exocrine pancreatic insufficiency. The group exhibited significantly elevated concentrations of MDA, which exceeded the upper level of the control in one half of the studied population. it is commonly accepted that patients with low plasma vitamin E concentration had decreased in vivo red cell survival times and elevated susceptibility to peroxide-induced hemolysis in vitro. Several authors established a threshold of vitamin E deficiency equivalent to 1,11 μmol α-tocopherol/mmol total lipids [26] or 11,6 μmol/l [27]. An increased rate of peroxide induced hemolysis has been associated with a fall of plasma vitamin E concentrations below 20,0 μmol/l. Extensive hemolysis occurred with α-tocopherol concentrations below 4,6 μmol/l.

Since vitamin E has been shown to scavenge lipid peroxyl radicals thereby blocking propagation of lipid peroxidation, the concentration of α-tocopherol not only in plasma but also in erythrocytes might affect the antioxidant potential of RBC. Previously, Winklhofer et al. [21] suggested that in CF patients, vitamin E is absorbed and transported efficiently enough to be delivered to erythrocytes in quantities similar to those of healthy subjects.

We observed very low concentrations of vitamin E in erythrocytes. In CF patients, it was one half of that found in the control. Our results are similar to those reported by James et al. [8], Peters and Kelly [28] but are lower than those shown by Winklhofer [21]. Increased MDA concentrations in RBC, apart from vitamin E depletion, may be due to some other causes including deficiency of enzymatic antioxidant activities.

Several authors reported in the erythrocytes of CF children a low activity of glutathione peroxidase, an enzyme that detoxifies hydroperoxides. Benabdeslam et al. [2] in RBC of CF patients found only 80% of GPx activity observed in the control. In accordance with the report of Carmagnol et al. [7] we show in our patients slightly but not significantly lower activity of this enzyme. Since selenocysteine is in an active site of GPx, a reduction of peroxidase activity in cystic fibrosis was often suggested to be associated with a decrease in blood selenium content, which occurs secondary to malabsorption. In the studies of Foucaud et al. [29] selenium content in plasma and erythrocytes, together with the activity of GPx, have been identified. Both parameters have shown significantly lower values in the CF group than in the control, but patients taking pancreatic enzymes had a higher content than the others. In the blood of our patients, the concentration of selenium was not measured, but deficiency of this micronutrient cannot be excluded.

Superoxidase dismutase, which catalyzed the dismutation of superoxide radicals to hydrogen peroxide, is considered to be an important part of the enzymatic antioxidant defense in red blood cells. In the erythrocytes of CF patients, the significant 2-fold increase in SOD activity was found by Gyurkovits et al. [25]. In other reports, an increase in the activity of SOD was not significant [2,7] or even observed [30,31]. The erythrocytes of our patients exhibited elevated activity of this enzyme as compared to the values found in the control group and the increase was statistically significant.

We observed in the red blood cells of CF patients decreased activity of catalase in comparison to controls. This is in concordance with the results obtained by Carmagnol et al. [7] but contradictory to Matkovics et al. [24]. In order to resolve the role of this enzyme in the erythrocytes antioxidant defense, more studies are needed.

In therapeutic concepts to reconstitute the balance between the free radical generation and antioxidant protection, an enhanced intake of pancreatic enzyme, together with an efficient antioxidant supply, are taken into consideration.

Despite regular treatment with pancreatic extracts, impaired nutritional status frequently persisted in CF children. Almost 40% of patients exhibited low albumin concentration and disturbed fatty acid status [32]. In the studies of Littlewood and MacDonald [33], protein deficiency and fetal nitrogen excretion were significantly reduced by the administration of pancreatic enzymes, but fat losses were not completely corrected. Pancreatic enzyme therapy considerably improves fat absorption but does not normalize it, even when the dosage is increased [34,35]. Soltani-Frisk et al. [36] and Lancelotti et al. [37] suggested that also in CF patients receiving modern pancreatic supplementation, residual steatorrhea results in fat malabsorption and low levels of fat soluble vitamin A, β-carotene and α-tocopherol. The authors indicated the necessity of supplying patients with high doses of α -tocopherol. The same was previously suggested by Winkhlofer et al. [21]. However, Benabdeslam et al. [32] observed that therapy with vitamins A and E did not normalize their blood levels. Wood et al. [31] suggested that concentrations of antioxidant defences of stable CF patients mainly α-tocopherol and β -carotene are lower than those of a healthy control. This occurred despite normal intakes of fat-soluble vitamins and supplementation of pancreatic enzymes.

Peters and Kelly [28], in the patients on individual established replacement pancreatic enzyme therapy, have shown normal erythrocyte vitamin E concentration with a supplement of 100 mg vitamin E /day. Doses of α-tocopherol prescribed in the international guidelines for children below 10 years old (100 mg daily) and for those above 10 years (200 mg/daily) and 2,5 mg of retinol/day failed to provide sufficient antioxidant protection. According to Madarasi et al. [38], the daily dose of these vitamins should be increased. Winklhofer et al. [21] recommend the restoration of normal vitamin E levels, the reduction of lipid peroxidation and the improvement of lung function at a recommended 400 IU of α-tocopherol daily with pancreatic enzymes and a fat-containing meal.

Some authors observed normalized oxidative stress when β-carotene status has been restored [39-44]. In CF children, a supplementation with a 0,69 mg/kg-1 of β -carotene three times per day with meals for 6 months resulted in correction of the β -carotene deficiency, in reduction of lipid peroxide level and in normalization LDL resistance to oxidation [45]. Winklhofer et al. [43,44] reported that oral supplementation with 0,5 mg/kg day of β -carotene restored the normal status of β -carotene within 3 weeks and reduced significantly the lipid peroxide level. The efficacy of long-term oral β-carotene supplementation was studied by Rust et al. [41,42]. They suggested that the dosage of 1mg β -carotene/ kg/ day (the maximum 50 mg/day) is necessary to achieve normal plasma β -carotene level in CF patients. During the treatment, a decrease of lipid peroxides content and improvement of total antioxidant capacity were observed. Moreover β -carotene supplementation significantly ameliorated pulmonary exacerbation improving the quality of life of patients [46].

According to some authors, β -carotene plays a unique role in cystic fibrosis [31,41]. An improvement of patient β -carotene status resulted in normalized oxidative stress, whereas for vitamin E and other antioxidants, it was not observed.

Our results confirmed the suggestion that in CF patients with exocrine pancreatic insufficiency, oxidative stress caused oxidative modification of proteins and enhanced peroxidation of lipids. This is accompanied by the lowering of antioxidant protection. We concluded that CF children with exocrine pancreatic insufficiency are susceptible to oxidative damage. Therefore, it seems that an adequate and balanced diet is essential for CF children to achieve and maintain a normal antioxidant status.

Acknowledgments

The authors thank Dr Dorota Sands and Dr Robert Piotrowski from the Department of Pediatrics at the Institute of Mother and Child in Warsaw for clinical information about patient management.

References

[1] Brown RK, Kelly FG: Role of free radicals in the pathogenesis of cystic fibrosis. *Thorax* 1994; 49: 738-742.

[2] Benabdeslam H et al.: Lipid peroxidation and antioxidant defenses in cystic fibrosis patients. *Clin Chem Lab Med* 1999; 37(5): 511-516.

[3] Brown RK et al.: Oxidative damage to DNA in patients with cystic fibrosis. *Free Rad Biol Med* 1995; 18(4): 801-806.

[4] Brown RK, Kelly FG: Evidence for increased oxidative damage in patients with cystic fibrosis. *Ped Res* 1994; 36(4): 487-493.

[5] Winklhofer-Roob BM: Oxygen free radicals and antioxidants in cystic fibrosis: the concept of an oxidant-antioxidant imbalance. *Acta Pediatr Suppl* 1994; 395: 49-57.

[6] Lands LC, Grey VL, Grenier C: Total plasma antioxidant capacity in cystic fibrosis. *Ped Pulm* 2000; 29:81-87.

[7] Carmagnol F et al.: Absence of modifications of the enzyme defense system against oxygen toxicity in cystic fibrosis. *Pediatr Res* 1983; 17: 181-182.

[8] James DR, Alfaham M, Goodchild MC: Increased susceptibility to peroxide-induced haemolysis with normal vitamin E concentrations in cystic fibrosis. *Clin Chim Acta* 1991; 204: 279-290.

[9] Bieri JG, Poukka RKH: In vitro haemolysis as related to rat erythrocyte content of α-tocopherol and polyunsaturated fatty acids. *J Nutr* 1970; 100: 557-564.

[10] Kramer K et al.: Influence of lipid peroxidation on beta-adrenoreceptors. *FEBS Lett.* 1986; 198(1): 80-84.

[11] Levine RL et al.: *The determination of carbonyl content in oxidatively modified proteins*. Methods in enzymology, Academic Press, London 1990; 186: 464-477.

[12] Wayner DD et al.: Quantitative measurement of the total peroxyl radical-trapping antioxidant of human blood plasma controlled peroxidation. *FEBS Lett* 1985; 187: 33-37.

[13] Zaman Z, Fielden P, Frost PG: Simultaneous determination of vitamins A and E and carotenoids in plasma by reversed-phase HPLC in elderly and younger subjects. *Clin Chem* 1993; 39(10): 2229-34.

[14] Beers RFJ, Sizer JW: A spectrophotometric method for measuring the breakdown of hydrogen peroxide by catalase. *J Biol Chem* 1952; 195: 33-34.

[15] Paglia DE, Valentine WN: Studies on quantitative and qualitative characterization of erythrocytes glutathione peroxidase. *J Lab Clin Med* 1967; 70: 158-169.

[16] Portal BC et al.: Altered antioxidant status and increased lipid peroxidation in children with cystic fibrosis. *Am J Clin Nutr* 1995; 61: 843-847.

[17] Brown RK et al.: Pulmonary dysfunction in cystic fibrosis is associated with oxidative stress. *Eur Respir J* 1996; 9: 334-339.

[18] Chelchowska M. et al.: Markers of oxidative damage in blood of children with cystic fibrosis. *Pol Merk Lek* 2002; 74: 123-125.

[19] Range SP et al.: Treatment of pulmonary exacerbations of cystic fibrosis leads to improved antioxidant status. *Eur Respir J* 1999; 13: 560-564.

[20] Langley RK et al: Reduced Free-Radical-Trapping capacity and altered plasma antioxidant status in Cystic Fibrosis. *Ped Res* 1993: 33(3): 247-250.

[21] Winklhofer-Roob BM et al.: Response to a single oral dose of all-rac-α-tocopheryl acetate in patients with cystic fibrosis and in healthy individuals. *Am J Clin Nutr* 1996; 63: 717-721.

[22] Chase HP, Long MA, Lavin MH: Cystic fibrosis and malnutrition. *J Pediatr* 1979; 95(3): 337-347.

[23] Sitrin MD et al.: Vitamin E deficiency and neurologic disease in cystic fibrosis. *Ann Inter Med* 1987; 107: 51-54.

[24] Matkovics B et al.: Altered peroxide metabolism in erythrocytes from children with cystic fibrosis. *Clin Chim Acta* 1982; 125: 59-62.

[25] Gyurkovits K et al.: A comparative study of superoxide dismutase (SOD), catalase (CAT), and lipid peroxidation (LP) in RBC from cystic fibrosis (CF) patients. *Eur J Pediatr* 1981; 137;115-118.

[26] Thurnham DI et al.: The use of different lipids to express serum tocopherol:lipid ratios for the measurement of vitamin E status. *Ann Clin Biochem* 1986; 23: 514-520.

[27] Sauberlich HE, Skala JH, Dowdy RP: In: *laboratory test for the assessment of nutritional status*. Florida: CRC Press 1974; 74-80.

[28] Peters SA, Kelly FG: Vitamin E supplementation in cystic fibrosis. *J Ped* 1996; 22(4): 341-345.

[29] Foucaud et al.: Selenium et vitamin E au course de la mucoviscidose. *Arch Fr Pediatr* 1988; 45:383-386.

[30] Wood LG et al.: Oxidative stress in cystic fibrosis: dietary and metabolic factors. *J Am Coll Nutr* 2001; 20(2): 157-165.

[31] Wood LG et al.: Improved antioxidant and fatty acid status of patients with cystic fibrosis after antioxidant supplementation is linked to improved lung function. *Am J Clin Nutr* 2003; 77: 150-159.

[32] Benabdeslam H et al.: Biochemical assessment of the nutritional status of cystic fibrosis patients treated with pancreatic enzyme extracts. *Am J Clin Nutr* 1998; 67: 912-918.

[33] Littlewood JM, MacDonald A: Rationale of modern dietary recommendation in cystic fibrosis. *J R Soc Med.* 1987; 80(15): 16-24.

[34] Fernandes J et al.: General aspects of nutrition in CF. *Acta Ped Scand Suppl* 1985; 317:5-8.

[35] Bouquet J, Sinaasapel M., Neijens HJ: Malabsorption in cystic fibrosis: mechanisms and treatment. *J Pediatr Gastroenterol Nutr* 1988; 7: S30-35.

[36] Soltani-Frisk S et al.: Water-miscible tocopherol is not superior to fat-soluble preparation for vitamin E absorption in cystic fibrosis. *Acta Pediatr* 2001; 90: 1112-1115.

[37] Lancelotti L et al.: Deficiency of vitamin E and A in cystic fibrosis is dependent of pancreatic function and current enzyme and vitamin supplementation. *Eur J Ped* 1996; 155: 281-285.

[38] Madarasi A et al.: Antioxidant status in patients with cystic fibrosis. *Ann Nutr Met* 2000; 44(5-6): 207-211.

[39] Lepage G et al.: Beta-carotene inhibits lipid peroxidation and improves peroxisomal function in cystic fibrosis. *FASEB J* 1993; 7: A39.

[40] Lepage G et al.: Supplementation with carotenoids corrects increased lipid peroxidation in children with cystic fibrosis. *Am J Clin Nutr* 1996; 64: 87-93.

[41] Rust P et al.: Long-term oral β-carotene supplementation in patients with cystic fibrosis-effects on antioxidative status and pulmonary function. *Ann Nutr Met* 2000; 44: 30-37.

[42] Rust Pet et al.: Effects of long-term oral β-carotene supplementation on lipid peroxidation in patients with cystic fibrosis. *Int J Vitam Nutr Res* 1998; 68: 83-87.

[43] Winklhofer-Roob BM: Response to oral β-carotene supplementation in patients with cystic fibrosis: a 16-month follow-up study. *Acta Ped* 1995; 84: 1132-1136.

[44] Winklhofer-Roob BM et al.: Enhanced resistance to oxidation of low density lipoproteins and decreased lipid peroxidation during β-carotene supplementation in cystic fibrosis. *Free Rad Biol Med* 1995; 18(5): 849-859.

[45] Renner S et al.: Effects of β-carotene supplementation for six months on clinical and laboratory parameters in patients with cystic fibrosis. *Thorax* 2001; 56(1): 48-52.

[46] Cobanoglu N et al.: Antioxidant effect of β-carotene in cystic fibrosis and bronchiectasis clinical and laboratory parameters of a pilot study. *Acta Pediatr* 2002; 91: 793-798.

In: Progress in Cystic Fibrosis Research
Editor: Margaret A. Harrison, pp. 99-115

ISBN 1-59454-232-5

Chapter V

Auxological and Endocrine Abnormalities in Cystic Fibrosis

Teresa Arrigo*, Concetta Sferlazzas, Fortunato Lombardo, Cristina Lucanto and Filippo De Luca
Department of Medical and Surgical Pediatrics, University of Messina, Italy

Abstract

Auxological abnormalities are frequently observed in Cystic Fibrosis (CF), as well as in other chronic pediatric diseases. In 20% of CF children the height is subnormal (at least -2 SDS) and bone age and puberty onset are delayed by a mean of 2 years. Final height tends to be below both the population mean and the target stature, owing to a decreased growth spurt. With respect to their mothers CF girls experience menarche approximately 1 year later and their menarcheal delay may be related to both genotype and disease severity. Other factors that may be implicated in the pathogenesis of growth and puberty retardation in CF are undernitrition, chronic hypoxia and respiratory acidosis. Although these children do not have classic growth hormone (GH) deficiency, the few available trials with recombinat human GH in CF have allowed encouraging conclusions in terms of both growth acceleration and clinical status, with no detrimental effects on pancreatic β-cell function.

Diabetes mellitus (DM) is the most frequent endocrine complication of CF. Its prevalence (10-15% in adulthood) is actually growing, due to the increasing longevity of CF patients. DM development is frequently preceded by a longstanding glucose intolerance status, that may be recorded in up to 40-50% of the subjects over the age of 18 years. CF related DM (CFRD) represents a peculiar form of DM, that affects patients with pancreatic exocrine insufficiency, differs from T1DM and shares a number of clinical and pathological similarities with T2 DM. Its pathophysiology has been clarified in the last years thanks to many prolonged follow-up studies, which allowed to reconstruct the natural history of glyco-metabolic status and β-cell function in CF from childhood to adulthood, with the following conclusions:

* Correspondence concerning this article should be addressed to Teresa Arrigo, University of Messina, Italy.

a) glucose tolerance (GT) tends to spontaneously and progressively deteriorate over time;
b) a concomitant spontaneous deterioration of β-cell function plays an important part in the pathogenesis of GT worsening and CFRD development, whereas insulin sensitivity changes are not signficantly involved;
c) no pathogenetic role is played by nutritional status;
d) ΔF508 homozygosis may predispose to the risk of CFRD, whereas N1303K mutation seems to play a protective role.

Osteopenia and osteoporosis are common especially in adults with severe disease and in those who have used corticosteroids.

Cystic fibrosis (CF) is no longer a disease confined to infancy and childhood. In the past, the occasional survival of a child beyond the age of 10 years was unusual and there were practically no authenticated adult cases [1]. Improved nutrition and intensive treatment of infections have changed the natural course of the disease and currently most people with CF survive their teen years and survival may be also into the fourth decade [2], with an average survival age of approximately 30 years [3,4]. The increased life span has brought new disease complications and attention has turned to complications which relate to older patients, such as diabetes mellitus and osteoporosis. Other emerging problems in the past few decades have been: impaired growth, delayed puberty and fertility issues. In particular, research has been directed towards factors which may maximize both survival and life quality in the longer term.

Growth Abnormalities

Failure to thrive is one of the presenting features of CF after the neonatal period and both weight gain and linear growth from birth until the time of diagnosis are well recognized to be poor [5]. For patients with CF, the issues arising from impaired growth are not merely aesthetic ones but concern to physical health and survival.

Usual Growth Pattern

At diagnosis approximately 40% of infants are below the 5th percentile for weight and lenght [6]. After diagnosis some catch-up growth is known to occur, possibly associated with aggressive management following diagnosis [6]. Despite this initial catch-up growth, however, height and weight deficits continue to be seen until the adolescence. At adolescence growth impairment becomes more severe than in mid-childhood and in the prepubertal years. At adolescence, in fact, growth pattern is characterized by a further deceleration in height velocity and skeletal maturation, associated with a delayed and reduced growth spurt. Compared to normal children, delay in age at peak height velocity is around 9-10 months in boys and 10-14 months in girls [5]. Since a negative relationship between age at peak height velocity and peak height velocity is generally observed even in a healthy population, CF patients with extreme delay in puberty fail to demonstrate a significant growth spurt [7]. Consequently the adult stature of CF patients is reduced and corresponds to 25th -42nd percentile for males and 25th- 44th percentile for females [5].

Aetiology and Pathogenesis

The major factors that have been found to possibly impair growth in CF are undernutrition, liver disease, chronic inflammation, diabetes mellitus (DM) and corticosteroid treatment [5]. It is likely that all these factors do so by attenuating the functional integrity of growth hormone (GH)/ insulin-growth-factor 1(IGF-1) axis through complex interactions [5].

Poor nutrition is the most important pathogenetic factor of growth stunting in CF. A fall in body mass index (BMI), in fact, is known to parallel with a decline in concentrations of IGF-1 and its principal binding protein (IGF- binding protein-3, IGFBP-3) [8]. Weight gain is of enormous importance to the overall prognosis in CF, as BMI correlates with overall survival and nutritional status influences the course of the disease [8]. Moreover, the attainment of a satisfactory weight gain has beeen shown to allow the prevention of height stunting and a dedicated CF dietitian is a fundamentally important member of a CF specialised team [9].

As well as poor nutrition, impaired liver function and insulin deficiency, recurrent infections may all contribute not only to reduced BMI but also to subnormal IGF-1 concentrations in CF [8].

Reduced IGF-1 levels have been found in CF patients during the development of liver impairment [10], but these findings have not been confirmed by other Authors [8,11].

Recurrent infections can have catabolic consequences, resulting in increased protein breakdown and diminished protein synthesis. These effects may be mediated by cytokines, which may have direct catabolic actions but may also interact with the IGF-1 axis. Cytokines, in fact, can affect IGFBP-3 production and IGF-1 actions at cellular levels [12].

Reduced concentrations of IGF-1 and IGFBP-3 are frequently observed during puberty in children with poorly controlled diabetes mellitus (DM). The progressive insulin deficiency documented in CF population during childhood [13] may, therefore, represent another important link between IGF-1 and IGFBP-3 abnormalities and the decline in BMI [14,15]. At the light of this possible association, the growth-stimulating effects of insulin therapy in relatively insulin-deficient patients should be considered in CF, even before the onset of DM [15].

Pharmacological doses of steroids are known to reduce linear growth, most often when the mean doses are above 5mg/m2/day or 0.25 mg/kg/day. The decrease in growth velocity is mediated by reduced GH secretion and decreased IGF-1 production. Therefore, it is generally accepted that systemic or inhaled corticosteroid treatment may play some role in conditioning the sub-optimal growth in many CF children. Although this possibility cannot be excluded, nevertheless it is to be underlined that children with CF, even if they are not treated with a glucocorticoid, have reduced height velocity and a delayed adolescent growth spurt [7].

Management

Low body weight and height have been clearly linked to worsened clinical outcome in CF; thus therapies designed to improve weight and growth are of paramount importance for the succesful treatment and increased survival rates of CF patients [16].

Although some studies have documented clinical improvement with enhanced nutritional intake [17], nutritional supplementations have not provided sustained or uniform results [18] and special dietary regimens have not eradicated the problem of poor growth [19].

Although CF children do not have classic GH deficiency, the anabolic and growth promoting effects of recombinant human GH have been repeatedly explored in the last years in CF children, by both open-labelled uncontrolled studies [20-23] and randomized controlled trials [16]. All these studies have documented significant improvements in height velocity and weight velocity for up to 2 years. In GH-treated patients improvements in lean mass and significant clinical benefits have been observed [16]. These studies, therefore, suggest a potential role of GH in short-term treatment of CF children with severe growth failure who have not shown adequate weight or height gain, in spite of good nutritional management [16].

However, the potential long-term benefits of GH therapy on body composition, bone density, adult height, quality of life and survival have yet to be ascertained. Additional questions that should be answered include the cost-effectiveness of this therapy and whether GH equally benefits children with good or poor baseline clinical status [16].

Furtherly, although no negative impact of this therapy on glucose tolerance (GT) has been hitherto reported in these short-term trials, screening for GT is highly recommended in CF patients before starting GH therapy. Moreover, considering the significant risk of glucose intolerance in CF, glyco-metabolic status of these patients should be periodically monitored during GH treatment.

Delayed Puberty

Delay in sexual development is recognized as a significant, although not universal, complication of CF [24]. Genital development in males has beeen reported to begin at an average age of 15.5 years [25]. In female patients menarche is frequently reported at between 13.3 and 14.9 years (Table 1). Menarcheal age (MA) in CF girls is generally retarded with respect to the normal population and exceeds the average MA of patients' mothers [24 – 29] and sisters [25].

Table 1. Data in literature on menarcheal age (years) in girls with CF, in their mothers and in controls

Reference	Girls with CF	CF mothers	Controls
Arrigo et al [29]	13.3 ± 1.1	12.2 ± 1.0	----
Stern et al [28]	14.2	---	12.9
Mitchell-Heggs et al [25]	14.4	---	12.9
Neinstein et al [27]	14.4 ± 1.4	---	12.9 ± 1.2
Moshang et al [24]	14.5 ± 1.6	13.0	12.9 ± 1.2
Johannesson et al [26]	14.9 ± 1.4	13.5 ± 1.6	13.0 ± 1.0

Aetiology and Pathogenesis

This maturational lag seems to be mediated by a transient dysfunction of the hypothalamo- pituitary-gonadal axis, with a significant delay in attaining pubertal levels of the gonadotropins and sex steroids [30]. The aetiological factors of this dysfunction, however, are still controversial. Undernutrition [30, 31], chronic infections, chronic hypoxia, ΔF508 homozygosity [26] and glyco-metabolic disorders [26] have been proposed as factors responsible for puberty abnormalities in CF.

According to the results of a very recent study a menarcheal delay of approximately one year exists between CF girls and their mothers, which is not related to either genotype or disease severity or glyco-metabolic status [29]. According to this study, the only variable that may significantly account for MA delay in CF is undernutrition. Menarche, in fact, was severely retarded in the girls with the lowest body mass percentile (BMP) and a close negative relationship was found between BMP and MA.

Undernutrition in CF is a frequent complication [6], which results from several aetiological factors: increased energy expenditure, decreased energy intake, malabsorption of ingested nutrients and chronic inflammation [33].

Undernutrition by itself can cause a transient hypogonadotrophic state, probably due to a diminished fat mass. The consequent decrease in leptin synthesis and secretion may, in turn, play some role in delaying puberty [34].

Many findings, however, indicate that nutritional status is not the only factor conditioning pubertal retardation in CF, since puberty is delayed even in patients with a good clinical and nutritional status [26]. Moreover adult female patients overall do well after puberty, even in case of persistent inanition.

Management

In conclusion, auxological, clinical and endocrine pattern of adolescents with CF may be similar to that observed in healthy subjects with constitutional delay of growth and puberty. As in that condition the most important aspects of management are explanation and reassurance, particularly about sexual drive and function. For male patients with major psychological problems, treatment with low dose testosterone for 3-6 months may be effective in advancing sex development and growth spurt, without compromising final height [35].

Fertility Issues

With the improved life expectancy and the increasing survival in CF, there is a growing need to deal with the desires of CF patients to become parents.

Hypothalamo-pituitary-gonadal axis function in CF is not considerably impaired whereas a transient impairment of gonadotropin and gonadal hormone secretion may be frequently observed during childhood and preadolescence. At adolescence, finally, CF subjects achieve essentially normal baseline and evoked gonadotropin release [36].

Female Fertility and Pregnancy

Unlike the males, there is no reproductive tract abnormalities in CF females. CF women theoretically may have abnormal cervical mucus (because of the reduction in water content), but there is no evidence of a reduced fertility in young female adults. Altough the global fertility rate in CF is unknown [37], pregnancy is possible and an increasing number of children are born to women with CF each year [32, 38]. However pregnancy in CF requires careful planning and the couple must be clearly informed about the potential risks of having a CF child. Moreover the patients must be informed about the risks of pregnancy with regard to their lung function and survival [39].

According to the results of recent investigations, pregnancy seems to be relatively safe for many women with CF [37, 40, 41] and does not seem to produce a greater overall rate of decline in patients'clinical status. Moreover, the decline in pulmonary fuction that occurs during pregnancy is usually re-gained post-partum [42, 43].

However, based on the available data, it is prudent to recommend that pregnancy be considered preferably in individuals with a milder disease [40]. In fact, maternal obstetric problems are rare and pregnancy does not worsen the disease in the patients who have an uncomplicated disease, whereas an increase risk of preterm birth and infant's associated complications have been reported in the women with severe lung imparement and/or other problems (diabetes, liver impairment). It is important that these groups of women with more severe disease are especially monitored and regarded as high-risk pregnancies [41].

The only absolute contraindications to pregnancy are pulmonary hypertension, cor pulmonale and spirometric indices <50% [32].

Pregnancy requires an additional 300 kcal per day and an overall weight gain of at least 11 kg during the entire gestation is recommended to assure good nutrition for the woman and the fetus [38]. It is necessary that weight and other nutritional parameters be closely followed during pregnancy and that aggressive intervention be initiated for those failing to increase weigth [40].

Alterations of glyco-metabolic status are known to be common in CF. Therefore it is not surprising that the prevalence of gestational DM in CF is higher than in the general population [44]. Consequently, a careful watch of glucose homeostasis levels is required during infection, delivery and in the post partum period [41]. DM has been associated with maternal deterioration during pregnancy. It is uncertain whether DM itself increases the risks of pregnancy or whether it is merely a marker of more advanced disease [40].

Finally, CF pregnancies require careful management in a Centre where there is a close working relationship between the CF physicial, the CF team and the obstetrician. The mother can be reassured that breastfeeding is possible, with normal breast milk composition [37].

Male Fertility

Almost 98% of CF males are infertile [37] secondary to obstructive azoospermia, because of abnormalities of the Wolfian duct derivates [45]. The head of the epididymis is usually spared, but absence and atrophy of the vas deferens tail and body of the epididymis and/or seminal vescicles are noted. In contrast, testicular volumes are normal, and Leydig cells appear normal in number and morphology, which allows a normal sexual function. Moreover active spermatogenesis is present within seminiferous tubules.

Since obstructive azoospermia cannot be surgically corrected and precludes natural conception, the alternatives for a CF male are adoption and assisted fertilisation. Sperm can be collected by microsurgical epididymal aspiration and delivered into the oocyte cytoplasm. According to recent reports a pregnancy rate of 62.5% can be achieved by this technique [46].

Due to its very high frequency, infertility represents a typical clinical feature of CF in males. Therefore it would be very important that CF boys are informed about their reproductive health during adolescence [47].

Osteoporosis

In 1979 Mischler et al documented the first evidence for reduced bone mineral density (BMD) in CF patients [48]. Other more recent studies have confirmed osteopenia and osteoporosis to be common, especially in adults with severe disease and in those who have used corticosteroids [49].

Osteoporosis increases the risk of fracture 2-3 folds for each standard deviation fall in the BMD below the mean for healthy population [50], which explains why atraumatic fractures of the axial and appendicular skeleton are becoming an important health problem in adolescents and adults with CF [51, 52]. Fractures in CF patients result in pain and disability. Structural chest wall changes following vertebral and rib fractures may result in an accelerated decline in lung function [49]. Moreover, thoracic fractures are clinically significant because they hinder sputum clearance and reduce quality of life. In addition, some Centres now consider symptomatic osteopenia to be a contraindication to transplantation [53].

Aetiology and Pathogenesis

Factors responsible for bone fragility in CF subjects include small bone size [54], inadequate gain in bone mass during growth and puberty [55] and excessive bone loss [56]. Other reasons for the observed BMD reduction in CF are poor nutritional intake, pancreatic failure, calcium and vitamin D malabsorption, reduced levels of physical activity, corticosteroid usage, pubertal delay, chronic respiratory acidosis and elevations in osteoclast activating cytokines [57].

The severity of CF disease is frequently found to be positively related to BMD reduction [58, 59]. The exact mechanisms by which the severity of CF affects BMD have not been completely clarified [53]. Patients with more severe disease are often nutritionally depleted, less active and may require more glucocorticoid therapy, all of which may influence BMD. An alternative hypothesis suggests that inflammatory cytokines, that are increased in CF individuals with chronic pulmonary infections, affect osteoblast and osteoclast activity, thus resulting in reduced BMD [53].

Bone demineralization in CF is probably conditioned by an imbalance between bone formation and degradation, resulting in net bone loss [56]. Bone turnover is significantly higher in ΔF508 homozygotes than in non-homozygotes [53], which confirms that bone mineralization in CF is poorer in the subjects with more severe disease. Moreover, it can be argued that there may be a genetic component in the aetiology of low BMD in CF.

Management

Treatment to prevent osteoporosis in the young patients with CF needs to be directed at increasing bone size, which may be obtained by increasing BMI and by limiting the catabolic condition [60]. Therefore, treatment should be directed at increasing the energy intake, correcting the malabsorption and limiting pulmonary infections [54]. Routine clinical management in prepubertal children with CF should also include judicious use of corticosteroid therapy and encouragement of regular physical activity and normal lifestyle [57]. The common treatment to prevent osteoporosis, using calcium and vitamin D supplementation, without targeting these other factors, may not improve bone mineralization in patients with CF [54]. Efforts to obtain and maintain normal bone mineralization in CF must begin early in chldhood [61].

Carbohydrate Metabolism Abnormalities

Epidemiology

The clinical picture of CF is frequently complicated by carbohydrate metabolism abnormalities, whose prevalence grows with age [62] and has dramatically increased in the last decades, probably due to these patients'increasing longevity.

Impaired glucose tolerance (IGT) occurs in approximately 50% of subjects older than 18 years and DM in as many as 15% of those after the age of 16 years [63]. DM prevalence increases up to 24% by the age of 20 years and up to 76% by the age of 30 years [64]. Usually DM occurs after the first decade of life, with a mean age at diagnosis reported to be around 20 years [62, 64].

A significantly higher proportion of the genotype homozygous ΔF508 has been repeatedly found in DM patients than in the whole CF population [63, 65, 66]. As this genotype is associated with pancreatic exocrine insufficiency and pancreatic exocrine insufficiency is associated with pancreatic endocrine dysfunction in CF, an association between this genotype and GT abnormalities is not surprising.

Aetiology and Pathophysiology

DM development in CF is considered to be the consequence of a progressive impairment of pancreatic β-cell function [66 – 68], that may precede the onset of IGT [69] and can be observed even in patients without glucose intolerance[70].

CF-related diabetes (CFRD) is a peculiar form of DM, that occurs almost exclusively in exocrine-insufficient patients [71] and is characterized by a slow onset, a non-ketotic nature and persistence of some insulin secretion [72]. Its aetiology is generally related to a progressive pancreatic fibrosis leading to progressive destruction of the pancreatic islet architecture [73].

CFRD shares a number of clinical and pathological similarities with type 2 DM [74], a disease that is predominantly associated with a significant increase in peripheral insulin resistance (IR). The role of IR in the pathogenesis of CFRD, however, has not been definitely confirmed, with several studies yelding inconsistent findings [70, 71, 75 – 78].

Thirteen years ago we started a longitudinal evaluation of GT, insulin secretion and peripheral insulin sensitivity (IS) in a cohort of CF patients originally selected on the basis of persistently normal fasting blood glucose levels [70], in order to evaluate the factors that can influence DM development in CF. Aim of our study was to evaluate whether eventual changes of GT over time may be associated with modifications of insulin secretion or sensitivity. A very recent paper has reported the 13-year observational data of our prospective study, comparing these data with baseline results [79]. From the 1st to the 2nd oral glucose tolerance test (OGTT) we have observed that: a) the prevalence of DM responses significantly increased over time; b) the areas beneath the respective glucose and insulin curves significantly increased (Fig.1) and decreased (Fig.2), respectively; c) IR and IS indices decreased and increased, respectively, even in the patients who developed DM. On the basis of these results we have concluded that: 1) the natural history of glyco-metabolic status in CF is characterized by deteriorating GT over time; 2) insulinopenia plays a prominent role in the pathogenesis of GT worsening; 3) IR does not play any significant part in the pathogenesis of DM development [79].

Clinical Consequences

The relationships between deteriorating GT and worsening clinical status over time in CF are not clear. It has been debated whether the age-related worsening of clinical conditions in these patients leads to metabolic derangements or whether the metabolic abnormalities precede and negatively influence the overall clinical course and prognosis of the disease [80].

According to the results of some prospective and multicenter studies [81, 82] CFRD seems to have a negative impact on pulmonary function and clinical outcome. These data, in fact, gave evidence that insulin deficiency leads to a direct decline in pulmonary function suggesting a cause and effect relationship between insulin deficiency and lung disease [81]. Moreover CFRD was shown to reduce patients'survival [82].

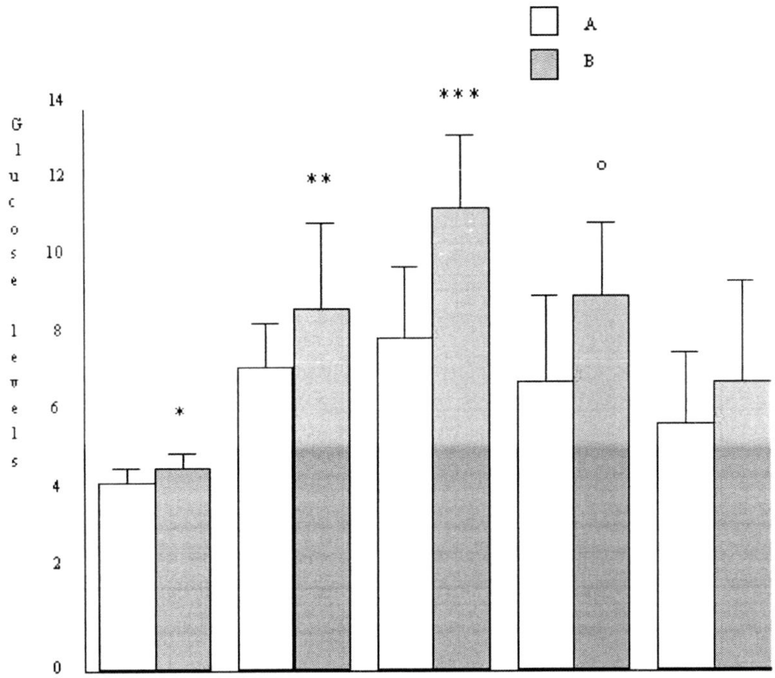

Fig. 1. Mean (+/- SD) glucose plasma levels (mmol/l) during the 1st (A) and the 2nd (B) oral glucose tolerance test (* $p< 0.05$ vs A; ** $p< 0.025$; *** $p< 0.0025$; ° $p< 0.005$).

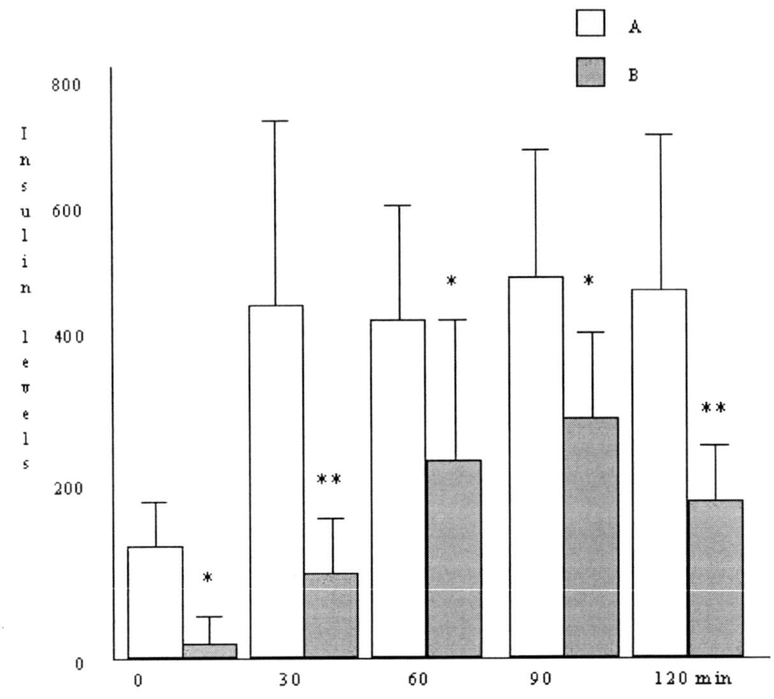

Fig. 2. Mean (+/- SD) insulin plasma levels (pmol/l) during the 1st (A) and the 2nd (B) oral glucose tolerance test (* $p< 0.0005$ vs A; ** $p< 0.0025$; ° $p< 0.005$).

It has been also suggested that an insulin-insufficient state, even without significant hyperglycemic symptoms, can create a disadvantageous metabolic environment and negatively influence overall health status [68, 69]. Another plausible hypothesis is that both deterioration of β-cell function and worsening of lung function may be two unrelated events occurring in the natural history of the adolescents and young adults with CF [79].

Metabolic Screening

Another important and unresolved question for physicians caring for CF patients is how and when screening for CFRD should be initiated [83]. According to a Consensus Conference for the identification of CFRD [84], urine analysis two or three times per year and fasting blood glucose and 2-hr post-prandial blood glucose measured every 2-4 years during late childhood and adolescence are recommended. More recently, routine measurements of glycosylated haemoglobin (HbA1c) levels (every 6 months) have beeen proposed as a screening and follow-up test for CFRD in patients > 12 years of age [83]. However, according to both cross-sectional [85] and longitudinal studies [68, 69], HbA1c measurements have not been shown to be sensitive markers of GT and are poor predictors of DM development in CF. Consequently, in our opinion, HbA1c measurement may be useful, in a screening program for early detection of hyperglycemia in CF, only if associated with post-prandial blood glucose determination and, eventually, OGTT.

Another simple investigation had been proposed as a screening procedure for early identification of patients at risk for glucose intolerance, i.e. the evaluation of first-phase insulin response to intravenous glucose. However, in our experience, this investigation cannot reliably identify those patients who will eventually develop overt DM and should not be used to screen for early glucose metabolism abnormalities in CF [86].

Finally, at present, it is possible to conclude that OGTT is still regarded by many as the gold standard method in the diagnosis of DM and GT abnormalities in CF [63].

Diabetic Complications

Compulsive glycemic control and regular screening for microangiopathy in CFRD patients is not as routine as in DM patients without CF. One viewpoint is that, because individuals with CF have a limited life span, secondary diabetic complications are not likely to be an issue.

With the increasing longevity of CF patients, cases of microvascular complications have emerged in recent years [87]. Retinopathy represents the most frequent complication, with a prevalence ranging from 16% to 23% according to follow-up duration [88]. Isolated cases of diabetic nephropathy have also been described [87], whereas clinically relevant diabetic neuropathy is rare and macrovascular complications remain exceedingly rare [63]. At the light of these evidences it is recommended that patients with CFRD will need to be screened for microvascular complications at least annually [63], although the limited available data suggest that microvascular complications are very rare within 10 years of CFRD.

Management

Specific treatment of CFRD is usually conditioned by the degree of the hyperglycemia and patient compliance. Dietary restrictions are not indicated, due to the high caloric requirements of these patients. The efficacy of oral hypoglycemic agents has not been proven.

As CFRD is an insulinopenic condition, insulin should be regarded as the choice therapy in the management of CFRD. A twice-daily regime of a mixture of short and intermediate acting insulin is a popular choice [63]. However insulin regimens should be tailored to suit patients'eating pattern and lifestyle.

After CFRD is diagnosed, monitoring is indicated in much the some way as in DM patients without CF. However, efforts in achieving tight glycemic control have to be weighed against the already busy and tedious treatment regimen that patients with CF have to adhere to [63]. It is reasonable to aim for an HbA1c of 6.5-7%, although many factors may prevent this. Intermittent insulin therapy may be also necessary in case of intermittent hyperglycemia during steroid administration, enteral feeding and infections [89].

References

[1] Schwachman H, Hulczychi LL, Khaw K. Studies on cystic fibrosis. A report of sixty-five patients over 17 years of age. *Pediatrics* 36: 689- 699; 1965.

[2] Dodge JA, Morison S, Lewis PA, Coles EC, Geddes D. Russell G, Littlewood JM, Scott MT. Incidence, population, and survival of cystic fibrosis in the UK, 1968-95. UK Cystic Fibrosis Survey Mangement Committee. *Arch Dis Child* 77: 493-496; 1997.

[3] Frederiksen B, Lanng S, Koch C, Hoiby N. Improved survival in the Danish center-treated cystic fibrosis patients: results of aggressive treatment. *Pediatr Pulmonol* 21: 153-158; 1996.

[4] Shale DJ. Predicting survival in cystic fibrosis. *Thorax* 52: 309; 1997.

[5] Patel L, Dixon M, David TJ. Growth and growth charts in cystic fibrosis. *J R Soc Med* 96 (Suppl 43): 35-41; 2003.

[6] Lai HC, Kosorok MR, Sondel SA, Chen ST, FitzSimmons SC, Green CG, Shen G, Walker S, Farrel PM. Growth status in children with cystic fibrosis based on the National Cystic Fibrosis Patient Registry data: evaluation of various criteria used to identify malnutrition. *J Pediatr* 132: 478-485;1998.

[7] Byard PJ. The adolescent growth spurt in children with cystic fibrosis. *Ann Hum Biol* 21: 229-240; 1994.

[8] Taylor CJ, Dalton A, Hardcastle J, Hardcastle PT, Evans S. Diagnosing cystic fibrosis: blood, sweat, and tears. *Arch Dis Child* 76:85-88; 1997.

[9] Collins CE, MacDonald-Wicks L, Rowe S, O'Loughlin EV, Henry RL. Normal growth in cystic fibrosis associated with a specialised centre. *Arch Dis Child* 81: 241-246; 1999.

[10] De Schepper J, Van Blerk M, Hachimi-Idrissi S, Dab I, Smitz J. Serum insulin-like growth factor-I determinations in patients with cystic fibrosis: influence of nutritional and liver status. *Clin Nutr* 11: 298-302; 1992.

[11] Laursen EM, Juul A, Lanng S, Hoiby N, Koch C, Muller J, Skakkebaek NE. Diminished concentrations of insulin-like growth factor I in cystic fibrosis. *Arch Dis Child* 72: 494-497; 1995.

[12] De Benedetti F, Meazza C, Martini A. Role of interleukin-6 in growth failure: an animal model. *Horm Res* 58 (Suppl 1): 24-27; 2002.

[13] Holl RW, Heinze E, Wolf A, Rank M, Teller WM. Reduced pancreatic insulin release and reduced peripheral insulin sensitivity contribute to hyperglycaemia in cystic fibrosis. *Eur J Pediatr* 154: 356-361; 1995.

[14] Taylor AM, Thomson A, Bruce-Morgan C, Ahmed ML, Watts A, Harris D, Holly JM, Dunger DB. The relationship between insulin, IGF-1 and weight gain in cystic fibrosis. *Clin Endocrinol* 51: 659-665;1999.

[15] Ripa P, Robertson I, Cowley D, Harris M, Maters IB, Cotterill AM. The relationship between insulin secretion, the insulin-like growth factor axis and growth in children with cystic fibrosis. *Clin Endocrinol* 56: 383-389; 2002.

[16] Hardin DS, Ellis KJ, Dyson M, Rice J, McConnell R, Seilheimer DK. Growth hormone improves clinical status in prepubertal children with cystic fibrosis: results of a randomized controlled trial. *J Pediatr* 139: 636-642; 2001.

[17] Dalzell AM, Shepherd RW, Dean B, Cleghorn GJ, Holt TL, Francis PJ. Nutritional rehabilitation in cystic fibrosis: a 5 year follow-up study. *J Pediatr Gastroenterol Nutr* 15: 141-145; 1992.

[18] National Institutes of Diabetes and Digestive and Kidney Diseases (NIDDK) and Cystic Fibrosis Foundation. Workshop on nutrition in cystic fibrosis. Bethesda (MD): CF Foundation Press;1993.

[19] Cystic Fibrosis Foundation. Cystic Fibrosis Foundation, Patient Registry 1998 Annual Data Report. Bethesda, MD: Cystic Fibrosis Foundation: 1999.

[20] Sachey AH, Taylor CJ, Barraclough M, Wales JKH, Pickering M. Growth hormone as a nutritional adjunct in cystic fibrosis: results of a pilot study. *J Hum Nutr Diet* 8: 185-191; 1995.

[21] Huseman CA, Colombo JL, Brooks MA, Smay JR, Greger NG, Sammut PH, Bier DM. Anabolic effect of biosynthetic growth hormone in cystic fibrosis patients. *Pediatr Pulmonol* 22: 90-95; 1996.

[22] Alemzadeh R, Upchurch L, McCarthy V. Anabolic effects of growth hormone treatment in young children with cystic fibrosis. *J Am Coll Nutr* 17: 419-424; 1998.

[23] Hardin DS, Stratton R, Kramer JC, Reyes de la Rocha S, Govaerts K, Wilson DP. Growth hormone improves weight velocity and height velocity in prepubertal children with cystic fibrosis. *Horm Metab Res* 30: 636-641; 1998.

[24] Moshang T, Holsclaw DS Jr. Menarchal determinants in cystic fibrosis. *Am J Dis Child* 134: 1139-1142; 1980.

[25] Mitchell-Heggs P, Mearns MJ, Batten JC. Cystic fibrosis in adolescents and adults. *Q J Med* 45: 479-504; 1976.

[26] Johannesson M, Gottlieb C, Hjelte L. Delayed puberty in cystic fibrosis despite good clinical status. *Pediatrics* 99: 29-34;1997.

[27] Neinstein LS, Stewart D, Wang CI, Johnson I. Menstual dysfunction in cystic fibrosis. *J Adolesc Health Care* 4: 153-157; 1983.

[28] Stern RC, Boat TF, Doershuk CF, Tucker AS, Primiano FP Jr, Matthews LW. Course of cystic fibrosis in 95 patients . *J Pediatr* 89: 406-411;1976.

[29] Arrigo T, De Luca F, Lucanto C, Lombardo M, Rulli I, Lombardo F. Nutritional, glycometabolic and genetic factors affecting menarcheal age in cystic fibrosis. *Diab Nutr Metab* 17; XX; 2004 (in press).
[30] Arrigo T, Rulli I, Sferlazzas C, De Luca F. Pubertal development in cystic fibrosis: an overview. *J Pediatr Endocrinol Metab* 16 (suppl 2): 267-270; 2003.
[31] Blecker U, Mehta DI, Davis R, Sothern MS, Suskind RM. Nutritional problems in patients who have chronic disease. *Pediatr Rev* 21: 29-32; 2000.
[32] Edenborough FP. Women with cystic fibrosis and their potential for reproduction. *Thorax* 56: 649-655; 2001.
[33] Hankard R, Munck A, Navarro J. Nutrition and growth in cystic fibrosis. *Horm Res* 58 (Suppl 1): 16-20; 2002.
[34] Simon D. Puberty in chronically diseased patients. *Horm Res* 57 (Suppl 2):53-56; 2002.
[35] Landon C, Rosenfeld RG. Short stature and pubertal delay in male adolescents with cystic fibrosis. Androgen treatment. *Am J Dis Child* 138: 388-391; 1984.
[36] Reiter EO, Stern RC, Root AW. The reproductive endocrine system in cystic fibrosis: 2. Changes in gonadotrophins and sex steroids following LHRH. *Clin Encdocrinol* 16: 127-137; 1982.
[37] Lyon A, Bilton D. Fertility issues in cystic fibrosis. *Pediatr Respir Rev* 3: 236-240; 2002.
[38] Hilman BC, Aitken ML, Constantinescu M. Pregnancy in patients with cystic fibrosis. *Clin Obstet Gynecol* 39: 70-86; 1996.
[39] Edenborough FP, Mackenzie WE, Stableforth DE. The outcome of 72 pregnancies in 55 women with cystic fibrosis in the United Kingdom 1977-1996. *BJOG* 107: 254-261; 2000.
[40] Frangolias DD, Nakielna EM, Wilcox PG. Pregnancy and cystic fibrosis. A case-controlled study. *Chest* 111: 963-969; 1997.
[41] Odegaard I, Stray-Pedersen B, Hallberg K, Haanes OC, Storrosten OT, Johannesson M. Maternal and fetal morbidity in pregnancies of Norwegian and Swedish women with cistic fibrosis. *Acta Obstet Gynecol Scand* 81: 698-705; 2002.
[42] Edenborough FP, Stableforth DE, Webb AK, Mackenzie WE, Smith DL. Outcome of pregnancy in women with cystic fibrosis. *Thorax* 50: 170-174; 1995.
[43] Olsen GL. Cystic fibrosis in pregnancy. *Semin Perinatol* 21: 307-312; 1997.
[44] Gilljam M, Antoniou M, Shin J, Dupuis A, Corey M, Tullis DE. Pregnancy in cystic fibrosis. Fetal and maternal outcome. *Chest* 118: 85-91; 2000.
[45] Kaplan E, Swachman H, Perlmutter AD, Rule A, Khan KT, Holsclaw DS. Reproductive failure in males with cystic fibrosis. *N Engl J Med* 279: 65-69; 1968.
[46] McCallum TJ, Milunsky JM, Cunningham DL, Harris DH, Maher TA, Oates RD. Fertility in men with cystic fibrosis - an update on current surgical practices and outcomes. *Chest* 118: 1059- 1062; 2000.
[47] Sawyer SM, Tully MM, Colin AA. Reproductive and sexual health in males with cystic fibrosis: a case for health professional education and training. *J Adolesc Health* 28: 36-40; 2001.
[48] Mischler EH, Chesney PJ, Chesney RW, Mazess RB. Demineralization in cystic fibrosis detected by direct photon absorptiometry. *Am J Dis Child* 133: 632-635; 1979.

[49] Conway SP, Morton AM, Oldroyd B, Truscott JG, White H, Smith AH, Haigh I, Osteoporosis and osteopenia in adults and adolescents with cystic fibrosis: prevalence and associated factors. *Thorax* 55: 798-804; 2000.

[50] Hui SL, Slemenda CW, Johnston CC Jr. Age and bone mass as predictors of fracture in a prospective study. *J Clin Invest* 81: 1804-1809; 1988.

[51] Aris RM, Renner JB, Winders AD, Buell HE, Riggs DB, Lester GE, Ontjes DA. Increased rate of fractures and severe kyphosis: sequelae of living into adulthood with cystic fibrosis. *Ann Intern Med* 128: 186- 193; 1998.

[52] Haworth CS, Freemont AJ, Webb AK, Dodd ME, Selby PL, Mawer EB, Adams JE. Hip fracture and bone histomorphometry in a young adult with cystic fibrosis. *Eur Resp J* 14: 478-479; 1999.

[53] Haworth CS, Selby PL, Webb AK, Dodd ME, Musson H, McL Niven R, Economou G, Horrocks AW, Freemont AJ, Mawer EB, Adams JE. Low bone mineral density in adults with cystic fibrosis. *Thorax* 54: 961-967; 1999.

[54] Laursen EM, Molgaard C, Michaelsen KF, Koch C, Muller J. Bone mineral status in 134 patients with cystic fibrosis. *Arch Dis Child* 81: 235-240;1999.

[55] Bhudhikanok GS, Wang MC, Marcus R, Harkins A, Moss RB, Bachrach LK. Bone acquisition and loss in children and adults with cystic fibrosis: a longitudinal study. *J Pediatr* 133: 18-27; 1998.

[56] Baroncelli GI, De Luca F, Magazzù G, Arrigo T, Sferlazzas C, Catena C, Bertelloni S, Saggese G. Bone demineralization in cystic fibrosis: evidence of imbalance between bone formation and degradation. *Pediatr Res* 41: 397- 403; 1997.

[57] Haslam RH, Borovnicar DJ, Stroud DB, Strauss BJ, Bines JE. Correlates of prepubertal bone mineral density in cystic fibrosis. *Arch Dis Child* 85: 166-171; 2001.

[58] Bhudhikanok GS, Lim J, Marcus R, Harkins A, Moss RB, Bachrach LK. Correlates of osteopenia in patients with cystic fibrosis. *Pediatrics* 97: 103-111; 1996.

[59] Grey AB, Ames RW, Matthews RD, Reid IR. Bone mineral density and body composition in adult patients with cystic fibrosis. *Thorax* 48: 589-593; 1993.

[60] Sood M, Hambleton G, Super M, Fraser WD, Adams JE, Mughal MZ. Bone status in cystic fibrosis. *Arch Dis Child* 84: 516-520; 2001.

[61] Henderson RC, Madsen CD. Bone density in children and adolescents with cystic fibrosis. *J Pediatr* 128: 28-34; 1996.

[62] Lanng S, Hansen A, Thorsteinsson B, Nerup J, Koch C. Glucose tolerance in patients with cystic fibrosis: five years prospective study. *BMJ* 311: 655-659; 1995.

[63] Yung B, Hodson ME. Diabetes in cystic fibrosis. *J R Soc Med* 92 (suppl 37): 35-40; 1999.

[64] Lanng S, Thorsteinsson B, Nerup J, Koch C. Diabetes mellitus in cystic fibrosis: a ten year prospective study. *Diabetologia* 43:107A; 2000.

[65] Hamdi I, Green M, Shneerson JM, Palmer CR, Hales CN. Proinsulin, proinsulin intermediate and insulin in cystic fibrosis. *Clin Endocrinol* 39: 21-6; 1993.

[66] Cucinotta D, De Luca F, Scoglio R, Lombardo F, Sferlazzas C, Di Benedetto A, Magazzù G, Raimondo G, Arrigo T. Factors affecting diabetes mellitus onset in cystic fibrosis: evidence from a 10-year follow-up study. *Acta Paediatr* 88: 389-393; 1999.

[67] Arrigo T, Cucinotta D, Conti Nibali S, Di Cesare E, Di Benedetto A, Magazzù G, De Luca F. Longitudinal evaluation of glucose tolerance and insulin secretion in non-

diabetic children and adolescents with cystic fibrosis: results of a two-year follow-up. *Acta Paediatr* 82: 249-253; 1993.

[68] De Luca F, Arrigo T, Di Benedetto A, Tedeschi A, Sferlazzas C, Crisafulli G, Di Cesare E, Romano G, Magazzù G, Cucinotta D. Four-year follow-up of glucose tolerance and beta-cell function in non-diabetic cystic fibrosis patients. *Horm Res* 44: 45-50; 1995.

[69] Cucinotta D, Arrigo T, De Luca F, Di Benedetto A, Lombardo F, Scoglio R, Sferlazzas C, Magazzù G. Metabolic and clinical events preceding diabetes mellitus onset in cystic fibrosis. *Eur J Endocrinol* 134: 731-736; 1996

[70] Cucinotta D, Conti Nibali S, Arrigo T, Di Benedetto A, Magazzù G, Di Cesare E, Costantino A, Pezzino V, De Luca F. Beta cell function, peripheral sensitivity to insulin and islet cell autoimmunity in cystic fibrosis patients with normal glucose tolerance. *Horm Res* 34: 33-38; 1990.

[71] Moran A, Pyzdrowski KL, Weinreb J, Kahn BB, Smith SA, Adams KS, Seaquist ER. Insulin sensitivity in cystic fibrosis. *Diabetes* 43: 1020-1026;1994.

[72] Knowles MR, Fernald GW. Diabetes and cystic fibrosis: new questions emerging from increased longevity. *J Pediatr* 112: 415-416; 1988.

[73] Lohr M, Goertchen P, Nizze H, Gould NS, Gould VE, Oberholzer M, Heitz PU, Kloppel G. Cystic fibrosis associated islet changes may provide a basis for diabetes. An immunocytochemical and morphometrical study. *Virchows Arch A Pathol Anat Histopathol* 414: 179-185; 1989.

[74] Dodge JA, Morrison G. Diabetes mellitus in cystic fibrosis: a review. *J Soc Med* 85 (suppl 19): 25-28; 1992.

[75] Lanng S, Thorsteinsson B, Roder ME, Nerup J, Koch C. Insulin sensitivity and insulin clearance in cystic fibrosis patients with normal and diabetic glucose tolerance. *Clin Endocrinol* 41: 217-223; 1994.

[76] Cucinotta D , De Luca F, Gigante A, Arrigo T, Di Benedetto A , Tedeschi A, Lombardo F, Romano G, Sferlazzas C. No changes of insulin sensitivity in cystic fibrosis patients with different degrees of glucose tolerance: an epidemiological and longitudinal study. *Eur J Endocrinol* 130: 253-258; 1994.

[77] Hardin DS, LeBlanc A, Lukenbough S, Seilheimer DK. Insulin resistance is associated with decreased clinical status in cystic fibrosis. *J Pediatr* 130: 948-956; 1997.

[78] Yung B, Noormohamed FH, Kemp M, Hooper J, Lant AF, Hodson ME. Cystic fibrosis-related diabetes: the role of peripheral insulin resistance and beta-cell dysfunction. *Diabet Med* 19: 221-226; 2002.

[79] Lombardo F, De Luca F, Rosano M, Sferlazzas C, Lucanto C, Arrigo T, Messina MF, Crisafulli G, Wasniewska M, Valenzise M, Cucinotta D. Natural history of glucose tolerance, beta-cell function and peripheral insulin sensitivity in cystic fibrosis patients with fasting euglycemia. *Eur J Endocrinol* 149: 53-59; 2003.

[80] Lanng S, Thorsteinsson B, Nerup J, Koch C. Influence of the development of diabetes mellitus on clinical status in patients with cystic fibrosis. *Eur J Pediatr* 151: 684-687; 1992.

[81] Rosenecker J, Hofler R, Steinkamp G, Eichler I, Smaczny C, Ballmann M, Posselt HG, Bargon J, von der Hardt H. Diabetes mellitus in patients with cystic fibrosis: the impact of diabetes melitus on pulmonary function and clinical outcome. *Eur J Med Res* 27: 345-350; 2001.

[82] Koch C, Rainisio M, Madessani U, Harms HK, Hodson ME, Mastella G, McKenzie SG, Navarro J, Strandvik B; Investigators of the European Epidemiologic Registry of Cystic Fibrosis. Presence of cystic fibrosis-related diabetes mellitus is thightly linked to poor lung function in patients with cystic fibrosis: data from the European Epidemiologic Registry of Cystic Fibrosis. *Pediatr Pulmonol* 32: 343-350; 2001.

[83] Hunkert F, Lietz T, Stach B, Kiess W. Potential impact of HbA1c determination on clinical decision making in patients with cystic fibrosis-related diabetes. *Diabetes Care* 22: 1008- 1010; 1999.

[84] Cystic Fibrosis Foundation Conference on CF-Related Diabetes Mellitus, Tyson Corner, VA, 11-12 January 1990. Cystic Fibrosis Foundation Consensus Conferences,1 :1-8; 1990.

[85] De Luca F, Arrigo T, Conti Nibali S, Sferlazzas C, Gigante A, Di Cesare E, Cucinotta D. Insulin secretion, glycosylated haemoglobin and islet cell antibodies in cystic fibrosis children and adolescents with different degrees of glucose tolerance. Horm Metab Res 23: 495- 498; 1991.

[86] Cucinotta D, De Luca F, Arrigo T, Di Benedetto A, Sferlazzas C, Gigante A, Rigoli L, Magazzù G. First-phase insulin response to intravenous glucose in cystic fibrosis patients with different degrees of glucose tolerance. *J Pediatr Endocrinol* 7: 13-17;1994.

[87] Lanng S, Thorsteinsson B, Lund-Andersen C, Nerup J, Schiotz PO, Koch C. Diabetes mellitus in Danish cystic fibrosis patients: prevalence and late diabetic complications. *Acta Paediatr* 83: 72-77; 1994.

[88] Yung B, Landers A, Mathalone B, Gyi KM, Hodson ME. Diabetic retinopathy in adult patients with cystic fibrosis-related diabetes. *Respir Med* 92: 871-872; 1998.

[89] Mackie AD, Thornton SJ, Edenborough FP. Cystic fibrosis-related diabetes. *Diabet Med* 20: 425-436; 2003.

In: Progress in Cystic Fibrosis Research
Editor: Margaret A. Harrison, pp. 117-129
ISBN 1-59454-232-5

Chapter VI

Agents that Enhance Mucociliary Clearance in the Treatment of Cystic Fibrosis Related Lung Disease

Peter Wark[1,*] *and Ashley P. Jones*[2]
[1]Brooke Laboratories, University of Southampton, Southampton General Hospital, UK
[2]Centre for Medical Statistics and Health Evaluation, School of Health Sciences, University of Liverpool, UK

Abstract

The genetic defect characterising cystic fibrosis (CF) leads to a failure to produce mature cystic fibrosis transmembrane regulator (CFTR) protein that plays a crucial role in regulating fluids and electrolytes in lung secretions, this results in impaired mucociliary clearance and is likely to play an important role in reducing the effectiveness of the innate immune response to pathogens. The consequence is recurrent endobronchial infection and inflammation that leads to progressive respiratory disease.

Treatments that enhance mucociliary clearance may reduce recurrent endobronchial infections and retard the development of respiratory disease. A number of agents have been developed for this purpose. Recombinant human DNase has the most experience where treatment in 12 randomised controlled trials of 2294 individuals demonstrated a small improvement in lung function at 1, 3, 6 months and two years compared to placebo with no significant increase in adverse events. Hypertonic saline (HS) has also been used; treatment against placebo shows an improvement in lung function though follow-up was only to 3 months. HS appears not to be as effective as DNase but also was well tolerated.

At this stage there is limited data available to determine the effect of treatments that enhance mucociliary clearance in CF, the most experience is with DNase that shows improvement in lung function though its long term impacts on mortality is unclear. Other

* Correspondence concerning this article should be addressed to Dr. Peter Wark, Brooke Laboratories, University of Southampton, Southampton General Hospital, Tremona Rd, Southampton SO16 6YD, UK. E-mail: p.wark@soton.ac.uk.

agents and the effects of combination therapy and treatment at different disease stages still require investigation.

Introduction

Cystic fibrosis (CF) is the most common genetic disorder afflicting Caucasian populations and since 1989 this defect has been known to occur as a consequence of mutations to the CF transmembrane conductance regulator (CFTR) [1] and while this leads to a multisystem disorder it is the effect on the lung that is the major cause of morbidity and mortality [2]. The aim of this review will be to relate the defect in CFTR to lung disease and its effect on mucociliary clearance (MCC) and explore treatments that enhance MCC and evaluate their effects on pulmonary disease in CF.

The Physiology of Airway Mucus Clearance

Airway Mucus Secretion and Clearance

The lung is exposed to a multitude of environmental stressors and has developed strategies to minimise the effects of infection and damage from inhaled particulate matter. Airway mucus secretion and clearance are key components of this innate immune defence. The airways are lined by pseudostratified columnar epithelium that are ciliated, interspersed with these cells are mucus-producing goblet cells and below the epithelium is mucus producing submucosal glands [3]. In the normal conducting airways this leads to a bilayer of airway surface liquid (ASL). The top layer is composed of airway mucus, while separating this layer from the epithelium is the periciliary liquid layer (PCL).

Mucus is an adhesive viscoelastic gel made of high molecular weight mucin monomers that are crosslinked by disulfide bonds. This produces a mesh like structure of polymers with moderate elasticity and viscosity that reflects in part the water content, monovalent and divalent ion concentrations [4]. A balance between these properties appears important to ensure adequate mucus clearance. In part the role of mucus appears to be to trap particulate matter and prevent contact with the epithelium, in airway inflammation it becomes mixed with bacteria and cellular debris, particularly Deoxyribose nucleic acid (DNA) and filamentous actin that act to increase the viscosity.

The PCL covers the ciliated epithelium and provides a low viscosity solution that allows cilia to beat rapidly [5] and thus acts upon the mucus layer above clearing it and any trapped debris proximally. The liquid volume and ionic composition of the PCL is also important to allow MCC and the defect in CFTR may play a crucial role at impairing this.

MCC occurs via an interaction of the following components allowing efficient MCC to occur in normal circumstances under 6 hours [5]:

(1) Ciliary beat frequency and effectiveness, that provides upward flow of the ASL
(2) The viscosity of the ASL with an interaction of the PCL upon the mucus layer acting as a secondary escalator. This is also dependent on the viscosity and elasticity of the mucus layer [6].

(3) The cough reflex. The efficiency of the cough reflex is inversely proportional to the viscosity of the ASL [7].

Innate Immune Defence Properties of the ASL

The ASL also exhibits antibacterial qualities containing substances such as lactoferrin, lysozyme, secretory leukoproteinase inhibitor and the defensins all of which are optimally activated in the isotonic environment of the healthy ASL [5]. These innate immune mediators are able to control introduced bacterial growth for 3-6 hours [8]. Under normal circumstances this would allow clearance of the bacteria by the mucociliary escalator, where there is impairment of MCC bacterial overgrowth occurs. This highlights the important interaction of MCC and the innate immune properties of the ASL.

The Defect in CFTR and its Impact on MCC

Several genetic defects in CFTR are responsible for the CF phenotype, essentially all lead to an inability to produce mature/ functioning CFTR protein. In the lungs the CFTR is present on the apical surface of ciliated epithelial cells as a transmembrane chloride secretory channel [9]. CFTR however also has the ability to regulate other ion channels, including the tonic inhibition of the epithelial sodium channel [10]. It is now felt that the major functional defect in CF is excessive absorption of sodium leading to excessive transport of sodium and with it chloride from the CF ASL [11]. While there is excessive absorption of sodium, impairment of CFTR also does not allow chloride and water to be added to the PCL, this depletes PCL volume and impairs MCC [11].

Airways Disease and Abnormal MCC in CF

The abnormal MCC in CF is thought to be a crucial factor in the development of endobronchial infection, which initiates a cycle of airway inflammation in response to infection, increased mucin secretion and cellular debris that further impairs MCC. Two hypotheses are current to explain this impairment of the lung's innate immune response to bacteria in CF, though both are not mutually exclusive. Firstly antibacterial factors such as defensins require a low sodium environment to work optimally and this is impaired in CF ASL [12]. Alternatively the inability to maintain an isotonic ASL fluid volume impairs MCC, bacteria overwhelm local innate immune defences and airway inflammation is initiated [8]. In support of this is the association of disorders of primary ciliary dyskinesia where the CFTR defect is not present but MCC is markedly impaired with the consequence of progressive bronchiectasis. These findings imply a crucial role for enhancing MCC as a means to retard the development of airways disease in CF.

Mucolytic Therapy

The aim of treatment with mucolytic agents is to alter the physical properties of mucus and to enhance mucociliary clearance. This has been attempted through the actions of agents that disrupt bonds within the mucus complex. The types of bonds occurring within mucus and the agents that may affect them are summarised in table 1. Each of these agents will be dealt with separately along with the mechanism of their action and their clinical effectiveness.

Table 1. Mucus bonds and sites of action for mucolytic agents*

Types of bonds	Site of bonds	Agents that disrupt
Covalent bonds	Glycoproteins are linked by intramolecular covalent bonds	Thiol reducing agents (N acetylcysteine)
Hydrogen bonds	Hydrogen ions link oligosaccharide side chains	Ionic agents (Hypertonic saline) Non-ionic agents (Dextran, mannitol, heparins)
Ionic bonds	Mucin macromoleculaes interact internally by their positive and negative charges	Ionic agents (Hypertonic saline) Non-ionic agents (Dextran, mannitol, heparins)
Van Der Waals forces	Interdigitation between oligosaccharides may occur	
Intermingling	The physical entanglement of the macromolecules themselves adds structure	
Extracellular DNA and F-actin	Released from cellular debris, both DNA and actin may form an additional network of structure.	Recombinant DNase Gelsolin

* Table adapted from information in King et al [4].

Recombinant Human DNase

Undegraded DNA is present in high quantities in the mucus of subjects with CF and is a major cause for the impairment in MCC [13]. The addition of DNase to CF sputum in vitro has been shown to cause a marked reduction in sputum viscosity [14]. This lead on to its clinical application and DNase is now the most widely used agent to increase MCC in CF.

The clinical effectiveness of DNase in CF has been systematically reviewed [15]. Twelve randomised controlled trials were included in the review with a total of 2294 participants. Ten studies compared rhDNase to placebo [16-25]. One trial compared daily rhDNase with hypertonic saline, and alternate day rhDNase [26] and one compared rhDNase to hypertonic saline [27]. In addition, three further papers [28-30] used the data from the included Fuchs trial to analyse the health care costs of using rhDNase

Seven studies lasted less than one month [16, 17, 19, 20, 22, 23, 27], one lasted three months [21], one lasted six months [18], one lasted nine months [31], one lasted one year [25] and the longest was two years [24].

Three trials included adult participants only [17, 20, 23]. The youngest patients were 5 years [31]. Severity of lung disease varied across the studies. Only two researchers studied participants with severe lung disease (FEV1 less than 40% predicted) [19, 21], in the other trials FEV1 ranged from 35-75% predicted. Only Wilmot et al [22] examined the effects of DNase on participants during treatment for a respiratory exacerbation.

Lung function was the primary end point in most trials. Mean change in FEV1 was examined at one month in 4 trials (DNase: n = 121, placebo: n = 127 [16, 17, 19, 20]). This was examined by meta-analysis [15]. The weighted mean difference (WMD) in percentage change in FEV1 was statistically significant, WMD 9.58 (95% CI 6.63, 12.52) (Figure 1). This result however must be interpreted with caution, as there was marked heterogeneity between the included trials. This may be due to the different doses used in these trials or due to the inclusion of trials with a marked degree of difference in severity of lung disease. In fact for participants with severe lung disease, short-term treatment with rhDNase did not improve FEV1 significantly, WMD –2.8 (-8.76,3.16)[19]. McCoy et al however looked at improvement in FEV1 in the group with severe lung disease and found a significant improvement after 3 months of treatment [21]. In stable patients with moderate lung disease treatment for 6 months with DNase 2.5mg daily slightly improved FEV1 by a mean (+/- SD) of 5.8 +/- 0.7. Disease severity may be an important predictor of a successful outcome with DNase. At the moment the evidence is strongest for an effect in those with moderate impairment in lung function (FEV1 40-75% predicted) as opposed to those with severe airflow limitation (FEV1 < 30%)[15] (Figure 2). The longest follow up was reported by Quan et al [24] (DNase n = 204, control: n = 206) who found a treatment benefit in percent predicted compared with placebo (mean +/- SE) of 3.2% +/- 1.2 in FEV1 (P =.006) demonstrating that this small benefit in lung function seen at 1 month appears to persists at least for two years, though this has not undergone longitudinal analysis.

A number of trials examined quality of life scores. Wilmott et al reported that the quality of life scores, showed no significant difference between the groups (in terms of improvement in cough and congestion, activity limitation, emotional well-being, fatigue, days of restriction to bed and general health perception) [22]. Fuchs et al reported that rhDNase once or twice daily improved the quality of life for patients during the six-month trial [18]. Ramsey reported that the frequency and magnitude of improvement across all quality of life questions was greater among patients receiving rhDNase [16] Ranasinha reported that only some variables in the quality of life score improved [17].

A significant reduction in the number of people experiencing respiratory exacerbations was not shown at three months with the age adjusted relative risk (RR) of having more than one respiratory exacerbation during the trial at 0.93 (95%CI 0.69 to 1.21)[21]. At six months Fuchs et al reported the effect of DNase on respiratory exacerbations as an age adjusted relative risk (RR) and 95% CI of having more than one exacerbation during the trial that required parenteral antibiotics of 0.72 (95% CI 0.52 to 0.98) and the twice daily group RR 0.63(95% CI 0.46 to 0.87). At two years Quan et al [24] reported the risk of having more than one exacerbation during the trial; but this was not statistically significant RR 0.71 (95% CI 0.49 to 1.02).

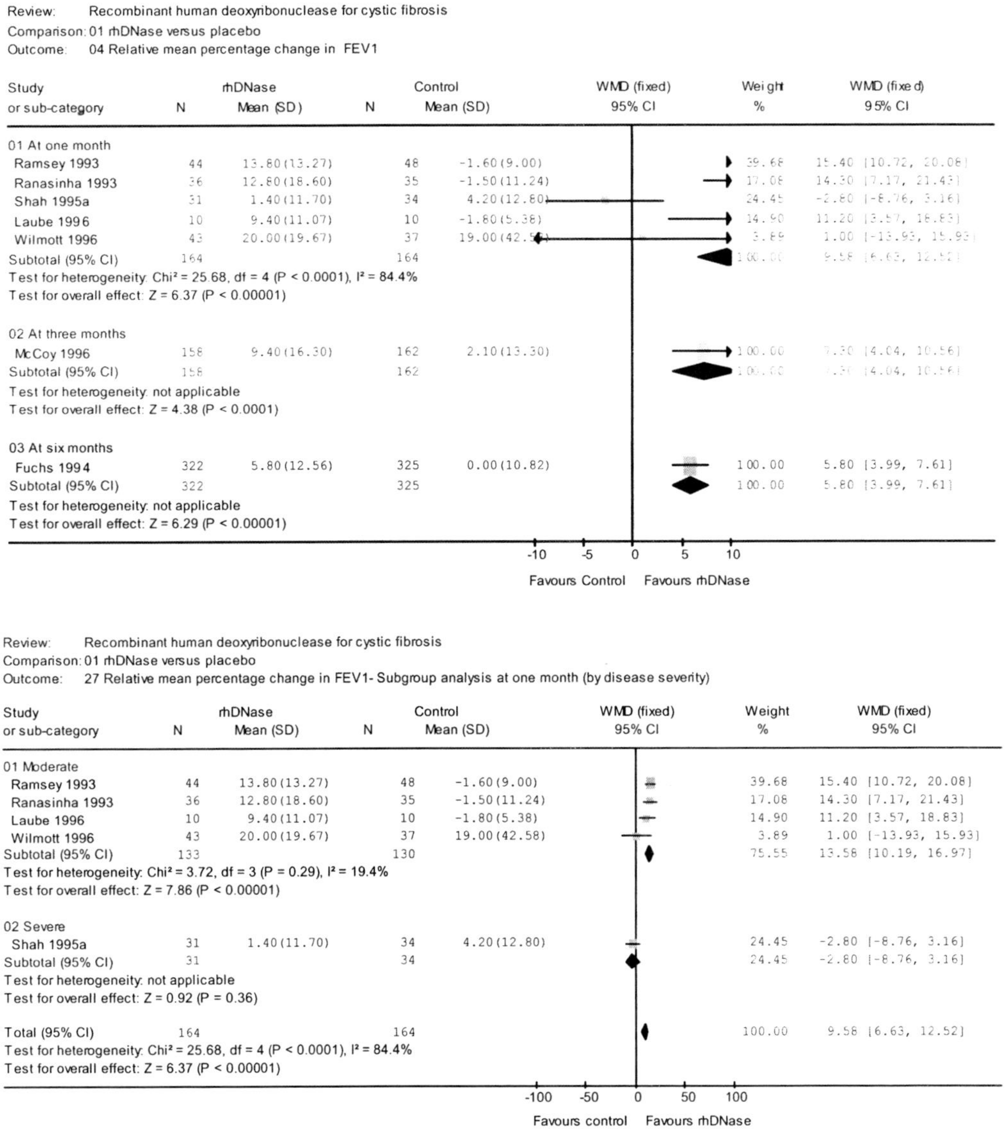

Fig. 1. WMD - weighted mean difference; RR - relative risk. Figure is reproduced with the permission of the Cochrane library of Systematic reviews [15].

Mortality was examined as an outcome at one month [16] [17, 19, 20, 22], three months [21], six months [18] and two years [24]. Given the relatively short durations and small numbers it is of no surprise that no statistical difference was seen in mortality.

Fuchs et al [18] found that 6 months treatment led to a reduction in exacerbations requiring hospitalisation. Participants treated with the once daily regimen spent 1.3 fewer days in hospital compared to placebo (p=0.06) and participants receiving twice daily rhDNase spent 1.0 fewer days in hospital compared to placebo (p< 0.05).

A change in weight is an important predictor of respiratory decline in CF and this was reported by Quan et al [24] who found at two years that the weight for age percentile decreased in both groups from baseline to the end of the trial and there was no statistical difference between the treatment groups.

None of the trials found an increase in the risk of haemoptysis [17-19], dyspnoea [17] [19] or pneumothorax [17-19, 22]. However treatment did consistently lead to an increase in voice alteration [16-19, 21, 22].

As DNase is an expensive medication that is used long term, cost of treatment is an important consideration. Three studies examined the cost of health care for participants involved in the trial of Fuchs [18]. The study by Oster [28] estimated that the mean total cost of respiratory tract infection related care was US$6443, US$4761 and US$5628 for the placebo, once daily and twice daily dosage regimens respectively. This cost included all outpatient antibiotic therapy as well as estimates of cost for any inpatient care. The estimates did not include the cost of DNase itself, as this was not marketed at the time of the trial. Once DNase was marketed, at a cost of US$27 per ampoule, they were able to estimate that the reduced cost of respiratory tract infection related care would be able to off set between 18.3% and 37.5% of the cost of therapy itself. Similarly, the Menzin study [29], analysed data from the Fuchs trial to estimate the reduction in cost of respiratory tract infection related care (excluding the cost of DNase itself) in the UK, France, Italy and Germany. Variations in medical practice in these countries led to a range of cost reductions from £434 (US$700) in the UK to a maximum of FF13, 872 (US$2100) in France.

Treatment with DNase leads to a small improvement in lung function that can be seen after the first month and appears to persist for at least the next two years. There is a reduction in the frequency of pulmonary exacerbations but no effect was seen on overall mortality. This benefit was seen in both adults and children but appears to be less in those with severe airflow obstruction (FEV1 % predicted < 40%). No serious adverse effects were noted in the trials.

Hypertonic Saline

Hypertonic saline (HS) in concentrations of > 3% saline breaks up the ionic bonds in the mucus gel, reducing crosslinking and viscosity [32]. In addition there may be effects on the water content of the ASL and an effect on separating DNA from mucins [4]. Use of HS in short term trials of radioisotope clearance in CF subjects demonstrates a clear benefit above placebo at increasing MCC [33].

A systematic review of HS in CF [34] has been carried which included fourteen randomised controlled trials involving 235 subjects with an age range of six to 46 years. The durations of the trials were limited to immediate effects on mucociliary clearance [33, 35] to a maximum of three months treatment [36]. Two trials compared HS to 0.9% saline as a placebo [37, 38]. Ballmann et al [27] compared the efficacy of three weeks of nebulised 5.75% saline (10mL) to 2.5mg recombinant DNase. Suri et al [26] compared hypertonic saline 7% (5mL) BD (twice daily) to rhDNase 2.5mg daily and 2.5mg alternate daily. Robinson et al [39] compared hypertonic saline 6% to 0.9% saline with matched voluntary cough, Mannitol 300mg, and placebo capsules with matched voluntary cough. Weller et al [40] compared hypertonic saline 7%(5mL) to Mistabron 20% (a mucolytic agent). Suri et al [26] compared hypertonic saline 7% (5mL) BD (twice daily) to rhDNase 2.5mg daily and 2.5mg alternate daily.

All the trials with the exception of Weller et al and Chadwick et al pre-treated participants with short acting beta-agonists [40, 41]. Riedler used the hypertonic saline as an adjunct to physiotherapy and an exercise programme and all participants had intravenous antibiotics [38]. Eng et al [37] had as an inclusion criteria, that participants perform physiotherapy at home and delivered hypertonic saline prior to the participants' regular physiotherapy session. The place of chest physiotherapy is likely to be an important contributor to mucolytic therapy but its role as a confounder was not addressed in any of the trials.

A change in lung function again was the most common outcome measured. Comparing HS 6% 10ml to isotonic saline Eng et al [37] after two weeks found a mean (SD) percentage increase in FEV1 from baseline of 15% [16] compared to 2.8% [13] with placebo (p=0.004). In addition they found significant improvements in symptoms for quality of sleep and feeling of cleared chest measured after one and two weeks of treatment. Both Riedler et al [38] and Eng et al [37] looked at a similar visual analogue scale for symptoms of cleared chest measured four days after treatment. The results of the two studies were pooled. This demonstrated a result favouring treatment with a weighted mean difference 0.97 (95%CI 0.35 to 1.60) [34]. No data was available on mortality or frequency of exacerbations.

In terms of adverse events In the Eng trial there were similar reports of increased cough and haemoptysis, one participant in the hypertonic saline group had to withdraw because of haemoptysis though it was not clear if this was directly related to treatment [37]. In the hypertonic saline group one participant complained of chest tightness and one of throat irritation, with none in the isotonic saline group complaining of these symptoms. Participants who received HS described higher scores for throat irritation on a VAS compared to isotonic saline control though the number describing throat irritation was not stated. Frequency of cough in those treated with HS could not be directly compared to the days when they received the isotonic saline control as to they were encouraged to cough on the control days to match the active day's cough so as not to confound the results of the mucociliary clearance data [33, 35].

Comparisons have also been made between treatment with HS and DNase. Suri et al in a crossover trial [26] measured the mean increase in FEV1 from baseline comparing hypertonic saline 3% 5mls (demonstrated a 3% increase in FEV1) to daily DNase (16% increase) and alternate daily DNase (14% increase) DNase with DNase leading to a significantly greater increase in lung function. However Ballmann et al [27] did not demonstrate a significant difference between hypertonic saline and DNase. Both Ballmann [27] and Suri [26]compared the number of participants who improved their FEV1 by 10% or more from baseline after treatment and the result from the pooled analysis found no significant difference between hypertonic saline and DNase, RR 0.75 (95%CI 0.49 to 1.15) [34]. Neither trial demonstrated a statistical difference in adverse events between the two treatments.

The Suri trial [26] found that participants when treated with either DNase regimen had a significant improvement in lung function from baseline, but when treated with HS there was an increase of only 3% from the baseline FEV1, less than the increase in FEV1 seen by Eng et al [37] and Ballmann [27]. In both of these later trials 10mL of hypertonic saline was used compared to 5mls used by Suri [26] and Weller [40], this raises the possibility that the effectiveness of treatment may also depend on the total volume of saline nebulised and this may account for the lower effect size. In addition Suri [26] found a wide variation in response to treatment with both DNase and hypertonic saline, with over 50% demonstrating an increase in FEV1 of greater than 10% with DNase and 35% with hypertonic saline. Thus despite the overall reduced effect seen with hypertonic saline on lung function, in individuals, both DNase and hypertonic saline have the potential to substantially improve lung function in the medium term. The wide variation seen in response to both hypertonic saline and DNase raises the possibility that there may be subgroups of people with CF who are more likely to respond to efforts to improve mucociliary clearance. It also suggests that some individuals may respond better to one treatment compared to the other and physicians may wish to consider this particularly in individuals who fail to respond to DNase. None of the trials were of sufficient duration or size to assess mortality.

Ballmann et al [27] and Suri [36](Suri 2001) compared cost of treatment between DNase and hypertonic saline. Ballmann et al [27] compared one month of hypertonic saline treatment with DNase and found HS was significantly less. Suri compared total health care cost for the treatments incorporating not just drug cost but also admission, outpatient review, cost of investigations and the cost of utilising community resources [36]. The total cost of daily DNase was £5694 Great Britain Pound (GBP)/9000 Euros compared to 4285GBP/6780 Euros incurred while on hypertonic saline, mean difference 1409GBP (95%CI 440 to 2318) or 2230 Euros (95%CI 696 to 3368).

In the trial by Weller et al [40] only 3mls of 7% HS was used and no substantial change was seen in peak expiratory flow.

Hypertonic saline has been shown in a concentration of 5% to 7% when delivered by an ultrasonic nebuliser to improve mucociliary clearance. In the medium term it does not appear to be associated with serious side effects, though bronchospasm can still occur despite pre-treatment with bronchodilators. While there is evidence that it improves lung function compared to control, this improvement appears to be less than seen with DNase.

Dry Powdered Mannitol

Hydrogen bonds and oligosaccharide side chains make up 80% of the mucin structure and agents such as dextran and dry powdered mannitol may disrupt these sites and have been shown to increase MCC [42]. One small clinical study has looked at the effects of dry powdered mannitol looking at radioisotope clearance in CF patients and comparing it to HS [39]. Both treatments demonstrated an increase in MCC though despite participants being pre-treated with terbutaline there was a tendency for those who received hypertonic saline to have a larger fall in FEV1 within five minutes of receiving hypertonic saline. It is likely further trials looking at the role of mannitol in CF MCC will be pursued.

Other Agents that may Increase MCC in CF

Short acting bronchodilators such as salbutamol and terbutaline increase MCC in normal subjects. The effect of inhaled terbutaline was assessed in a small number of individuals with CF but was found to have less effect on MCC than it did in individuals who did not have CF [43].

The electrolyte defect in CFTR has also been targeted by treatment with inhaled amiloride, a sodium channel blocker with the aim to favourably alter the sodium and water balance in CF ASL. Treatment of individuals with CF with inhaled amiloride led to increased MCC [44] but the effect on lung function was disappointing [45] and has now been found to be clearly less effective than DNase.

The thiol reducing agent N-acetylcysteine has been used to treat patients with chronic obstructive pulmonary disease and non-CF bronchiectasis though its clinical effectiveness remains uncertain. N-acetylcysteine disrupts disulphide mucus bonds and reduces mucus viscosity; it may also increase mucus chloride content [4]. At this stage no controlled clinical trials of N-acetylcysteine have been carried out.

Triphosphate nucleotides (Uridine triphosphate) are novel approach to enhance MCC. These agents act via epithelial P2Y2 receptors to stimulate chloride and water secretion into the PCL [46]. The stable nucleotide INS 365 has been trialled in adults and children with CF and moderate airflow obstruction [47]. Doses of nebulised INS 365 above 40mg led to an increase in symptoms of wheeze and chest tightness and a fall in FEV1. Unfortunately no consistent effect of treatment was seen in terms of sputum production and mucus production and sputum weight.

Conclusions

Treatments that may enhance MCC in CF are likely to remain important targets for intervention particularly as this defect is so closely linked to recurrent endobronchial infection and its consequences of airway inflammation and worsening lung function. Currently DNase is the only treatment that has found widespread clinical use in CF. While treatment improves lung function within one month and for up to two years with a possible reduction in the frequency of pulmonary exacerbations, these changes have not been profound and the overall impact on mortality remains unclear. Less evidence is available for HS but it appears also to improve lung function at least in the short term, though it is probably not as effective as DNase. Individual patient responses to treatment may be important and as it remains clinical practice to trial CF patients on these agents to determine response before committing to long term treatment it may be possible to select those individuals most likely to respond to one or both of these of these interventions. For both DNase and HS more information is needed on long-term efficacy, particularly in terms of lung function, pulmonary exacerbations and mortality. Dry powdered mannitol is the only other agent that currently the evidence would suggest is deserving of evaluation in clinical trials. In addition possible combination therapy approaches with combinations or all of these agents may be worth exploring and provide benefits above monotherapy alone.

Targeting airway inflammation and secretion of mucus in CF remain important strategies in treating CF lung disease. Agents that block inflammatory cytokines (Il-13, IL-8, IL-9), second messengers (p38 MAP kinase) and the serine proteases released by neutrophils may all have beneficial effects on airway inflammation in CF and therefore reduce mucus secretion and decrease the DNA content in the ASL and are currently undergoing pre-clinical trials. Until treatment is available that reverses the defect present in CFTR, strategies to improve MCC will be worth exploring in the treatment of CF lung disease.

References

[1] Cutting, G. R. 1994. Genotype defect: Its effect on cellular function and phenotype expression. *Semin Respir Crit Care Med* 15:356-363.

[2] Marshall, S. G., M. Rosenfield, and B. W. Ramsey. 2000. In M. E. Hodsen and D. M. Geddes, editors. *Cystic Fibrosis*, 2nd ed. Arnold, London. 204-217.

[3] Davies, J. R., and I. Carlstedt. 2001. Respiratory Tract Mucins. In M. Salathe, editor. *Cilia and Mucus*. Marcel Dekker, New York. 167-178.

[4] King, M., and B. K. Rubin. 2002. Pharmacological approaches to discovery and development of new mucolytic agents. *Adv Drug Deliv Rev* 54:1475-1490.

[5] Knowles, M. R., and R. C. Boucher. 2002. Mucus clearance as a primary innate defence mechanism for mammalian airways. *J Clin Invest* 109:571-577.

[6] Matsui, H., and e. al. 1998. Evidence for pericilary liquid layer depletion, not abnormal ion composition in the pathogenesis of cystic fibrosis airways disease. *Cell* 95:1005-1015.

[7] Zahm, J. M., and e. al. 1989. The role of mucus sol phase in clearance by simulated cough. *Biorheology* 26:747-752.

[8] Cole, A. M., P. Dewan, and T. Ganz. 1999. Innate antimicrobial activity of nasal secretions. *Infect Immun* 67:3267-3275.

[9] Bear, C. E., N. Li, R. J. Kartner, T. J. Bridges, M. Jensen, J. R. Ramjeesingh, and J. R. Riordan. 1992. Purification and functional reconsitution of the cystic fibrosis transmembrane conductance regulator. *Cell* 68:809-818.

[10] Stutts, M. J., C. M. Canessa, J. C. Olsen, M. Hamrick, J. A. Cohn, B. C. Rossier, and R. C. Boucher. 1995. CFTR as a cAMP dependent regulator of sodium channels. *Science* 269:847-850.

[11] Boucher, R. C. 2002. An overview of the pathogenesis of CF lung disease. *Adv Drug Deliv Rev* 54:1359-1371.

[12] Goldman, M. J., G. M. Anderson, E. D. Stolzenberg, U. P. Kari, M. Zasloff, and J. M. Wilson. 1997. Human beta-defensin-1 is a salt sensitive antibiotic that is inactivated in cystic fibrosis. *Cell* 88:553-560.

[13] Lethem, M. I., S. L. James, C. Marriott, and J. F. Burke. 1990. The origin of DNA associated with mucus glycoproteins in cystic fibrosis sputum. *Eur Respir* J 3:19-23.

[14] Shak, S., D. J. Capon, R. Hellmiss, S. A. Marsters, and C. L. Baker. 1990. Recombinant human DNase I reduces the viscosity of cystic fibrosis sputum. *Proc Natl Acad Sci* 87:9188-9192.

[15] Jones, A. P., C. E. Wallis C.Kearney. 2004. Recombinant human deoxyribonuclease for cystic fibrosis. *In the Cochrane Database Syst Rev* 1:CD001127.

[16] Ramsey, B. W., S. J. Astley, M. L. Aitken, W. Burke, A. A. Colin, H. L. Dorkin, and e. al. 1993. Efficacy and safety of short-term adminstration of aerosolized recombinant human deoxyribonuclease in patients with cystic fibrosis. *Am Rev Respir Dis* 148:145-151.

[17] Ranasinha, C., B. Assoufi, S. Shak, D. Christiansen, H. J. Fuchs, D. Empey, and e. al. 1993. Efficacy and safety of short-term administration of aerosolised recombinant human DNase I in adults with stable stage cystic fibrosis. *Lancet* 342:199-202.

[18] Fuchs, H. J., D. Borowitz, D. Christiansen, E. Morris, M. Nash, B. Ramsey, and e. al. 1994. Effect of aerosolized recombinant human DNase on exacerbations of respiratory symptoms and on pulmonary function in patients with cystic fibrosis. *N Eng J Med* 331:637-642.

[19] Shah, P. I., A. Bush, G. J. Canny, A. A. Colin, H. J. Fuchs, D. M. Geddes, and e. al. 1995. Recombinant human DNase I in cystic fibrosis patients with severe pulmonary

disease: a short-term, double-blind study followed by six months open-label treatment. *Eur Respir J* 8:954-958.

[20] Laube, B. L., R. M. Auci, D. E. Shield, D. H. Christiansen, M. K. Lucas, H. J. Fuchs, and e. al. 1996. Effect of rhDNase on airflow obstruction and mucocilary clearance in cystic fibrosis. *Am J Respir Crit Care Med* 153:752-760.

[21] McCoy, K., S. Hamilton, and C. A. C. Johnson. 1996. Effects of 12-week administration of dornase alfa in patients with advanced cystic fibrosis lung disease. *Chest* 110:889-895.

[22] Wilmott, R. W., R. S. Amin, A. A. Colin, A. De Vault, A. J. Dozor, H. Eigen, and e. al. 1996. Aerosolized recombinant human DNase in hospitalized cystic fibrosis patients with acute pulmonary exacerbations. *Am J Respir Crit Care Med* 153:1914-1917.

[23] Dodd, M. E., A. J. Moorcroft, C. S. Haworth, S. Francis, J. Miles, N. Clayton, and e. al. 2000. The effect of rhDNase on exercise performance and gas trapping in adults with cystic fibrosis: a randomised controlled trial [abstract]. 13th International Cystic Fibroisis Congress, Stockholm. 147.

[24] Quan, J. M., H. A. W. M. Tiddens, J. P. Sy, S. G. McKenzie, M. D. Montgomery, P. J. Robinson, and e. al. 2001. A two-year randomized, placebo controlled trial of dornase alfa in young patients with cystic fibrosis with mild lung function abnormalities. *J Pediatr* 139:813-820.

[25] Robinson, T., A. N. Leung, W. H. Northway, F. G. Blankenberg, F. Chan, D. A. Bloch, and e. al. 2002. Composite CT/PFT score: an outcome measure which markedly improves sensitivity to change in early cystic fibrosis lung disease [abstract]. *Pediatr Pulomol* Suppl 2:298.

[26] Suri, R., C. Metcalfe, B. Lees, R. Grieve, M. Flather, C. Normand, and e. al. 2001. Comparison of hypertonic saline and alternate-day or daily recombinant human deoxyribonuclease in children with cystic fibrosis: a randomised trial. *Lancet* 358:1316-1321.

[27] Ballmann, M., and H. von der Hardt. 2002. Hypertonic saline and recombinant human DNase: a randomised cross-over pilot study in patients with cystic fibrosis. *J Cyst Fibr* 1:35-37.

[28] Oster, G., D. Huse, M. J. Lacey, M. M. Regan, and H. J. Fuchs. 1995. Effects of recombinant human DNase therapy on healthcare use and costs in patients with cystic fibrosis. *Ann Phacotherapr* 29:459-464.

[29] Menzin, J., G. Oster, L. Davies, M. F. Drummond, W. Greiner, C. Lucioni, and e. al. 1996. A multinational economic evaluation of rhDNase in the treatment of cystic fibrosis. International Journal of Technology Assessment in Healthcare. *Int J Tech Ass Healthcare* 12:52-61.

[30] von der Schulenburg, J. M. G., W. Greiner, and H. von der Hardt. 1995. Socioeconomic evaluation of the influence of rhDNase on the costs of treating respiratory tract infections in patients with cystic fibrosis. *Med Klinik* 90:220-224.

[31] Suri, R., L. J. Marshall, C. Wallis, C. Metcalfe, A. Bush, and J. K. Shute. 2002. Effects of recombinant human DNase and hypertonic saline on airway inflammation in children with cystic fibrosis. *Am J Respir Crit Care Med* 166:352-355.

[32] King, M., B. Dasgupta, R. P. Tomkiewicz, and N. E. Brown. 1997. Rheology of cystic fibrosis sputum after in vitro treatment with hypertonic saline alone and in combination with rhDNase. *Am J Respir Crit Care Med* 156:173-177.

[33] Robinson, M., A. Hemming, J. Regnis, A. Wong, D. Bailey, G. Bautotvich, P. T. P. Bye, and e. al. 1997. Effect of increasing doses of hypertonic saline on mucociliary clearance in patients with cystic fibrosis. *Thorax* 52:900-903.

[34] Wark, P. A., and V. McDonald. 2004. Nebulised hypertonic saline for cystic fibrosis. In: The Cochrane Library (Issue 1).

[35] Robinson, M., J. Regnis, D. L. Bailey, M. King, G. Bautovich, and P. T. P. Bye. 1996. The effects of hypertonic saline, amiloride and cough on mucociliary clearance in patients with cystic fibrosis. *Am J Respir Crit Care Med* 153:1503-1509.

[36] Suri, R., R. Grieve, C. Normand, C. Metcalfe, S. Thompson, C. Wallis, and e. al. 2002. Effects of hypertonic saline, alternate day and daily rhDNase on healthcare use, costs and outcomes in children with cystic fibrosis. *Thorax* 57:841-846.

[37] Eng, P. A., J. Morton, J. A. Douglass, J. Riedler, J. M. Wilson, and C. F. Robertson. 1996. Short term efficacy of ultrasonically nebulised hypertonic saline in cystic fibrosis. *Pediatr Pulomol* 21:77-83.

[38] Riedler, J., T. Reade, B. Button, and C. F. Robertson. 1996. Inhaled hypertonic saline increases sputum expectoration in cystic fibrosis. *J Paediatr Child Health* 32:48-50.

[39] Robinson, M., E. Daviskas, S. Eberl, J. Baker, H. Chan, S. Anderson, and e. al. 1999. The effect of inhaled mannitol on bronchial mucus clearance in cystic fibrosis patients: a pilot study. *Eur Respir J* 14:678-685.

[40] Weller, P., D. Ingram, M. Preece, and D. Matthew. 1980. Controlled trial of intermittent aerosol therapy with sodium 2-mercaptoethane sulphonate in cystic fibrosis. *Thorax* 35:42-46.

[41] Chadwick, S. L., S. J. Moss, J. Bott, D. M. Geddes, and E. W. F. W. Alton. 1997. Effect of hypertonic, isotonic saline and water challenges on the airways of cystic fibrosis patients. *Thorax* 52(Suppl 6):A43.

[42] Daviskas, E., S. Anderson, S. Eberl, H. K. Chan, and G. Bautotvich. 1999. Inhalation of dry poder mannitol improves clearance of mucus in patients with bronchiectasis. *Am J Respir Crit Care Med* 159:1843-1848.

[43] Mortensen, J., A. Hansen, M. Falk, I. K. Nielsen, and S. Groth. 1993. Reduced effect of inhaled beta 2 adrenergic agonists on lung mucociliary clearance in patients with cystic fibrosis. *Chest* 103:805-811.

[44] App, E. M., M. King, R. Helfsrieder, D. Kohler, and H. Matthys. 1990. Acute and long-term amiloride inhalation in cystic fibrosis lung disease. A rational approach to cystic fibrosis therapy. *Am Rev Respir Dis* 141:605-612.

[45] Knowles, M. R., N. L. Church, W. E. Waltner, J. R. Yankaskas, P. Gilligan, M. King, L. J. Edwards, R. W. Helms, and R. C. Boucher. 1990. A pilot study of aerosolized amiloride for the treatment of lung disease in cystic fibrosis. *N Eng J Med* 322:1189-1194.

[46] Brown, H. A., E. R. Lazarowski, R. C. Boucher, and T. K. Harden. 1991. Evidence that UTP and ATP regulate phospholipase C through a common extracellular 5'-nuleotide receptor in human airway epithelial cells. *Mol Pharmacol* 40:648-655.

[47] Noone, P. G., N. Hamblett, F. Accurso, M. L. Aitken, M. Boyle, and e. al. 2001. Safety of aerosolised INS 365 in patients with mild to moderate cystic fibrosis: results of a phase I multi-centre trial. *Pediatr Pulomol* 32:122-128.

In: Progress in Cystic Fibrosis Research
Editor: Margaret A. Harrison, pp. 131-149

ISBN 1-59454-232-5

Chapter VII

Molecular Genetics of Hispanic Cystic Fibrosis

Lee-Jun C. Wong* * *and Özgül Alper

Institute for Molecular and Human Genetics, Georgetown University Medical Center, Washington DC, USA

Abstract

Cystic fibrosis (CF) is a common autosomal recessive disease in Caucasian population. Although more than 900 mutations have been reported, the most common mutation, deltaF508, accounts for about 70% of all CF mutant alleles in Northern Europeans. The disease frequency in Hispanic population is much less and deltaF508 mutation accounts for about 50% of CF alleles in Hispanic population. Most commercially available mutation testing panels detect 85-95% of Caucasian CF mutations, but vary from 33% to 58% in Hispanic CF. To improve the detection rate in Hispanic CF patients, the entire coding and flanking intron regions of CFTR gene were screened by temporal temperature gradient gel electrophoresis followed by sequencing. Novel mutations were identified and the detection rate increases to 97%. Identification of CFTR mutations is important in confirming the disease diagnosis and providing appropriate genetic counseling.

Key words: Hispanic CF, *CFTR* mutation, TTGE, mutation detection of CF.

Abbreviations

CF	Cystic fibrosis
CFTR	cystic fibrosis transmembrane conductance regulator gene

---

* Correspondence concerning this article should be addressed to Lee-Jun C. Wong, Ph.D., Institute for Molecular and Human Genetics, Georgetown University Medical Center, M4000, 3800 Reservoir Rd, NW, Washington, DC 20007. Tel: 202 444 0760, Fax: 202 444 1770, Email: wonglj@georgetown.edu. Present address: Akdeniz University, School of Medicine, Department of Medical Biology-Genetics, Antalya,Turkey

TTGE	Temporal temperature gradient gel electrophoresis.

1. Introduction

Cystic fibrosis (CF; OMIM# 219700), caused by mutations in cystic fibrosis transmembrane conductance regulator (*CFTR*, MIM#602421) gene, is the most common life shortening autosomal recessive disease in Caucasian population. It occurs much less frequently in Hispanic population. The molecular genetics of Hispanic CF is not well characterized, such that a significant proportion of Hispanic *CFTR* mutations have not been identified. With the increase in Hispanic population in the United States, in order to provide more accurate newborn screening, effective molecular diagnosis, appropriate genetic counseling, and proper patient management, the determination of *CFTR* mutation spectrum and clinical correlation in this patient population is becoming more and more important. In this chapter, we review the recent advances in molecular genetic studies of Hispanic CF, identification of novel and rare mutations, clinical features associated with novel genotypes, and the importance of comprehensive mutational analysis.

2. Clinical Diagnosis and Molecular Genetics of CF

The diagnosis of cystic fibrosis (CF) is based on (a) the presence of at least one characteristic clinical feature including persistent infection of the airways, airway obstruction, nasal polyps, meconium ileus, pancreatic insufficiency, failure to thrive, steatorrhea, salt loss syndromes, or male infertility due to congenital bilateral absence of vas deferens, (b) positive family history or positive newborn screening, (c) laboratory evidence of a *CFTR* abnormality such as elevated sweat chloride concentration or identification of deleterious mutations in *CFTR* gene.

The *CFTR* gene contains 27 exons encompassing approximately 250 kb of DNA on chromosome 7q31.2 [1]. The gene is transcribed into a mature messenger RNA of 6.5 kb which encodes for a protein of 1480 amino acids and a molecular mass of 168 kDa [1, 2]. The CFTR protein is a member of ATP binding cassette (ABC) transporter family of membrane proteins. The CFTR protein forms a regulated cell membrane chloride channel with two transmembrane spans, each containing 6 transmembrane segments, two nucleotide-binding folds (binding to ATP), and a regulatory R domain for phosphorylation by cAMP dependent protein kinase.

Since the discovery of the gene [1, 2], more than 900 mutations have been identified throughout the gene [3]. Mutations in the *CFTR* gene are categorized into four classes according to their pathogenic mechanisms [4]. Class I mutations are severe nonsense mutations, splicing abnormalities and frameshift mutations that produce little or no functional CFTR protein. Class II mutations produce defective protein that is not properly processed post-translationally to reach the apical membrane where the protein will function. Class III mutations generate mutant CFTR protein that reaches the plasma membrane but the channels are not properly regulated. Class IV mutations produce correctly localized CFTR protein with altered activity. Individual mutations may have more than one effect. The nature of the mutation correlates with the severity of the disease including pancreatic insufficiency and degree of sweat chloride abnormality.

The vast majority of the disease-associated mutations involve one or a few nucleotides. Only about 1 percent are genomic large deletions or insertions [4]. Approximately 44 percent of disease causative mutations are missense mutations. Frameshift, splice site, nonsense, and in-frame mutations account for 22%,16%,14 %, and 2% of the overall mutations, respectively [4]. In general, nonsense, frameshift, and splice site mutations are severe mutations predicted to be deleterious because they either produce truncated CFTR protein or no wild type protein. To determine the functional consequence of missense mutations is much more difficult, and there are gold standard procedures to assess the consequence of a missense mutation [4].

3. Incidence of CF and Prevalent Mutations

Cystic fibrosis is one of the most common life threatening autosomal recessive diseases affecting primarily Caucasian populations. In the United States, CF occurs at a frequency of 1 in 2,000 to 3,000 Caucasians [4], but at a much lower rate in Hispanic (1 in 9,200), Native American (1 in 10,900) [5], African American (1 in 15,000), and Asian American live births (1 in 31,000) [6].

The spectrum of *CFTR* mutations varies among different populations, ethnic backgrounds, and geographical locations [7]. The most common mutation, ΔF508, accounts for about 70% of all *CFTR* mutant alleles in Northern Europeans, but it accounts for only about 50% of CF alleles in Hispanics and Spaniards [8]. This ΔF508 mutation has not been found in some Asian patients [9, 10], [11]. Similarly, the frequency of W1282X mutation is about 1 to 2% in Caucasians but is as high as 60% in Ashkenazi population [12, 13]. The most common mutation, 1898+5G>T, in Taiwanese CF accounts for 33% of the mutant alleles in this CF patient population [9], but it is present in only 0.1% of Caucasian CF patients in the United States [8]. Five common mutations account for 97% of Ashkenazi Jewish CF chromosomes [14, 15], 24 most frequent recurrent mutations account for about 80% of Northern European and Northern American Caucasian CF chromosomes [12], 15 mutations account for 75% of African American CF chromosomes [5], and as many as 75 mutations account for 90% of Spanish CF chromosomes [16]. Therefore, there is broad mutation spectrum within the same population and variations among different populations.

4. Mutation Detection Rate

Genetic testing for CF is necessary in order to (a) confirm the diagnosis of the disease, particularly when clinical presentation is atypical, (b) evaluate an individual's carrier status, (c) determine the carrier or affected status of a fetus, and (d) provide accurate genetic counseling for at-risk family members. Thus, it is important to know the incidence and the mutation spectrum in a particular patient population. For the molecular diagnosis of CF, usually a panel of recurrent mutations is analyzed. Depending on the ethnic background of the patient, the mutation detection rate varies. Most of the commercially available mutation panels are designed to detect most of the recurrent *CFTR* mutations in Caucasians and Ashkenazi Jewish patient populations. Inclusion of additional specific mutations improved the mutation detection rate in African Americans to 75% [5]. Recently, other panels have also been modified to increase the detection rate of *CFTR* mutations in other ethnic groups [8]. A pan-ethnic panel containing 86 mutations had a CF mutation detection rate of 62% in African Americans, 58% in Hispanics, 38% in Asians, and 81% in Native Americans in the United States compared to 85% in Caucasians and 95 % in Ashkenazi populations [8]. In general, in Caucasian and Ashkenazi Jewish population where the detection rate is already high, increase the number of mutations tested does not increase the detection rate significantly. Whereas in Asian and Hispanic populations where the detection rate is low, identification of mutations that are prevalent in these particular populations will greatly facilitate the design of mutation panels for routine molecular diagnosis.

5. Prevalent Mutations in Hispanic CF

The U.S. Census Bureau (http://www.census.gov) projects that by 2010 the Hispanic population may become the second largest racial/ethnic group in the United States [17]. In California, already, 50% of live births are to Hispanics, largely of Mexican origin and 6% are to African Americans [18]. Each year in California we expect 33 % of all new CF cases are expected to be Hispanic and 2% to be African American. Similar increase in Hispanic population in states such as Texas and Florida has been observed.

The ethnic origin of Hispanic populations is diverse. The term "Hispanic" generally refers to individuals from Latin America including the Caribbean, and Central and Southern America, with varying contribution from European settlers, native people, and Africans [19]. Thus, the prevalent mutations in the Hispanic patient pool in southern California may not represent that in Hispanics in Florida or New York [19-21].

Several investigations focused on molecular genetics of Hispanics CF patients. Analysis of 97 unrelated Mexican CF families for mutations in *CFTR* gene identified a total of 34 different mutations accounting for 74.6% of the CF chromosomes [22]. A study of CF in three Latin American countries; Mexico, Colombia, and Venezuela, analyzing 16 known *CFTR* mutations found differences in mutation detection rate and mutation prevalence among the three countries. In these three patient populations, 57.8, 45.8, and 33.3% of CF mutant alleles were accounted for by 15, 9, and 2 distinct known mutations, respectively, indicating the heterogeneity among different Hispanic patient groups in Latin American countries [23]. In all Hispanic CF populations, the most prevalent mutation is ΔF508del, which accounts for 29.2, 29.6, 35.4, 41-48, 47.7, 57, 53, and 56.4% of CF mutant alleles in Chile, Venezuela, Columbia, Mexico, Brazil, Argentina, Spain, and Southern Italy, respectively [7, 16, 22-26]. The second most prevalent mutation in most Hispanic CF patient populations analyzed is G542X, which varies between 3 and 8%.

In the United States, molecular genetic studies of Hispanic CF are limited. Screening for 23 common mutations in 65 Hispanic CF patients with Mexican, Central and South American origins in the southwestern part of the United States identified 58% of CF mutant chromosomes, in which, the most prevalent mutation, ΔF508, accounted for 46% of the CF alleles [21]. However, only 32.2% of the overall US Hispanic CF patients had ΔF508 in a large study [8]. This study includes Puerto Ricans, Cubans and patients with Caribbean origin, in addition to Central and South American origins.

Depending upon the number of known mutations screened, the detection rate for Hispanic CF varies from around 30% to about 80% in the United States. The detection rate can be improved by using indirect mutation detection followed by sequence analysis to identify the mutations.

6. Methods for Mutation Detection

6.1. Detection of Known Mutations

Many molecular methods have been used routinely for the detection of known *CFTR* mutations. Allele specific oligonucleotide (ASO) dot blot analysis is a frequently used method, particularly for simultaneous detection of multiple point mutations. Usually, the DNA regions containing the mutation are amplified using multiple pairs of PCR primers in a multiplex PCR reaction. The PCR products are dotted onto positively charged nylon membrane and hybridized with either the wild type or mutant ASO probes [15]. The advantage of this method is cost effective and ability for multiplexing. The disadvantage is the usage of radioactive material to label the probes. Reverse ASO dot blot is based on the same principle except that the ASO's are dotted on the membrane and hybridized with labeled PCR products [27]. Restriction fragment length polymorphism (RFLP) analysis is often used to analyze one mutation at a time. It is simple but the disadvantage is the inability for multiplexing and the requirement of a differential diagnostic restriction site for the distinction between mutant and wild type sequences. It is not suitable if multiple mutations are to be analyzed simultaneously. Allele refractory mutation system (ARMS) uses allele specific primers to amplify either the wild type or the mutant allele followed by gel analysis [28]. This method eliminates the RFLP procedures, but requires the optimization of ARMS PCR conditions. More recently, several rapid and automated mutation detection methodologies have been developed.

The one-step PCR coupled with fluorescent detection using either molecular Beacon [29] or TaqMan probes [30] were used in the allele discrimination assay. The principle is based on the discriminatory binding of a target sequence specific fluorescent probe to either the wild type or the mutant PCR product. The probe contains a fluorescent reporter group and a quencher. When the probe binds to the target sequence (Molecular Beacon) and is cleaved by the 5'>3' exonuclease of *Taq* polymerase, the reporter and the quencher are separated and emit fluorescent light which reflects the target sequence (wild type or mutant). The advantage of this method is one-step amplification and detection, but the reagent and the equipment can be expensive. A commercially available CF mutation detection kit is available from Applied Biosystems Inc. that uses oligo ligation assay (OLA) (http://www/appliedbiosystems.com). Because of the allele specific ligation, the capability of labeling each probe with different fluorescent molecule, and the design of amplicons with various lengths followed by separation (sequence coded separation, SCS), as many as 30 fragments (3 different colors each with 10 amplicons with different sizes can be run per lane (or per capillary electrophoresis run). This method is rapid and high throughput.

6.2. Screening of the *CFTR* Gene for Unknown Mutations

More than 900 CFTR mutations have been reported (http://www.genet.sickkids.on.ca/cftr/). It is not practical to screen for all known mutations. Although direct DNA sequencing is considered as the gold standard, it is tedious and expensive. Thus, indirect mutation scanning methods are developed to detect unknown mutations [31]. Single strand conformational polymorphism (SSCP) analysis is a commonly used simple method. It is based on the effect of mutations on the folding and hence the mobility of the DNA in the gel [32]. The mutation detection rate of SSCP is only about 50-80%. Heteroduplex analysis is similar to SSCP; however it relies on the formation of heteroduplexes between mutant and wild type DNA. It requires mixing with the wild type DNA in order to detect homozygous mutations. The detection rate is also low. Denaturing gradient gel electrophoresis (DGGE) is based on the melting behavior of the double stranded wild type or mutant DNA fragments [33]. The DNA fragments electrophorese through a gradient of chemical denaturant (urea) that separates partially melted homoduplex and heteroduplex DNA species. This method was used to screen *CFTR* mutations in Asian and African American CF patients at a detection rate greater than 90% [5, 34]. The disadvantage of this method is the requirement of a GC- clamp attached to one of the PCR primers. This method is modified by replacing the chemical denaturant gradient with temperature gradient and eliminating the GC-clamp by increasing the size of the DNA fragment and taking the advantage of the internal GC stretches [35, 36]. Such modified temporal temperature gradient gel electrophoresis (TTGE) method was used to detect the unknown *CFTR* mutations in Hispanic CF patients and improved the detection rate to greater than 94% [36].

Recently, more rapid and high throughput automated methods have been developed. This includes denaturing high performance liquid chromatography (dHPLC) and capillary gel electrophoresis [37]. These methods also depend on temperature denaturant and melting behavior of the DNA fragments. However, the separation time is greatly reduced, from hours in polyacrylamide gel to minutes in dHPLC and capillaries. More sophisticated is the development of SEQUENOM's MassARRAY™ Analyser that uses matrix-assisted laser desorption/ionization time-of-flight mass spectrometry (MALDI-TOF MS). This novel technology is accurate, fast, and high throughput [38], however, the equipment is expensive.

7. Mutational Analysis of Hispanic CF

Table 1 summarizes the molecular studies of Hispanic CF in Central and Southern American countries, Spain, Southern Italy, and various US Hispanic CF populations. The data demonstrate the broad mutation spectrum with high heterogeneity. This table also lists the methodologies used to screen for mutations and the number of mutations analyzed or identified. Most studies used ASO dot blot method for the detection of multiple known mutations [8, 21-24, 26, 36]. The overall detection rate by screening with defined number of known mutations is usually below 70%. Scanning of all 27 coding exons using SSCP raised the detection rate from 56% to 74.6% in Mexican patients [22]. DGGE analysis improves the detection rate to 85% in Southern Italy and to 90% in Spain [16, 26]. Study of Hispanic CF patients in California using TTGE achieved a detection rate greater than 94% [36, 39], It is apparent that mutations in California Hispanic CF are quite diverse. A total of 76 distinct mutations have been discovered. It is worth noting that 3849+10 kbC>T alternative splice mutation, and the newly identified 3876delA, 406-1 G>A, 1288insTA, 2105-2117del13insAGAAA, H199Y, W1204X, P205S, ΔF311, W1089X, 663delT, R75X, and Q98R are among the 12 most frequent *CFTR* mutations found only in California Hispanic patients that are currently not in the commercially available test panels (Tables 1 and 2) [39]. We recommend that these mutations be analyzed in Hispanic CF patients. A pan-ethnic 86-mutation panel identified 58% of the Hispanic mutant alleles in the United States [8], whereas the same mutation panel identified approximately 75% of Hispanic CF mutant alleles in Southern California and 80% of the Hispanic CF mutant alleles in California [36, 39]. These results suggest that there is heterogeneity among Hispanic patient populations in the United States. The *CFTR* mutation spectrum of Hispanics in New York and southeastern states may differ from that in California and southwestern states. Figure 1 illustrates the *CFTR* mutations identified in California Hispanic patients. The mutations spread along the entire *CFTR* gene. The majority is frameshift, nonsense, or splice site mutation. Exons 13, 4, 17B, 11, 10, 20, and 7 appear to be hot spots.

8. Characteristics of Novel *CFTR* Mutations in Hispanic CF and Clinical Correlation

Data from our most recent comprehensive studies of California Hispanic CF indicate that the majority (Figure 1, 32/43=74%) of the rare and newly identified mutations are class I mutations that are due to splicing, frame shift, or nonsense mutations that result in truncated CFTR proteins without functional activity. Similarly, the majority (35/46=76%) of the mutations found only in Hispanics are class I mutations (Table 2). Whereas, 47 out of the 86 pan-ethnic mutations (54.6%) are class I mutations. Class I mutations are associated with severe clinical phenotype. Most of the California Hispanic CF patients are pancreatic insufficient. These results are consistent with the previous observation that Hispanic CF cases are more severe than Caucasian cases.

Several mutations are worth noting. Five patients were found compound heterozygous for 3894+10kbC>T mutation in 62 Hispanic CF patients from Southern California, accounting for 4% of the mutant alleles [36, 40]. We later found a Hispanic CF patient homozygous for this mutation. Thus, the frequency of 3894+10kb C>T mutation in Southern California Hispanic CF is significantly higher than that in the general US CF population (0.6%) [40]. The average age of diagnosis of this group of patients is 3.1 years, which is much younger than that reported for CF patients of other ethnicities with the same mutation. Both pancreatic sufficient and pancreatic insufficient patients were observed. It is concluded that the 3894+10kbC>T mutation is associated with variable, progressive, but potentially mild CF phenotype. This mutation may also have different tissue-specific pathogenic effect, since the majority of the patients are pancreatic sufficient [40].

Table 1. *CFTR* gene mutations found in worldwide Hispanic population.

Country/Study	US	US	CA-US	Mexico	Spain	S Italy	Brazil	SW US	Mexico	Columbia	Venezuela	Argentina	Chile
# of chromosomes	248/74	124	728	194	1280	396	154	129	190	48	54	228	72
# of mutations found	70/86	32	48	12-34	75	8-13	84	23	15	9	2	10	2
Detection rate (%)	58	94	94	75	90	85	55	58	80	46	33	67	
Method	Panels	TTGE	Panels, TTGE	SSCP, mHET	RFLP, DGGE, SSCP	ASO, DGGE		ASO	R-ASO	R-ASO	R-ASO	RFLP, ASO	
Reference number	8	36	39	22	16	26	7	21	23	23	23	24	7
Mutation													
ΔF508	32.3	51.6	571	40.72	53.2	56.4		46	47.8	35.4	29.6	57	29.2
G542X	2.8	4	4.9	6.18	8.43	5.7		5.4	4.4	6.3	3.7	3.9	
ΔF507	2.4		1.7	2.57	0.78								
3120+1G>A	2	1.6	1.2										
R334W	2	1.6	0.7		1.64			1.6					
F311del	1.4		0.4										
S549N	1.2	2.4	1	2.57					1.1				
R1162X	1.2	0.8	1.2		1.64			1.6				0.4	
N1303K	1.2	0.8	0.5	2.06	2.65	6.8			1.1	2.1		1.7	
W1282X	1.2	0.8	0.5	0.51	0.78	3.8		0.8		2.1		3.1	
W1089X	1.2	0.8	0.5										
G1244E	1.2	0.8				1.3							
R553X	1.2		0.5	0.51	0.31	1.1		0.8				0.4	4.2
D1270N	1.2												
G85E	0.8	0.8	1	0.51	0.94								
1677delTA	0.8												
3849+10kbC>T	0.4	4	1.3	0.51	0.39			2.3	2.2				
I148T	0.4	1.6	0.1	1.54	0.08	0.7							
G551D	0.4	0.8	0.4		0.31								
2183AA>G	0.4		0.6	1.03		1.9							
711+1G>T	0.4		0.4		1.71	1.3							
1078delT	0.4		0.4										
2789+5G>A	0.4		0.3		0.86								
Y1092X	0.4		0.3	0.51									
1812-1G>A	0.4		0.3										
1898+1G>A	0.4		0.1										

Table 1. *CFTR* gene mutations found in worldwide Hispanic population. (Continued)

Country/Study	US	US	CA-US	Mexico	Spain	S Italy	Brazil	SW US	Mexico	Columbia	Venezuela	Argentina	Chile
# of chromosomes	248/74	124	728	194	1280	396	154	129	190	48	54	228	72
# of mutations found	70/86	32	48	12-34	75	8-13	84	23	15	9	2	10	2
Detection rate (%)	58	94	94	75	90	85	55	58	80	46	33	67	
Method	Panels	TTGE	Panels, TTGE	SSCP, mHET	RFLP, DGGE, SSCP	ASO, DGGE		ASO	R-ASO	R-ASO	R-ASO	RFLP, ASO	
Reference number	8	36	39	22	16	26	7	21	23	23	23	24	7
2869insG	0.4												
R352Q	0.4												
3876delA		5.65	1.8										
406-1G>A		1.6	1.6	1.54									
R1066C		1.6	0.7										
935delA		1.6	0.1										
R75X		0.8	0.5	1.54									
P205S		0.8	0.5										
1949del84		0.8	0.4										
2108delA		0.8	0.1										
3199del6		0.8	0.1										
Q98R		08											
1288insTA*			0.8										
W1204X			0.7										
2105-2117del13insAGAAA			0.7										
1717-1G>A			0.6			2.3						0.9	
Q98X			0.5										
663delT			0.5										
3272-26>G			0.4										
S492F			0.4										
R117H			0.3										
Q890X			0.3										
621+1G>T			0.3										
2184delA			0.3										
712-1G>T			0.3										
1924del7			0.3										

Table 1. *CFTR* gene mutations found in worldwide Hispanic population. (Continued)

Country/Study	US	US	CA-US	Mexico	Spain	S Italy	Brazil	SW US	Mexico	Columbia	Venezuela	Argentina	Chile
# of chromosomes	248/74	124	728	194	1280	396	154	129	190	48	54	228	72
# of mutations found	70/86	32	48	12-34	75	8-13	84	23	15	9	2	10	2
Detection rate (%)	58	94	94	75	90	85	55	58	80	46	33	67	
Method	Panels	TTGE	Panels, TTGE	SSCP, mHET	RFLP, DGGE, SSCP	ASO, DGGE		ASO	R-ASO	R-ASO	R-ASO	RFLP, ASO	
Reference number	8	36	39	22	16	26	7	21	23	23	23	24	7
2184insA			0.3										
3500-2A>T			0.3										
R1158X			0.1										
R347P			0.1										
S1255X			0.1										
3821delT			0.1										
S945L			0.1										
G1061R			0.1										
2307insA			0.1										
A561E			0.1										
I1027T			0.1										
3271delGG			0.1										
3171delC			0.1										
Q179K			0.1										
F1016S			0.1										
124-146del23bp*			0.1										
2289-2298del10ins5 *			0.1										
296+2T>A*			0.1										
360-365insT*			0.1										
379-381insT*			0.1										
3960-3961delA*			0.1										
4016insT						1.8							
R1185X						1.3							
L1065P						1.3							

* indicate novel mutations recently found in Hispanic population.

Abbreviations: TTGE, temporal temperature gradient gel electrophoresis; SSCP, single strand conformation polymorphism; mHET, multiplex heteroduplex analysis; ASO, allele specific oligonucleotide; RFLP, restriction fragment length polymorphism; DGGE, denaturing gradient gel electrophoresis; R-ASO, reverse allele specific oligonucleotide; RDB, reverse dot blot.

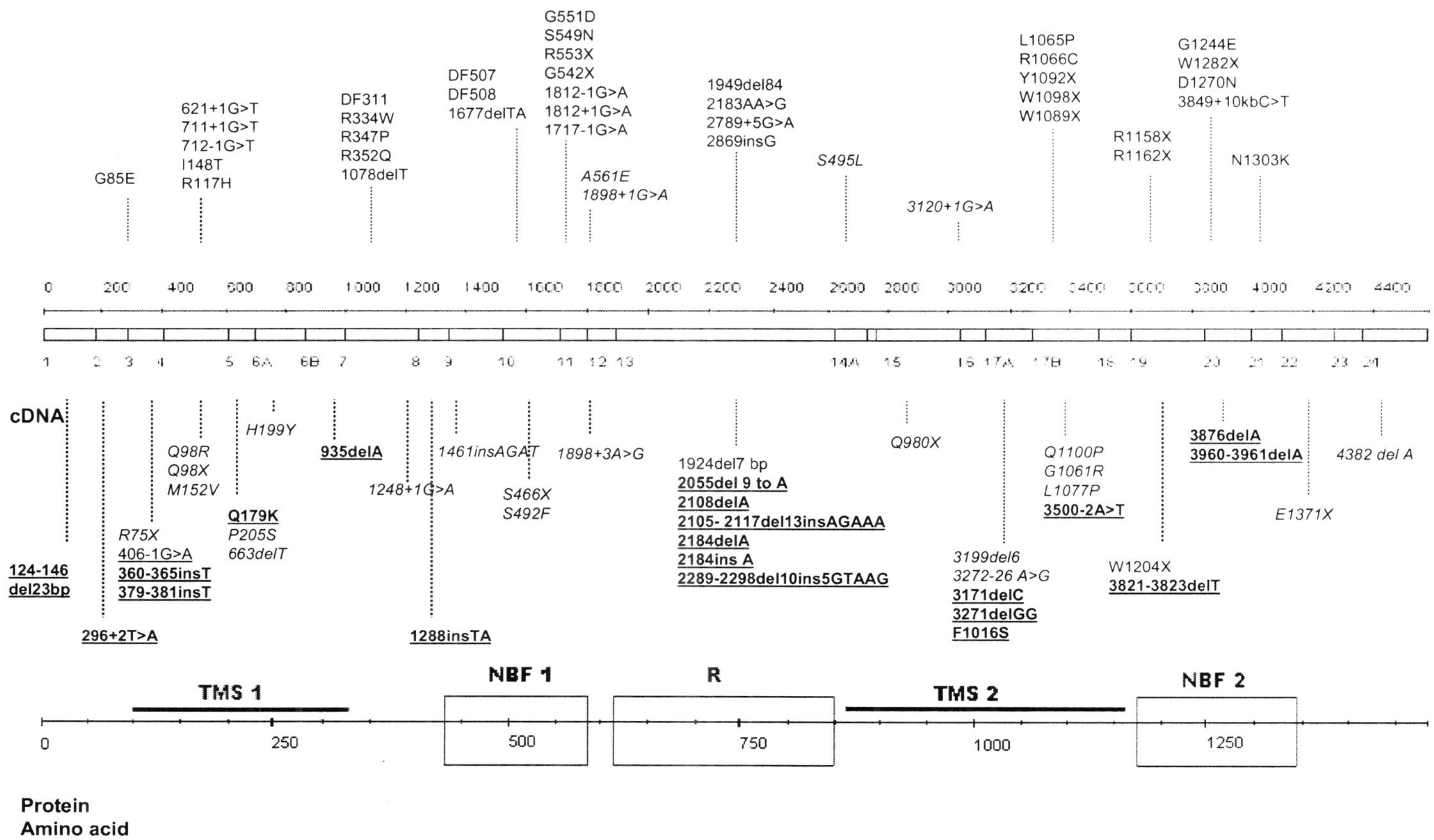

Figure 1. The mutation spectrum of *CFTR* gene found in Hispanic patients. The mRNA is at the middle with exons numbered and the cDNA nucleotides numbered every 200. The line at the bottom illustrates the functional domains of the CFTR protein: two transmembrane spans (TMS1 and TMS2), two nucleotide binding folds (NBF1 and NBF2), and the regulatory domain (R). The amino acids are numbered every 250. The mutations on the top have been reported by other studies, the mutations below the cDNA were identified in our laboratory. The novel mutations found in Hispanic population were in bold and underlined. The missense mutations are in italic and the remaining frameshift, splice site, and nonsense mutations are in regular style.

Table 2. Mutations found only in California Hispanic population.

Mutation	Class
124-146del 23bp	I
296+2T>A	I
R75X	I
406-1G>A	I
360-365insT	I
379-381insT	I
712-1G>T	I
Q98R	II-V
Q98X	I
M152V	II-V
Q179K	II-V
P205S	II-V
663delT	I
H199Y	II-V
935delA	I
F311del	I
1078delT	I
1248+1G>A	I
1288insTA	I
1461insAGAT	I
S466X	I
S492F	II-V
1898+3A>G	I
1924del7bp	I
2055del9toA	I
2108delA	I
2105-2117del13insAGAAA	I
2184delA	I
2184insA	I
2289-2298del10ins5	I
S945L	II-V
Q890X	I
3272-26A>G	I
3171delC	I
3271delGG	I
F1016S	II-V
W1089X	I
Q1100P	II-V
G1061R	II-V
L1077P	II-V
3500-2A>T	I
W1204X	I
3821-3823delT	I
3876delA	I
3960-3961delA	I
E1371X	I
4382del A	I

In search of *CFTR* mutations in California Hispanic CF population, we found a novel mutation 3876delA was present in 5.7% (7/124) of Southern California Hispanic CF patients [36]. It is the third most frequent mutation, next to ΔF508 and G542X mutations [36]. This mutation, 3876delA, is a deleterious frameshift mutation resulting in a truncated CFTR protein lacking most part of the nucleotide binding domain 2 (NBD2) [41]. Since ATP hydrolysis at NBD2 terminates a burst of activities associated with opening the channel, loss of NBD2 would confer a loss of the gating control [41, 42]. Clinical evaluation of seven patients compound heterozygous with this mutation confirmed that 3876delA is a severe mutation. The age of diagnosis ranged from 3 weeks to 7 months [41]. In all cases, high levels of sweat chloride (84-142 mmol/L) were detected. All seven patients had severely impaired pulmonary function, repetitive respiratory tract infection, and were pancreatic insufficient [41]. Since this mutation was not detected after extensive search for CF mutations in Spanish, European, Ashkenazi Jewish, and African-American populations, and most of the Hispanic CF patients are descendants of people from Mexico and South America, the 3876delA mutation may be derived from native Mexicans [4, 5, 14, 16, 41].

The next most frequent Hispanic *CFTR* mutation is 406-1G>A. This mutation was found in 12/728 (1.6%) California Hispanic CF mutant alleles [39], but was not detected in any other large-scale studies world-wide except the Mexican studies [7, 22]. The 406-1G>C or G>T mutation has been reported in the database (http://www.genet.sickkids.on.ca/cftr/), but not G>A mutation [36]. The patients who carried 406-1G>A mutation were all from Mexico. This mutation also accounts for1.5% of Mexican CF mutant alleles [22]. The data suggest that the 406-1G>A mutation is probably derived from native Mexicans.

Another novel mutation, 1288insTA, was found in 6 California Hispanic CF patients, including one homozygote and five compound heterozygotes [39, 43]. All six patients carrying this mutation are from Mexico. This is a frameshift mutation results in a truncated CFTR protein that is lacking the regulatory domain, the second nucleotide-binding fold, and the second transmembrane span. All six patients had severe clinical phenotype with elevated sweat chloride, pancreatic insufficiency, and reduced pulmonary function [43].

The 2105-2117del13insAGAAA novel mutation was discovered in a Hispanic family from Mexico with three affected children [44]. This mutation was subsequently found in three additional unrelated families [39, 43]. Four of these patients were compound heterozygous with ΔF508. The clinical phenotype of this mutation is consistent with severe impairment of the CFTR function.

Others remarkable are 663delT and 935delA in exons 5 and 6, found in 4 and 2 unrelated Hispanic families, respectively [45, 46]. These frameshift mutations produce truncated proteins that lack more than three quarters of the cystic fibrosis transmembrane regulator protein are expected to be null. A patient compound heterozygous for these two mutations was reported to have a severe clinical course [45].

9. Association of CFTR Mutations with Other Diseases

Although the major clinical manifestation of mutations in *CFTR* gene is classical cystic fibrosis, mild *CFTR* variants in which there is sufficient residual CFTR activity to prevent the manifestation of classical CF such as pancreatic insufficiency and lung disease, maybe the cause of idiopathic chronic pancreatitis rhinosinusitis, asthma, or congenital bilateral absence of vas deferens (CBAVD) [47-51]. Thus, even though CF is a single gene disorder, clinical phenotype may be heterogeneous. In addition, the presence of nuclear modifier genes may complicate the clinical diagnosis [52]. Thus, genetic heterogeneity may result in variant cystic fibrosis phenotypes in the absence of *CFTR* mutations [53]. In any case, if there is any suspicion, comprehensive mutational analysis of the *CFTR* gene using one of the mutation scanning methods such as TTGE should be conducted in order to confirm or rule out the involvement of *CFTR* mutations in a disease.

Since CF is a common genetic disease, it is possible that a family may have CF in addition to another genetic disease. We have reported a CF patient who also has mitochondrial disease [54]. The patient was compound heterozygous for a mild R347P and a ΔF508 *CFTR* mutations [54]. She did not manifest classical CF symptoms except chronic cough and thick mucus plugs. She was not diagnosed with CF until 18 years of age. Her clinical manifestation includes mostly neuromuscular symptoms including movement disorders that lead to the diagnosis of mitochondrial disease. She harbored two novel mutations in mitochondrial encoded tRNA genes. Thus, CF patients may carry mutations in other genes [54].

While counseling women with family history of CF, other factors such as advanced maternal age should also be considered. We recently described a family with a CF affected child. Since one of the CF mutant allele was unidentified, the prenatal genetic counseling and diagnosis were focused on finding of the other CF mutant allele, although the advanced maternal age was also discussed. The fetus turned out to carry two normal *CFTR* alleles, but it had trisomy 21 [55]. This case emphasizes the importance of thorough consideration of all factors that may affect the pregnancy outcome during the prenatal genetic counseling, even though the major concern may be CF.

CFTR is a large gene. Numerous mutations have been found throughout the gene. It is not unusual for an affected CF female to have affected children with discordant phenotype. The affected males are usually infertile. Most infertile males with congenital bilateral absence of vas deferens (CBAVD) carry mutations in *CFTR* gene [56, 57]. These males may be asymptomatic for CF. *In vitro* fertilization (IVF) or surgical procedures are usually used to overcome the male infertility. Since CBAVD is associated with mutations in the *CFTR* gene and the offspring of the infertile males are at an increased risk for CF, mutational analysis of CFTR is always recommended for infertile couples [58, 59]. However, standard screening methods testing for 23-87 *CFTR* mutations are not sufficient to detect all the mutations in infertile men. As a matter of fact, studies have shown that a substantial number of infertile men have *CFTR* mutations that are undetectable by routine screening [60]. This was seen in a couple who had difficulty conceiving, underwent IVF that resulted in a triplet with discordant CF phenotype. Comprehensive mutational analysis revealed that the man carried two *CFTR* mutations; R553X and R117C. The woman carried ΔF508. One of the triplet who had classical CF had ΔF508 and R553X. The other two of the triplet who had mild CF symptoms had ΔF508 and R117C. Thus, comprehensive *CFTR* mutational analysis is essential on infertile couple if the male has CBAVD despite the negative family history of CF. This is particularly important in Hispanic families because the *CFTR* mutation detection rate of the commercially available panels for Hispanics is already lower than that for Caucasians, and they are not designed to detect mutations in CBAVD.

10. Conclusion

In conclusion, *CFTR* mutation spectrum in Hispanic CF differs from Caucasian CF. The detection rate of currently available mutation panels varies depending upon the number of mutations analyzed and the geographic origin of the patient. Therefore, if CF mutant alleles cannot be identified using mutation panels, more comprehensive whole gene scanning by indirect mutation screening method such as DGGE and TTGE, coupled to direct DNA sequencing should be performed. These methods provide a detection rate greater than 97%. Diagnosis of CF may be complicated by other genetic conditions. If necessary, thorough molecular analysis should always be performed to confirm or rule out the involvement of *CFTR* mutations in the disease condition.

Databases

CFTR: OMIM #602421, CF: OMIM #219700; GDB120584; Genbank: M55106-M55131; HGMD: CFTR http://www.genet.sickkids.on.ca/cftr/ (CFTR Mutation Database)

References

[1] Riordan JR, Rommens JM, Kerem B, Alon N, Rozmahel R, Grzelczak Z, Zielenski J, Lok S, Plavsic N, Chou JL, et al. Identification of the cystic fibrosis gene: cloning and characterization of complementary DNA. *Science* 1989;245:1066-73

[2] Kerem B, Rommens JM, Buchanan JA, Markiewicz D, Cox TK, Chakravarti A, Buchwald M, Tsui LC. Identification of the cystic fibrosis gene: genetic analysis. *Science* 1989;245:1073-80

[3] CF Foundation. *Cystic Fibrosis Foundation Patient Registry.*2002 Annual Data to the center Directors.Bethesda, Maryland. Run courtesy of Marci Sontag, 2003.

[4] Welsh MJ, Romsey BW, Accurso F, Cutting GR. *Cystic fibrosis.* In: Scriver CR BA, Sly WS, Valle D, ed. *Metabolic and Molecular Bases of Inherited Disease*, 8 ed. Vol III. NewYork: McGraw-Hill, 2001; 5121-5188.

[5] Macek M, Jr., Mackova A, Hamosh A, Hilman BC, Selden RF, Lucotte G, Friedman KJ, Knowles MR, Rosenstein BJ, Cutting GR. Identification of common cystic fibrosis mutations in African-Americans with cystic fibrosis increases the detection rate to 75%. *Am J Hum Genet* 1997;60:1122-7

[6] Hamosh A, Fitz-Simmons SC, Macek M, Jr., Knowles MR, Rosenstein BJ, Cutting GR. Comparison of the clinical manifestations of cystic fibrosis in black and white patients. *J Pediatr* 1998;132:255-9

[7] Bobadilla JL, Macek M, Jr., Fine JP, Farrell PM. Cystic fibrosis: a worldwide analysis of CFTR mutations--correlation with incidence data and application to screening. *Hum Mutat* 2002;19:575-606

[8] Heim RA, Sugarman EA, Allitto BA. Improved detection of cystic fibrosis mutations in the heterogeneous U.S. population using an expanded, pan-ethnic mutation panel. *Genet Med* 2001;3:168-76

[9] Wong LJ, Alper OM, Wang BT, Lee MH, Lo SY. Two novel null mutations in a Taiwanese cystic fibrosis patient and a survey of East Asian CFTR mutations. *Am J Med Genet* 2003;120A:296-8

[10] Alper OM, Shu SG, Lee MH, Wang BT, Lo SY, Lin KL, Chiu YL, Wong LJ. Detection of novel CFTR mutations in Taiwanese cystic fibrosis patients. *J Formos Med Assoc* 2003;102:287-91

[11] Schrijver I, Karnsakul W, Ramalingam S, Sankaran R, Limwongse C, Moss R, Gardner P. Novel contributions to the Asian CFTR mutaton spectrum: genotype and phenotype in Thai patients with cystic fibrosis. *Am J Med Genet* 2004;in press

[12] Cystic Fibrosis Genetic Analysis consortium. Population variationof common cystic fibrosis mutations. *Hum Mutat* 1994;4:167-177

[13] Shoshani T, Augarten A, Gazit E, Bashan N, Yahav Y, Rivlin Y, Tal A, Seret H, Yaar L, Kerem E, et al. Association of a nonsense mutation (W1282X), the most common mutation in the Ashkenazi Jewish cystic fibrosis patients in Israel, with presentation of severe disease. *Am J Hum Genet* 1992;50:222-8

[14] Abeliovich D, Lavon IP, Lerer I, Cohen T, Springer C, Avital A, Cutting GR. Screening for five mutations detects 97% of cystic fibrosis chromosomes and predicts carrier frequency of 1:29 in the Jewish Ashkenozi population. *Am J Hum Genet* 1992;51:951-956

[15] DeMarchi JM, Caskey CT, Richards CS. Population-specific screening by mutation analysis for diseases frequent in Ashkenazi Jews. *Hum Mutat* 1996; 8:116-125

[16] Casals T, Ramos MD, Gimenez J, Larriba S, Nunes V, Estivill X. High heterogeneity for cystic fibrosis in Spanish families: 75 mutations account for 90% of chromosomes. *Hum Genet.* 1997;101:365-370

[17] Day JC. *Population Projections of the United States by Age, Sex, Race, and Hispanic Origin*:1995 to 2050.: U.S. Bureau of the Census, Current Population Reports, P25-1130, U.S. Government Printing office, Washington, DC., 1996.

[18] Services CoH. Center for Health Statistics Vital Query System, Birth Records. California Department of Health Services,http://www.applications.dhs.ca.gov/vsq/default.asp, 2003.

[19] Arzimanoglou, II, Tuchman A, Li Z, Gilbert F, Denning C, Valverde K, Zar H, Quittell L, Arzimanoglou I. Cystic fibrosis carrier screening in Hispanics. *Am J Hum Genet* 1995;56:544-7

[20] Grebe TA, Doane WW, Richter SF, Seltzer WK, Jain KD. A rational approach to cystic fibrosis mutation analysis in Hispanics: reply to Arzimanoglou et al. *Am J Hum Genet* 1996;59:269-72

[21] Grebe TA, Seltzer WK, DeMarchi J, Silva DK, Doane WW, Gozal D, Richter SF, Bowman CM, Norman RA, Rhodes SN, et al. Genetic analysis of Hispanic individuals with cystic fibrosis. *Am J Hum Genet* 1994;54:443-6

[22] Orozco L, Velazquez R, Zielenski J, Tsui LC, Chavez M, Lezana JL, Saldana Y, Hernandez E, Carnevale A. Spectrum of CFTR mutations in Mexican cystic fibrosis patients: identification of five novel mutations (W1098C, 846delT, P750L, 4160insGGGG and 297-1G-->A). *Hum Genet* 2000;106:360-5

[23] Restrepo CM, Pineda L, Rojas-Martinez A, Gutierrez CA, Morales A, Gomez Y, Villalobos MC, Borjas L, Delgado W, Myers A, Barrera-Saldana HA. CFTR mutations in three Latin American countries. *Am J Med Genet* 2000;91:277-9

[24] Chertkoff L, Visich A, Bienvenu T, Grenoville M, Segal E, Carniglia L, Kaplan JC, Barreiro C. Spectrum of CFTR mutations in Argentine cystic fibrosis patients. *Clin Genet* 1997;51:43-7

[25] Bernardino AL, Ferri A, Passos-Bueno MR, Kim CE, Nakaie CM, Gomes CE, Damaceno N, Zatz M. Molecular analysis in Brazilian cystic fibrosis patients reveals five novel mutations. *Genet Test* 2000;4:69-74

[26] Castaldo G, Fuccio A, Cazeneuve C, Picci L, Salvatore D, Raia V, Scarpa M, Goossens M, Salvatore F. Detection of five rare cystic fibrosis mutations peculiar to Southern Italy: implications in screening for the disease and phenotype characterization for patients with homozygote mutations. *Clin Chem* 1999;45:957-62

[27] Chehab FF, Wall J. Detection of multiple cystic fibrosis mutations by reverse dot blot hybridization: a technology for carrier screening. *Hum Genet* 1992;89:163-8

[28] Ferrie RM, Schwarz MJ, Robertson NH, Vaudin S, Super M, Malone G, Little S. Development, multiplexing, and application of ARMS tests for common mutations in the CFTR gene. *Am J Hum Genet* 1992;51:251-62

[29] Tyagi S, Bratu DP, Kramer FR. Multicolor molecular beacons for allele discrimination. *Nat Biotechnol* 1998;16:49-53

[30] Glaab WE, Skopek TR. A novel assay for allelic discrimination that combines the fluorogenic 5' nuclease polymerase chain reaction (TaqMan) and mismatch amplification mutation assay. *Mutat Res* 1999;430:1-12

[31] Nollau P, Wagener C. Methods for detection of point mutations: performance and quality assessment. IFCC Scientific Division, Committee on Molecular Biology Techniques. *Clin Chem* 1997;43:1114-28

[32] Orita M, Iwahana H, Kanazawa H, Hayashi K, Sekiya T. Detection of polymorphisms of human DNA by gel electrophoresis as single-strand conformation polymorphisms. *Proc Natl Acad Sci U S A* 1989;86:2766-70

[33] Myers RM, Fischer SG, Lerman LS, Maniatis T. Nearly all single base substitutions in DNA fragments joined to a GC-clamp can be detected by denaturing gradient gel electrophoresis. *Nucleic Acids Res* 1985;13:3131-45

[34] Macek M, Jr., Mercier B, Mackova A, Miller PW, Hamosh A, Ferec C, Cutting GR. Sensitivity of the denaturing gradient gel electrophoresis technique in detection of known mutations and novel Asian mutations in the CFTR gene. *Hum Mutat* 1997;9:136-47

[35] Wong LJ, Liang MH, Kwon H, Park J, Bai RK, Tan DJ. Comprehensive scanning of the entire mitochondrial genome for mutations. *Clin Chem* 2002;48:1901-12

[36] Wong LJ, Wang J, Zhang YH, Hsu E, Heim RA, Bowman CM, Woo MS. Improved detection of CFTR mutations in Southern California Hispanic CF patients. *Hum Mutat* 2001;18:296-307

[37] Ravnik-Glavac M, Atkinson A, Glavac D, Dean M. DHPLC screening of cystic fibrosis gene mutations. *Hum Mutat* 2002;19:374-83

[38] Bocker S. SNP and mutation discovery using base-specific cleavage and MALDI-TOF mass spectrometry. *Bioinformatics* 2003;19 Suppl 1:I44-I53

[39] Kharrazi M, Alper OM, Young S, Pearl M, Graham S, Lorey F, Sherwin J, Wong LJ. Cystic fibrosis transmembrane regulator mutations in Hispanic Californians with cystic fibrosis. *Am J Hum Genet* 2003;supplement 73:413

[40] Liang MH, Wertz KK, Bowman CM, Hsu E, Shapiro B, Wong LJ. 3849 + 10 kb C --> T splicing mutation in Hispanic CF patients. *Mol Genet Metab* 1998;64:213-6

[41] Wang J, Bowman MC, Hsu E, Wertz K, Wong LJ. A novel mutation in the CFTR gene correlates with severe clinical phenotype in seven Hispanic patients. *J Med Genet* 2000;37:215-8

[42] Carson MR, Travis SM, Welsh MJ. The two nucleotide-binding domains of cystic fibrosis transmembrane conductance regulator (CFTR) have distinct functions in controlling channel activity. *J Biol Chem* 1995;270:1711-7

[43] Alper OM, Wong LJC, Young S, Pearl M, Graham S, Sherwin J, Nussbaum E, Nielson D, Platzker A, Davies Z, Lieberthal A, Chin T, Shay G, Hardy K, Kharrazi M. Identification of novel and rare mutations in California Hispanic and African American cystic fibrosis patients. *Hum Mutat* 2004;24:353

[44] Wong LJ, Wang J, Woo M, Hsu E, Bowman CM. A novel mutation detected by temporal temperature gradient gel electrophoresis led to the confirmative prenatal diagnosis of a Hispanic CF family. *Prenat Diagn* 2000;20:807-10

[45] Wong LJ, Wang J, Bowman CM. Two novel frame shift mutations of CFTR causing null alleles in a patient with a severe course of CF. *Am J Med Genet* 2001;102:389-90

[46] Wang J, Bowman CM, Wong LJ. A novel CFTR frame-shift mutation, 935delA, in two Hispanic cystic fibrosis patients. *Mol Genet Metab* 2000;70:316-21

[47] Cohn JA, Bornstein JD, Jowell PS. Cystic fibrosis mutations and genetic predisposition to idiopathic chronic pancreatitis. *Med Clin North Am* 2000;84:621-31, ix

[48] Cohn JA, Friedman KJ, Noone PG, Knowles MR, Silverman LM, Jowell PS. Relation between mutations of the cystic fibrosis gene and idiopathic pancreatitis. *N Engl J Med* 1998;339:653-8

[49] Claustres M, Guittard C, Bozon D, Chevalier F, Verlingue C, Ferec C, Girodon E, Cazeneuve C, Bienvenu T, Lalau G, Dumur V, Feldmann D, Bieth E, Blayau M, Clavel C, Creveaux I, Malinge MC, Monnier N, Malzac P, Mittre H, Chomel JC, Bonnefont JP, Iron A, Chery M, Georges MD. Spectrum of CFTR mutations in cystic fibrosis and in congenital absence of the vas deferens in France. *Hum Mutat* 2000;16:143-56

[50] Lazaro C, de Cid R, Sunyer J, Soriano J, Gimenez J, Alvarez M, Casals T, Anto JM, Estivill X. Missense mutations in the cystic fibrosis gene in adult patients with asthma. *Hum Mutat* 1999;14:510-9

[51] Wang X, Moylan B, Leopold DA, Kim J, Rubenstein RC, Togias A, Proud D, Zeitlin PL, Cutting GR. Mutation in the gene responsible for cystic fibrosis and predisposition to chronic rhinosinusitis in the general population. *Jama* 2000;284:1814-9

[52] Cohn JA, Noone PG, Jowell PS. Idiopathic pancreatitis related to CFTR: complex inheritance and identification of a modifier gene. *J Investig Med* 2002;50:247S-255S

[53] Groman JD, Meyer ME, Wilmott RW, Zeitlin PL, Cutting GR. Variant cystic fibrosis phenotypes in the absence of CFTR mutations. *N Engl J Med* 2002;347:401-7

[54] Wong L-JC, Liang M-H, Kwon H, Bai RK, Alper O, Gropman A. A CF patient with two novel mutations in mitochondrial DNA: mild disease led to delayed diagnosis of both disorders. *Am J Med Genet* 2002;113:59-64

[55] Wong LJ, Herbert WS, Zhang YH, Hsu E, Wong IH, Wladyka C, Woo M, Bowman CM. Prenatal genetic counseling on a woman with advanced maternal age and a family history of a known genetic disease. *Changhua J Med* 2002;7:75-81

[56] Dohle GR, Halley DJ, Van Hemel JO, van den Ouwel AM, Pieters MH, Weber RF, Govaerts LC. Genetic risk factors in infertile men with severe oligozoospermia and azoospermia. *Hum Reprod* 2002;17:13-6

[57] Dohle GR, Veeze HJ, Overbeek SE, van den Ouweland AM, Halley DJ, Weber RF, Niermeijer MF. The complex relationships between cystic fibrosis and congenital bilateral absence of the vas deferens: clinical, electrophysiological and genetic data. *Hum Reprod* 1999;14:371-4

[58] Spurgeon D. Men using IVF inadequately screened for cystic fibrosis. *Bmj* 1999;318:1720B

[59] Meschede D, Dworniczak B, Nieschlag E, Horst J. Genetic diseases of the seminal ducts. *Biomed Pharmacother* 1998;52:197-203

[60] Mak V, Zielenski J, Tsui LC, Durie P, Zini A, Martin S, Longley TB, Jarvi KA. Proportion of cystic fibrosis gene mutations not detected by routine testing in men with obstructive azoospermia. *Jama* 1999;281:2217-24

In: Progress in Cystic Fibrosis Research
Editor: Margaret A. Harrison, pp. 151-169
ISBN 1-59454-232-5

Chapter VIII

Pregnancy in Cystic Fibrosis-Scandinavian Experience

Marie Johannesson *

Uppsala CF center, Uppsala University Hospital, Uppsala, Sweden

Abstract

More women with cystic fibrosis (CF) now reach reproductive age and wish to become pregnant. Although women with CF have reduced fertility, many of them can become mothers. In a study including all Norwegian and Swedish women with CF (n=132), 46% of them expressed a wish to become mothers. Of these women 75% succeeded in becoming pregnant. Out of 80 pregnancies, 85% were spontaneous and 15% conceived through assisted reproductive techniques (ART) This is a spontaneous pregnancy rate over 50 %.

Thirty-three of these pregnancies were later examined in a retrospective study. The most frequent complication among these pregnancies was preterm delivery (24 %). Lung function did not deteriorate during pregnancy, even though the need for intravenous antibiotics was doubled compared with the year before and after pregnancy. The weight gain in pregnancy was on average 10.3 kg. Gestational diabetes developed in four patients.

Caesarean sections were performed in 24%, and 79% were breastfed. No child had congenital malformation and no one had an Apgar score < 7 at 5 minutes. One child with a birth weight of 4.1 kg died three months after birth from sudden infant death syndrome. No evidence of CF was found in this child or the 32 others included in the study. The 32 children who lived at one year of age were all growing well and normal when looking at mental and neurological development.

Our conclusion is in accordance with previous retrospective studies on pregnancy and CF. Women with mild to moderate disease may safely go through pregnancy. In those with severe disease, preterm delivery is common. Our results indicate that the most useful predictor of preterm delivery in women with cystic fibrosis is a low FEV1(<60%) before pregnancy and a low weight gain during pregnancy. A pregnancy ought to be

* Correspondence concerning this article should be addressed to Prof. Marie Johannesson, Uppsala CF center, Uppsala University Hospital, Uppsala, Sweden E-mail: marie.johannesson@akademiska.se.

carefully planned since several studies have shown that pregnancy is well tolerated if good medical care is provided, and the woman with CF is in a stable good condition Women with CF should be advised against pregnancy after lungtransplantation.

Problems arise when we counsel women with moderate disease since there are no absolute guidelines of physiological, functional and nutritional impairment that predict successful pregnancy. An international prospective study is needed. Such a study should form the basis for management guidelines that would be widely accepted both obstetrically and medically.

Introduction

Cystic fibrosis (CF) is the most common autosomal recessive hereditary lethal disease in the Caucasian population [1]. Early diagnosis, intensive treatment and follow-up by specialist centres have improved the prognosis markedly for CF patients. The average life expectancy in Scandinavia is now more than 30 years [2]. The care of CF patients (total number 700) in Norway and Sweden is centralised into one national and four centers in the major cities. At these centers the patients are cared for by multiprofessionel teams including medical doctors, nurses, physiotherapists, dieticians, social workers and psychologists. The patients who live near the centers are seen monthly at a CF center whereas the patients who live further away have their primary medical care provided by the local hospital in close association with one specific CF center ("shared care"). Today, many women with CF live into their reproductive years in good health and have the opportunity to choose motherhood [3-5].

The disease occurs in one of 3-5000 humans in the Scandinavian countries with one in 40 being carriers of the CF gene [3,6].

It is commonly held that women with CF have problems with infertility [7,8]. It is well known that they have menarcheal delay, menstrual irregularities, tenacious cervical mucus and ovulation difficulties [9,10]. Infertility has been attributed to impermeable cervical plugs occluding the cervical os [9]. Malnutrition has previously been seen as a major problem for these patients probably both affecting menarcheal age and fertility [7,8]. But even with optimal nutrition, growth and menarche are delayed [11]. Physiological and/or psychological stress in these chronically ill women may influence ovulation and fertility [12]. In addition, CFTR mRNA recently found in areas of rat hypothalamus are involved in regulation of sexual maturation and reproduction [13].

The question at present, both for the woman and her physician, is how the CF disease will affect her pregnancy and how the pregnancy will affect her health. Previous studies from Europe have described CF pregnancies: 24 live births from Germany [14] and 48 live births from UK [15].

The risk for deterioration of health during pregnancy in women with CF is considered minimal if good medical care is provided and the women are in a stable good condition [16,17]. However, pregnancy complications have been reported, and pregnancy may complicate the disease [15,18-21]. Certain physiological changes in the body during normal pregnancy has to be taken into account when caring for pregnant CF women.

Physiological Changes in the Body During Pregnancy in Relation to Cystic Fibrosis

Respiratory

Normal pregnancy is a state of compensated respiratory alkalosis. Effective exchange of CO2 from the fetus to mother requires the PCO2 to be higher in the fetus than in the mother. Progesterone stimulates the respiratory centers in the brain to produce hyperventilation early in pregnancy. Secondarily to this, a majority (60-70 %) of normal healthy women complain of dyspnea during pregnancy [22,23]. Inspiratory capacity increases significantly due to flaring of the lower ribs and widening of the rib cage. This might become a problem for CF patients who are very tense in their thoracic musculature. Relaxation of smooth muscles in the tracheobronchial tree secondary to hormonal changes decreases total pulmonary resistance in late pregnancy. This might be beneficial for the patients who have more obstructive airway disease. However, at the end of pregnancy, residual volume decreases secondary to elevation of the diaphragm. This may create regions with low ventilation-perfusion ratios which adversely affect gas exchange [22,23]. All these physiological changes can cause a CF woman with poor lung function to deteriorate during pregnancy. Even so, noninvasive ventilatory support has been used succesfully in such cases [24].

Cardiovascular System

The cardiac output increases by about 40 % at week 20, and the blood volume increases around 40 % with a peak at week 30 secondary to new placental circulation as well as general vasodilatation [25]. An additional increase in blood volume and cardiac output is seen during labor and delivery. Pulmonary hypertension is considered to be a contraindication to pregnancy due to this increase in cardiac work [26].

Pancreas

In healthy women, the number of B-cells and size of Langerhan islets increases during pregnancy [27]. It is not known if this also happens in women with CF and pancreatic insufficiency (PI). Glucose provides the major fuel requirement for the fetus. Placental hormones create a state of "insulin resistance" with increased levels of insulin associated with decreased cellular response [28]. Blood glucose levels should be carefully monitored in CF women since they might more readily develop gestational diabetes. In one study of pregnant women with CF, the prevalence of gestational diabetes was 14 % [21] which is higher than in the general population [29,30].

Liver

The gallbladder empties more slowly during pregnancy, and a certain degree of cholestasis is considered physiological during pregnancy [31]. This can cause problems for CF patients since they may already have impaired bile secretion [32].

Gastrointestinal Tract

Decreased motility and increased absorption of water and salt in the gastrointestinal (GI) tract is noticed during normal pregnancy. This may give rise to constipation in healthy individuals [31]. Pregnant CF women may suffer more from this since many already have problems with the GI tract [33]. CF women may also suffer from the increased gastroesophageal reflux commonly seen during pregnancy [31,33].

Nutrition

A pregnancy demands approximately 300 extra kcal per day [34]. A weight gain during pregnancy above 11 kg is recommended to reassure good nutrition for the woman and the fetus [35]. Many patients with CF have problems with this extra energy requirement. However, it is necessary to provide a pregnant CF woman with all nutritional support available since it is known that many of the CF women who fail to gain weight adequately may give birth prematurely [7,35]. It is also very important to remember that a deficiency of essential fatty acids (EFA) is seen in healthy women during pregnancy and lactation [36]. This may aggravate the already deranged EFA status of CF women, and thereby worsen CF symptoms [37]. It should also be remembered that certain minerals and vitamins, such as iron and folic acid, need to be provided during pregnancy for optimal fetal health [38].

Immunity

The balance in the immune system changes from cellular to humoral response in order to protect the fetus during a pregnancy [39]. This is probably the reason why pregnant women are considered to be of greater risk at certain infections [40]. Some autoimmune diseases, like multiple sclerosis and rheumatoid arthritis, may benefit from this while other autoimmune diseases may worsen [39,41,42]. So far, we do not know how this change in immunity affects women with CF. In a recent animal study, it was shown that pregnancy increased the severity of chronic Pseudomonas aeruginosa lung infection in immunomodulated mice, and that pregnant mice had a higher degree of inflammation compared to nonpregnant animals [43]. Elevated cortisol levels which are seen during pregnancy [28,44] might be beneficial since there are indications that CF is a ”proinflammatory state” [45], and many CF patients also have bronchial hyper reactivity [46].

Pharmacology

Physiological changes during pregnancy change the pharmacokinetics of many drugs. The increase in maternal plasma volume creates a larger volume of distribution, and more rapid renal clearance is seen secondary to increased filtration rate [31,47,48]. Plasma binding may change as well as intestinal absorption. The hepatic metabolism is usually not affected [31]. So far, we have too little knowledge concerning the use of recombinant DNAse during pregnancy, wherefore this inhalation should be avoided. Tetracycline may cause discoloration of decidious teeth, and ciprofloxacin should be avoided since this drug has given irreversible arthropathy in animal studies [47]. Nonsteroidal antiinflammatory drugs may cause constriction of the ductus arteriosus and predispose to necrotizing enterocolitis if given late in pregnancy [48]. So far, aminoglycosides have mostly been avoided during pregnancy in CF women due to fear of fetal ototoxicity. There are no studies showing this complication in humans [47-49]. However, it appears safe not to give them during the first trimester. Most other CF drugs, including antibiotics, can be used with relative safety during pregnancy [47-49]. This is important to remember, since CF women might experience exacerbation of their disease during pregnancy. No pharmacological studies on pregnant CF women have been performed so far, therefore we do not know if pregnant CF women need higher or lower doses of antibiotics. Looking at the change in pharmacokinetics among healthy pregnant indviduals, CF women probably need higher doses of antibiotics during pregnancy [47-49].

Delivery

Vaginal delivery with optimal pain relief and oxygen supply is recommended for both healthy women and for women with CF and cardiac disease [22,25,35]. Bronchodilators should be used during delivery if necessary. Caesarean section should only be used for obstretic indications. If caesarean section is necessary, emphasis should be placed on rapid mobilization and postoperatively active physiotherapy.

Lactation

Deficiency of EFA is seen in healthy women during pregnancy and lactation [36]. This is important to remember when deciding if breastfeeding should be encouraged for a CF woman who might already have nutritional problems [50]. The breast milk from CF women usually supply the energy needs of the nursing infants [50]. Analysis of breastmilk has shown a normal content of protein and sodium, but somewhat lower levels of linoleic acid [51,52].

Prevalence and Outcome of Pregnancies in Norwegian and Swedish Women with Cystic Fibrosis

The aim of our first study was to report the prevalence and outcome of pregnancies in women with CF in Norway and Sweden [53].

Living women with CF in Norway and Sweden 18 years and older were included in the study (n=132). The number of women according to the year of birth is given in Figure One. The median age of the women was 26 years (range 18- 61). All pregnancies in the period from 1977 to 1998 were registered.

The Norwegian women answered a written questionnaire about reproductive issues. The questionnaire was sent by mail to the women with information concerning the study. In those patients not replying, interviews were performed by phone. Medical information was obtained from their medical records.

The information from the women with CF in Sweden was obtained from medical records and interviews done by the CF specialist at their local CF center. The questions used in the interviews were similar to the ones in the questionnaire used in Norway.

For the older women (n-10) there were problems obtaining complete medical information prior to centralisation of CF care (before 1985).

The information on fertility and abortion in the general population was obtained from the official statistics of both countries [54].

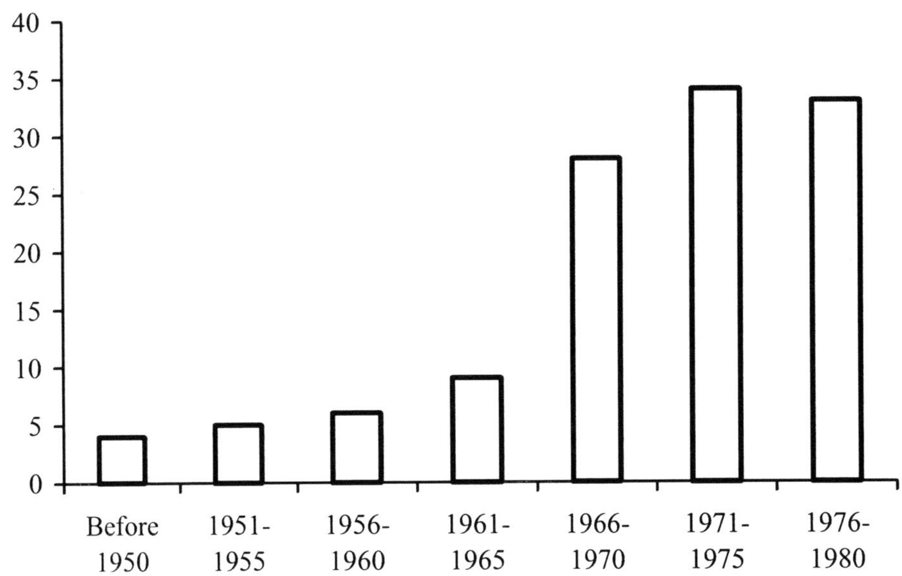

Figure 1. The number of living women with CF from Norway and Sweden according to the year of birth

Of the 132 women identified, 61 women (46%) expressed a previous or current wish to become pregnant.

Among the women (n=71, 54%) who did not want to have children, the interviews revealed various reasons: difficulties in finding a permanent partner, no extra energy to raise a child, fear of complications in pregnancy or fear of inheritance of the CF disease.

There were no differences in age or clinical status between these two groups, although in Sweden, we were unable to find complete medical information for the 10 older patients prior to centralised CF care.

The reproductive history and outcome of the women conceiving is shown in Figure Two. As seen, fifteen women (25%) were never able to conceive. Among the 46 women who became pregnant, 80 pregnancies were reported. Twelve of the pregnancies (15%) were achieved with assisted reproductive techniques (ART) such as intrauterine insemination (n=7) and in vitro fertilisation (n=5). To our knowledge, all the male partners were fertile.

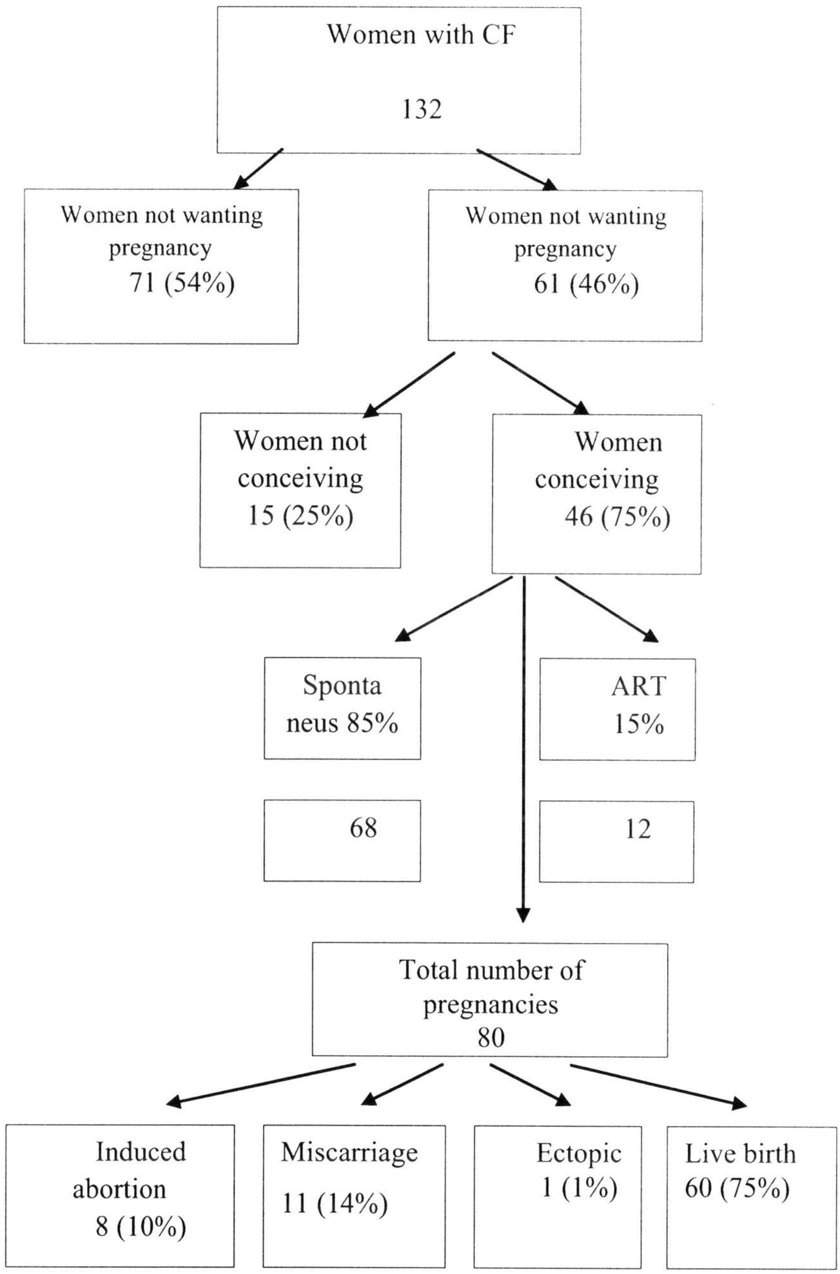

Figure 2. The reproductive history and outcome of pregnancy in living women with CF from Norway and Sweden.

The women who became pregnant without ART did so without delay. No teenage pregnancies occured during this time period.

The outcome of these pregnancies was as follows: in eight (10%) the women changed their mind and applied for induced abortions. These were mostly young women living in unstable relationships. Eleven (14%) of the pregnancies were disrupted by miscarriage and one woman experienced an extrauterine pregnancy. The remaining 60 (75%) pregnancies resulted in live born infants. None of the children had cystic fibrosis.

Maternal and Fetal Morbidity in Pregnancies of Norwegian and Swedish Women with Cystic Fibrosis

The aim of our second study was to evaluate maternal and fetal outcome of the pregnancies [55]. Women with CF with a completed pregnancy from the national CF center in Norway and two Swedish centers (Gothenburg and Stockholm) in the period 1977-1998 were included in the study (n=23). Information was obtained from medical records and maternal health cards. The data from the children were accessed from the medical records from pediatric in and outpatient clinics. The children were followed up for at least one year. Unfortunately, we were not able to include all completed pregnancies previously reported [53]. From Norway all completed pregnancies were included, while in Sweden we only had access to follow-up data of mother and children from two CF centers.

The medical information concerning the mothers included: genotype, pancreatic function, body weight, body mass index (BMI), presence of CF related diabetes or liver disease, lung function measured as forced vital capacity (FVC) and forced expiratory volume in one second (FEV1) both expressed as percent predicted for age, height and sex (% FVC,% FEV1) [56], microbiological flora of the respiratory tract. The need for intravenous antibiotic (IV ABX) use was noted for nine months before and nine months after the pregnancies.

Details of these parameters were collected at three different periods:

(1) pre-pregnancy: last recorded measure before pregnancy,
(2) at delivery: last recorded measure prior to delivery,
(3) post pregnancy: one year after birth.

Obstetric data and maternal and neonatal complications and outcome were recorded after birth. Information on social stability and family life was also included.

Statistical Analysis

The two-sample Student t-test and Chi squared test with Yates correction were used to compare the different groups. P-values < 0.05 were considered statistically significant.

The study group comprised 23 women with CF with a median age at time of the study of 32 years (range 24-50). Thirteen of the women were Swedish and 10 Norwegian.

The CF disease was diagnosed in early childhood in 13 cases (57 %), while in 7 (30%) the diagnosis was established after 20 years of age.

Genotyping showed that nine women were homozygous for delta F 508, four had mixed mutation and 10 were either heterozygotes or had no known mutation even though clinical criteria and sweat test established the CF diagnosis.

Twenty-one of the women (91%) had diagnosed pancreatic insufficiency before pregnancy and received enzyme replacement therapy. The mean BMI was 20.7 (range 16.5-23.7) before pregnancy. Two women had IDDM diagnosed in childhood (in both cases it was classified as CF related). In two other women, the CF disease had severe impact on their liver function. One woman had liver affection diagnosed at ten years of age, another had experienced a successful liver transplant four years prior to pregnancy.

The 23 women completed 33 pregnancies. One mother gave birth to four children, 7 mothers had two children, the remaining 15 mothers had one completed pregnancy each. The first pregnancy occurred at a median age of 27 years (range 21-35). Five women conceived by assisted reproduction.

Lung function before pregnancy showed a mean (range) of FEV1 76 (40-110) % and FVC of 94 (49-121) %. The change in maternal lung function during pregnancy was non-significant as shown in Table 1.

The bacteriological investigation of sputum indicated that in 21 of the 33 pregnancies, the women were chronically colonized with Pseudomonas aeruginosa whereas in 16 pregnancies, Staphylococcus aureus was demonstrated. A nonpathogenic flora was identified in six pregnancies.

As an indication of severe pulmonary infection, the number of intravenous antibiotic courses during a 9 months period was recorded and compared with the number required in a similar period before and after pregnancy. The women were given an average of 2.4 courses of intravenous antibiotics during pregnancy (Table 1). This was nearly double the use compared with the year before and the year after pregnancy. One mother had a reactivation of tuberculosis during pregnancy. She was given tuberculostatic drugs from gestational week 27 and delivered a normal baby in week 35.

Table 1. Influence of pregnancy on maternal characteristics

	Prepregnancy	Pregnancy	1 year postpregnancy
Pregnancies (n)	33	33	33
Body weight (kg)			
mean	54.9	65.2	57.9
range	(40.0-75.7)	(49.0-88.0)	(39.0-77.5)
Lung function			
% FEV1.0 mean	76	78	70
range	(40-110)	(42-100)	(40-102)
% FVC			
mean	94	93	92
range	(49-121)	(55-118)	(59-114)
Courses of iv abx (n) (per 9 months)			
mean	1.5	2.4	1.3
range	(0-5)	(0-8)	(0-6)

The mean (range) body weight and BMI before the first pregnancy were 54.9 kg (40.0-75.7) kg and 20.7 (16.5-23.7) kg/m2 respectively. The weight gain in pregnancy ranged from -1.1 kg to 26 kg, the mean being 10.3 kg (Table 1). In 19 pregnancies no additional nutrition was given. Intravenous parenteral nutrition was required during nine of the pregnancies and supplemental nasogastric feeding needed in the remaining 5 pregnancies.

The 14 women who required extra nutritional support were all pancreatic insufficient.

All together, 6 pregnancies were complicated by diabetes. In addition to the two women with diabetes from childhood, four others developed gestational diabetes which resolved after delivery.

The mother with liver disease from childhood had a decline in liver function shown by an increase of the liver transaminases by 50 % during pregnancy. A specific drug (ursodeoxycholic acid) was given, and the liver function tests normalised. She suffered from premature contractions, and the baby was delivered by Caesarean section in the 28th gestational week due to fetal bradycardia. The lung function of this mother was not severely affected. Otherwise the pregnancies did not appear to alter liver function in the other mothers including the woman post liver transplantation.

Pregnancy complications: The most common complication was preterm delivery. Eight out of 33 (24%) children were born before the 37th gestational week, two were born very prematurely in the 26-27th gestational week.

Table 2 shows the maternal and fetal details of the deliveries. In 5 of the 8 preterm deliveries, the mothers had conceived by assisted reproductive techniques (ART), while all the women who delivered by term became pregnant spontaneously.

Obstretic complications other than preterm delivery were rare. Only two patients experienced minor vaginal bleedings and two suffered from pyelonephritis in mid-trimester. No preeclampsia, no growth retardation or fetal death was observed.

The prepregnant lung function was significantly lower among the mothers delivering preterm indicating that this group was more severely affected by their disease than those delivering at term. Among our patients with FEV1 <60 %, 67% (4 of 6) delivered preterm compared to 15% for those with FEV1 > 60%. The women with IDDM and liver disease were in the group delivering preterm (table 2).

Oddly enough, the two mothers with the very preterm deliveries had FEV1 values above the average of the total group. Both conceived by ART. The women giving birth preterm did not have more exacerbations requiring intravenous antibiotic therapy in pregnancy than those delivering at term.

Twenty-three of the 33 births were normal vaginal deliveries. One baby was born after a forceps delivery, another after a vacuum. Eight (24%) children were delivered by Caesarean section, 6 were elective cases due to maternal complication. Only two Caesarean sections were performed due to signs of severe fetal distress. These were the most preterm deliveries (26-27th gestational week).

The 23 women gave birth to 33 healthy children. The two very premature infants born in 26-27th gestational week had a birth weight below 1,5 kg. One baby weighing 500g suffered from respiratory distress syndrome, sepsis and cerebral haemorrhage. However, the baby was healthy at one year of age. All the other children had a birth weight above 2 kg with a mean of 3,2 kg. No child had congenital malformations and no one had an Apgar score < 7 at 5 minutes. One child with a birth weight of 4,1 kg died three months after birth from sudden infant death syndrome. No evidence of cystic fibrosis was found in this child or the 32 others included in the study. The 32 children who lived at one year of age were all growing well and normal when looking at mental and neurological development.

Table 2. The reproductive history and outcome of pregnancy in living women with CF from Norway and Sweden.

No. of pregnancies	Preterm	Term	Total
	8	25	33
Mean gestational age (weeks)	32.8	39.3	37.7
Mean infant birth weight (kg)	2.0	3.4	3.2
Delivery by caesarean section (n)	3 (38%)*	5 (20%)	8 (24%)
Infant breast feeding (n)	4 (50%)	22 (88%)*	26 (79%)
Before pregnancy			
Pancreatic insufficient (n)	8 (100%)	23 (92%)	31 (88%)
IDDM	2 (25 %)*	0 (0%)	2 (6 %)
Liver disease	2 (25 %)*	0 (0 %)	2 (6 %)
ART (n)	5 (63%)*	0 (0%)	5 (15%)
Mean courses of intravenous antibiotics (n) one year before pregnancy	3.0	1.7	2.0
Mean body weight (kg)	59.5	56.4	57.2
Mean BMI (kg/m2)	21.7	20.7	20.9
Mean %FEV1.0	63%*	80%	76%
Mean %FVC	84%	97%	94%
During pregnancy			
Mean weight gain (kg)	5.5	11.8*	10.3
Courses of intravenous antibiotics (n)	3 (38%)	14 (56%)	17 (51%)
Gestational diabetes (n)	0	4 (17%)	4 (12%)
Pregnancy complications (n)	2 (25%)	2 (8%)	4 (12%)

* $p<0,05$ (chi square)

Twenty six of the 33 babies (79%) were breastfed. However, the breast feeding was stopped before three months. The mothers who delivered preterm were less likely to breastfeed their babies (Table 2).

All the women lived in stable relationships with the fathers to their children before and one year after the pregnancies.

Discussion

The results from our first study indicate that CF women of today have less infertility problems than previously described [9]. Among the 61 women wishing to become pregnant, 64 % had already succeeded without ART. This is in contrast to the 20% reported in 1973 by Kopito et al. [9], but in accordance with the 67 % observed in 1995 by Sawyer et al. [57]. The higher fertility rate today is probably a reflection of better overall treatment.

More than half of the women did not want to have children. Several of the Scandinavian women with CF are still young and have no wish for a family at present time. Others fear for the future for themselves and their children.

Studies have shown that women with CF with moderate to severe lung disease (forced expiratory volume 1 second (FEV1) <50%), colonisation with Burkholderia cepacia, pancreatic insufficiency, poor nutrition and diabetes mellitus produce more preterm infants and do worse themselves [18-21].

However, it has also been shown that these women may tolerate pregnancies better than expected [21].The risk for deterioration of health during pregnancy for CF patients is considered small if good medical care is provided and the women are in a stable clinical condition [16,17]. Pre-pregnancy lung function and body weight appear to be useful indicators for the outcome of both mother and child [21].

However, as will be discussed later, there are no prospective studies of pregnancies in women with CF done so far. This is important to remember for caregivers and takers.

The ethical issues regarding whether women with CF should become mothers or not are complicated [58]. It is also important to explain the mode of inheritance of cystic fibrosis. Genetic counselling should be given since the disease is autosomal recessive. If the male partner has no known mutations, the risk of having a CF child is extremely small [59]. However, the child of a CF mother will always be a carrier of one CF mutation.

These potential problems and concerns indicate that patients with CF and their doctors need updated information.

Ten percent of the pregnancies among the women in our study were terminated by abortion. This is less than the induced abortion rate in the Norwegian female population [54], being 20 % of all pregnancies. This may indicate that the Scandinavian women with CF are very motivated when they become pregnant. Moreover, in a Canadian study with 111 pregnancies the therapeutic abortion rate in 1990 was reported to be 22% [21]. In a recent English report 30% chose therapeutic abortion [15], while only 16% of the women in a German study [14], however these data may be misleading due to reporting bias.

The miscarriage rate of 15% in the women with CF is approximately as expected in the general population, and within the 2,6 – 21,4% range reported previously [15].

Extra uterine pregnancy was only observed in one out of 80 pregnancies, which is similar to the frequency in the general population. It might be speculated that women with CF should have an increased risk of this condition. However, the ciliary epithelium of the Fallopian tubes in these women appears to function normally. Extra uterine pregnancies have not been a common problem reported in other studies [15,21], and there are no published studies looking specifically at the fallopian tube function in women with CF.

Due to the high spontaneous pregnancy rate found among the women in our study, we recommend that women with CF, who are sexually active and do not want a baby ,use contraceptive methods. All barrier methods (e.g diaphragm and condom) are safe for the woman but relatively unreliable. Intrauterine contraceptive device (IUCD) can also be used, but should be avoided in nullipara as in healthy women. It has been debated whether oral combination contraceptives are suitable for women with CF. Concern has been raised about worsening of lung function due to the gestagen component of oral contraceptives, impaired glucose tolerance and the risk of intrahepatic cholestasis [60-62]. So far, no studies have proven them to be harmful, therefore they can be recommended for CF women without other complications, such as severe liver disease [60-63].

There is some evidence that oral contraceptives may be less effective during antibiotic treatment [61,62]. Women are advised to use barrier methods during and for seven days after an antibiotic course. Barrier methods are also recommended to minimise risk of acquiring or transmitting infection especially candida.

In our second study 23 women with CF attending three centers in Scandinavia were followed during 33 successful pregnancies [55]. This group of women might reflect a healthier subgroup of the CF population since 30 % were diagnosed late, and the national maternal death registers in Norway and Sweden have not recorded a single mother with CF dying during the last 20 years.

The group of women who gave birth prematurely had more severe CF with poorer lung function and more CF related complications including diabetes and liver disease. Although their nutritional status was good at the start of pregnancy, their weight gain was less than in the term group even after correction for the gestational length (Table 2). In contrast, they did not require more intravenous antibiotic treatment than the term group.

The most important predictor of the severity of CF disease appears to be the prepregnant lung function [21]. The women had %FEV1 from 40 to 110 % and %FVC from 49 to 121 % before pregnancy, but in 16 women (70 %) the lung function was only slightly affected (%FEV1>60). Pregnancy per se did not seem to affect the lung function.

Compared to studies from other European countries, the Scandinavian women seemed to maintain a better lung capacity during pregnancy [14,15]. In the reports from UK [15,19] a loss of 13% of FEV1 and 11% of FVC during pregnancy was observed. This difference might be due to milder disease in our group of women (30% of the women were diagnosed after 20 years of age) or difference in the way data was reported. However, the need for intensified antibiotic treatment during pregnancy found in our study might also be of significance.

As mentioned in the introduction, results from an animal study showed that pregnancy increased the severity of chronic Pseudomonas aeruginosa lung infection in immunomodulated mice, and that pregnant mice had a higher degree of inflammation compared to nonpregnant animals [43]. This could explain why the women in study II needed more antibiotics during pregnancy. Another interpretation of the increased use of antibiotics during pregnancy could also be more intensive surveillance of the women and increased willingness from the women's side to use antibiotics to protect the growing fetus.

Increased need for antibiotics has not been reported in previous studies [14,15,21].

Another explanation for stable lung function among our women may be that they had a larger weight gain (+10,3 kg) during pregnancy compared to the other European studies [14,15]. The weight gain during pregnancy showed a 19% increase, which is within the normal range. Pregnancy did not seem to affect body weight measured one year after birth.

Impaired glucose tolerance is common in patients with CF [63,64]. Among the CF women who were not diabetic prior to pregnancy (n=21), four developed gestational diabetes (19%). OGTT is recommended for pregnant CF women at 20 weeks gestation, and careful watch of glucose homeostasis is required during infection, delivery and in the post partum period.

The risk of preterm delivery was increased in the women with CF compared with normal pregnant population (24% versus 6%) [54]. Three of the 8 preterm births occurred in women who had low lung function pre-pregnancy (FEV1.0 < 60%) and who had required assisted reproduction to conceive. They had a history of CF related complications before pregnancy. The need for additional nutrition support was higher in the mothers of the preterm group than in the women going through a full term pregnancy, but the need for intravenous courses of antibiotics did not differ between the groups.

Our results indicate that the most useful predictor of preterm delivery in women with CF is a low FEV1.0 (<60%) before pregnancy and a low weight gain during pregnancy.

Concerning the mode of delivery, 24% of the children were delivered by Caesarean section. After evaluating the birth records and the mothers' status, it seemed that half of these children could without doubt have been born by vaginal delivery. Previously it has been feared that mothers with CF would not have the lung capacity to undergo a normal vaginal birth. Today with optimal care and follow-up in pregnancy this should not be necessary.

Conclusion

In conclusion, women with CF today seem to have a better chance of getting pregnant with a successful outcome than previously. In study I, 75% of the women with CF who wanted to become pregnant managed to conceive. Sixty of 72 continued pregnancies (83%) resulted in a liveborn infant. However, various assisted techniques was required in 15% of the pregnancies. In women not planning a pregnancy, the use of contraception should be stressed.

In study II it was shown that pregnancy appeared to be safe for some women with CF. Maternal obstretic complications were rare and pregnancy did not worsen the disease in those who were otherwise healthy.

Those with FEV1.0 <60% and complicated disease (diabetes, liver affection and asthma) may have an increased risk of preterm birth and associated complications of the infant. It is important that these groups of women are especially monitored and regarded as high-risk pregnancies.

So far, the experience concerning lung transplantation and pregnancy is limited. Therefore women with CF post lung transplantation should be advised against pregnancy. It appears as if female lung transplant recipients have an increased risk of rejection of the transplanted lung during or after pregnancy compared to other solid organ transplant patients [65-67]. This finding requires further studies.

The known side effects of the classic immunosuppresive medicines-cyclosporine A, azathioprine and steroids on the fetus are high incidence of low birth weight and prematurity More novel immunosuppresive agents such as mycophenolate mofetil (MMF) might increase the risk for birth defects and/or spontaneous miscarriage [66,68].

All together, it is very hard to advise women with CF about pregnancy. There are both medical and ethical aspects that need to be addressed.

Problems arise when we counsel women with moderate disease since there are no absolute guidelines for physiological, functional and nutritional impairment that predict successful pregnancy.

We also have to remember also that being a mother to a newborn baby is very time consuming.

This might be one of the reasons why we see deterioration in lung function one year after pregnancy in our second study (Table 1).

In the management of patients with CF, a team approach is needed. Up-to-date guidelines on how to handle and advise women with CF in fertile age should be available for health care providers dealing with these women. With optimal care, a successful outcome of pregnancy for the mother with CF and her child is possible. Intensified support after delivery should not be forgotten.

Modern obstetric practice uses ratified guidelines for the management of common medical conditions occurring in pregnancy. One example would be the management of pregnancy in women with diabetes mellitus. Common guidelines exist for this condition that apply throughout Western obstetric practice and are useful not only to professionals but also patients themselves. As the number of pregnancies in women with CF increases the time has come for the development of similar guidelines. Such guidelines should be developed from robust data which only a prospective study of pregnancy in women with CF could provide.

A survey of the medical literature suggests that there is no consensus view on the best way to manage pregnant women with CF. In particular, the literature at the moment is contradictory on the best obstetric and medical management of women with CF, especially those who have poor lung function, pancreatic insufficiency or colonization with Burkholderia cepacia complex.

A recent large and statistically powerful American study [17] suggested that women with CF who became pregnant did not have a worse outcome compared with women who did not, irrespective of the severity of their disease. European data casts doubt on this assertion [15,19]. Physicians and obstreticians in Europe dealing with sub-sets of CF patients, for example, those with pancreatic insufficiency, lung function below FEV1 of 50% or colonization with Burkholderia cepacia complex, believe that they are a special case with specific complications–both obstetric and medical. The American study mentioned above [17] suggested no significant interaction between pancreatic insufficiency, Burkholderia cepacia complex colonization or the presence of insulin dependent diabetes mellitus.

The real issue is what happens to sub-sets of CF patients when they carry their pregnancies to term. Had the American study been analysed only for women who proceeded to delivery the results of the various sub-sets might have been different. The problem with all current studies on pregnancy and cystic fibrosis are that they are retrospective. Hence the need for a prospective study.

An international prospective study is needed since no single country has sufficient numbers of CF women who become pregnant during a reasonable timeframe such that statistical rigor can be applied to the data , for example, for the prevalence of perinatal mortality, premature labour, congenital anomalies or the long term survival in certain subsets of patients with CF. Such an international prospective study should form the basis for management guidelines that would be widely accepted both obstetrically and medically.

References

[1] Boat T, Welsh MJ, Beaudet AL. Cystic Fibrosis. In: Scriver CR, Beaudet AL, Sly WS, Valle D, (eds.): *The Metabolic Basis of Inherited Disease*. 6th edn. New York: McGraw-Hill, 1989: 2649-2680.

[2] Fredriksen B, Lanng S, Koch C, Höiby N. Improved survival in the Danish center-treated cystic fibrosis patients: results of aggressive treatment. *Pediatr Pulmonol* 1996; 21: 153-8.

[3] Fluge G.Cystisk Fibrose i Helseregion, Vest. (Cystic Fibrosis in the Western health region in Norway). *Tidsskrift Nor Laegeforen* 2000; 120:568-71.

[4] Fredriksen B, Lanng S, Koch C, Höiby N. Improved survival in the Danish center-treated cystic fibrosis patients: results of aggressive treatment. *Pediatr Pulmonol* 1996; 21: 153-8.

[5] Willet MJ, Ellis AG. Reproductive health in women with cystic fibrosis. *Hosp Med* 1999; 60:863-7.

[6] Dahl N, Grandell U, Martinsson T et al Frequency of four cystic fibrosis mutations in a Swedish population. *Acta Paediatr* 1993; 82:609.

[7] Kotloff RM, FitzSimmons SC, Fiel SB. Fertility and pregnancy in patients with cystic fibrosis. *Clin Chest Med* 1992; 13:623-35.

[8] Stead RJ, Hodson ME, Batten JC, Adams J, Jacobs HS. Amenorrhea in cystic fibrosis. *Clin Endocrinol* 1987; 26: 187-95.

[9] Kopito LE, Kosasky HJ, Shwachman H. Water and electrolytes in cervical mucus from patients with cystic fibrosis. *Fertil Steril* 1973; 24: 512-16.

[10] Johannesson M, Csemiczky G, Landgren, B-M, Hjelte L, Gottlieb C. Female patients with cystic fibrosis suffer from reproductive endocrinological disorders despite good clinical status. *Hum Reprod* 1998; 13: 2092-7.

[11] Johannesson M, Gottlieb C, Hjelte L. Delayed puberty in girls with cystic fibrosis despite good clinical status. *Pediatrics* 1997; 99: 29-34.

[12] Speroff L, Glass RH, and Kase NG. *Amenorrhea. In Clinical Gynecological endocrinology and infertility*. Speroff L, Glass RH, Kase NG, (eds.) 5th edition. Williams &Wilkins, Baltimore, 1994: pp 401.

[13] Johannesson M, Bogdanovic N, Sandberg et al: Cystic Fibrosis mRNA expression in rat brain: cerebral cortex and preoptic area. *Neuroreport*. 1997;8: 535-539.

[14] Metz OW, Metz S. Schwangerschaft und Geburt bei Mukoviszidose – Resultate der Deutschland-Studie. *Klin Padiatr* 1992; 204: 145-9.

[15] Edenborough FP, Mackenzie WE, Stableforth DE. The outcome of 72 pregnancies in 55 women with cystic fibrosis in the United Kingdom 1977-1996. *Br J Obstet Gynaecol* 2000; 107: 254-61.

[16] FitzSimmons SC, Fitzpatrick S, Thompson B, Aitkin M, Fiel S, Winnie G, Hilman B. A longitudinal study of the effects of pregnancy on 325 women with cystic fibrosis. 10th North American Cystic Fibrosis Conference. *Pediatr Pulmonol* 1996; 13: 99-101.

[17] Goss CH, Rubenfeld GD, Otto K, Aitken ML. The effect of pregnancy on survival in women with cystic fibrosis. *Chest* 2003; 124:1460-68.

[18] Frangolias DD, Nakielna EM, Wilcox PG. Pregnancy and Cystic Fibrosis. A Case-Controlled Study. *Chest* 1997; 111: 963-9.

[19] Edenborough FP, Stableforth DE, Webb AK, Mackenzie WE, Smith DL. Outcome of pregnancy in women with cystic fibrosis. *Thorax* 1995; 50: 170-4.

[20] Jankelson D, Robinson M, Parsons S, Torzillo P, Peat B, Bye P. Cystic fibrosis and pregnancy. *Aust NZJ Obstet Gynaecol* 1998; 38: 180-4.

[21] Gilljam M, Antoniou M, Shin J, Dupuis A, Corey M, Tullis E. Pregnancy in Cystic Fibrosis. Fetal and Maternal outcome. *Chest* 2000; 118: 85-91.

[22] Elkus R, Popovich J. Respiratory physiology in pregnancy. *Clinics in Chest Medicine* 1992; 13:555-565.

[23] Weinberger SE, Weiss SC, CohenWR, Woodrow Weiss J, Sott Johnson T. State of the art: Pregnancy and the lung. *Am Rev Resp Dis* 1980; 121:559-581.

[24] Butler, JA, Esmond GM, Mickelsons C, Empey DW. Pregnancy assisted by nasal intermittent positive pressure ventilation in a patient with cystic fibrosis. *J Royal Soc Med* 1997; 90:222-223.

[25] Mogensen L Cardiac considerations related to pregnancy. *J Intern Med* 1994; 235:383-385.

[26] McAnulty JH, Metcalfe J, Ueland K Cardiovascular disease. *In Medical Complications During Pregnancy* 1988 Eds: Burrow GN, Ferris TF. 3rd edition WB Saunders, Philadelphia

[27] Puavilai G, Drogny EC, Domont LA, Bauma G. Insulin receptors and insulin resistance in human pregnancy: evidence for a post receptor defect in insulin action. *J Clin Endo Metab* 1982; 54:247-253.

[28] Speroff L, Glass RH, Kase NG. *The endocrinology of pregnancy*. 1994. In Clinical Gynecological endocrinology and infertility. Eds: Speroff L, Glass RH, Kase NG. 5th edition. Williams &Wilkins, Baltimore, USA.

[29] Pausi K, McFarland KF. Management of diabetes in pregnancy. *Am Fam Physician* 1997; 55:2731-2738.

[30] Coustan D. Screeing and testing for gestational diabetes Obstet *Gynecol Clin North Am* 1996; 23:126-136.

[31] McFayden IR. *Maternal changes in normal pregnancy*. 1989. In Obstretics. Eds: Turnbull SA, Chamberlain G. Churchill Livingstone, Edinburgh, London, Melbourne and New York.

[32] Lindblad A. Liver *disease in cystic fibrosis*. PhD thesis, May 1998 Gothenburg Sweden.

[33] Eggermont E. Gastrointestinal manifestations in cystic fibrosis. *Eur J Gastro Hepatol* 1996; 8:731-738.

[34] King JC, Butte NF, Bronstein MN, Kopp LE, Lindquist SA. Energy metabolism during pregnancy: influence of maternal energy status. *Am J Clin Nutr* 1994;59 (suppl) :439S-445S.

[35] Hilman BC, Aitken ML, Constantinescu M. Pregnancy in patients with cystic fibrosis. *Clin Obstet Gynecol* 1996; 39:70-86.

[36] Holman RT, Johnson SB, Ogburn PL. Deficiency of essential fatty acids and membrane fluidity during pregnancy and lactation. *Proc Natl Acad Sci* 1991; 88:4835-4839.

[37] Strandvik B. Relation between essential fatty acid metabolism and gastrointestinal symptoms in cystic fibrosis. *Acta Paediatr Scand Suppl* 1989; 363:58-65.

[38] Colie CF. Medications in pregnancy. *Curr Opinion Obstretics & Gynecology* 1996; 8:398-402.

[39] Wegmann TG, Lin H, Guilbert L, Mosmann TR Bidirectional cytokine interactions in the maternal-fetal relationship: is succesful pregnancy a TH2 phenomenon? *Imm Today* 1993; 14:353-356.

[40] Brabin BJ. Epidemiology of infection in pregnancy. Rev Inf Dis 1985; 7:579-603.

[41] Da Silva JAP, Spector TD. The role of pregnancy in the course and aetiology of rheumatoid arthritis. *Clin Rheum* 1992; 11:189-194.

[42] Duquette P, Girard M. Hormonal factors in susceptibilty to multiple sclerosis. *Curr Op Neur Neurosurg* 1993; 6:195-201.

[43] Moser C, Johannesson M, Song ZJ, Hougen HP, Kharazmi A, Hoiby N. Altered cytokine response and increased degree of lung pathology in pregnant C3HIHeN mice

with chronic Pseudomonas aeruginosa lung infection. *The Netherlands Journal of Medicine* 1999; 54 (s): Abstract 184.

[44] Nolten WE, Rueckert PA Elevated free cortisol index in pregnancy: possible regulatory mechanisms: *Am J Obstet Gynecol* 1981; 139:492-498.

[45] Khan TZ, Wagener JS, Bost T, Martinez J, Accurso FJ, Riches DW. Early pulmonary inflammation in infants with cystic fibrosis. *Am J Resp Crit Care Med* 1995; 151:1075-1082.

[46] Bisgaard H, Pedersen SS, Nielsen KG, Skov M, Laursen EM, Kronborg G, Reimert CM, Höiby N, Koch C. Controlled trial of inhaled budesonide in patients with cystic fibrosis and chronic bronchopulmonary Pseudomonas aeruginosa infection. *Am J Resp &Crit Care Med* 1997; 156:1190-1196.

[47] Dashe JS, Gilstrap LC. Antibiotic use in pregnancy. *Obstet Gyn Clin North Am* 1997; 24:617-629.

[48] Edwards MS. Antibacterial therapy in pregnancy and neonates. *Clin Perinatol* 1997; 24:251-266.

[49] Koren G, Pasuszak A, Ito S. Drugs in pregnancy. *New Engl J Med* 1998; 338:1128-1137.

[50] Kent NE, Farquharson DF. Cystic fibrosis in pregnancy. *Can Med Assoc J* 1993; 149: 809-13.

[51] Alpert SE, Cormier AD. Normal electrolyte and protein content in milk from mothers with cystic fibrosis: an explanation for the initial report of elevated milk sodium concentration. *J Pediatr* 1983; 102:77-80.

[52] Bitman J, Hamosh M, Wood DL, Freed LM, Hamosh P. Lipid composition of milk from mothers with cystic fibrosis. *Pediatr* 1987; 80: 927-932.

[53] Ödegaard I, Stray-Pedersen B, Hallberg K et al. Prevalence and outcome of pregnancies in Norwegian and Swedish women with cystic fibrosis. *Acta Obstet Gynecol Scand* 2002 Aug; 81(8):693-697.

[54] Statistics Norway. *Fertility and abortion statistics* 2000.www.statistics.no/abort.

[55] Ödegaard I, Stray-Pedersen B, Hallberg K, Haanes O, Storrosten O, Johannesson M. Maternal and Fetal Morbidity in Pregnancies of Norwegian and Swedish women with Cystic Fibrosis. *Acta Obstet Gynecol Scand* 2002 Aug; 81(8):698-705.

[56] Quanjer, PhH. Standardized lung function testing. Report from Working Party Standardisation of lung function tests". European Community for Coal and Steel. *Bull Europ Physiopath Resp* 1983; 19:Suppl 5:45-51

[57] Sawyer SM. Reproductive health in young people with cystic fibrosis. *Curr Opin Pediatr* 1995; 7: 376-80.

[58] Ödegaard I, Johannesson M. *Bör patienter med cystisk fibros skaffa barn? Sett från medicinskt och etiskt perspektiv.* [Should patients with cystic fibrosis become parents? Patient's own choice following matter-of-fact information is significant]. Lakartidningen 1996; 96: 3901-2.

[59] Goodchild MC, Watson E. *Diagnostic methods and screening.* In: Hodson ME, Geddes DM, (eds.): Cystic Fibrosis. London: Chapman Hall, 1995: 175-211.

[60] Penketh ARL, Wise A, Mearns MB, Hodson ME, Batten JC. Cystic Fibrosis in adolescents and adults *Thorax* 1987; 42: 526-532

[61] Fizpatrick SB, Stokes DC, Rosenstein BJ, Terry P, Hubbard VS. Use of oral contraceptives in women with cystic fibrosis. *Chest* 1984; 86: 863-7.

[62] Orme M, Back DJ. Oral contraceptive steroids - pharmacological issues of interest to the prescribing physician. *Adv Contracept* 1991; 7: 325-31.

[63] Lanng S, Thorsteinsson B, Erichsen G et al. Glucose tolerance in cystic fibrosis. *Arch Dis Child* 1991; 66:612-616.

[64] Lanng S Diabetes mellitus in cystic fibrosis. *Eur J Gastro Hepatol* 1996; 8:744-47.

[65] Gertner G, Coscia L, McGrory C, Morlitz M, Arment V. Pregnancy in lung transplant recipients. *Prog Transplant* 2000; 10:109-12.

[66] Knoop C. Letters to the editor. *J Cystic Fibrosis* 2002; 1:295-6.

[67] Armenti VT, Radomiski JS, Moritz MJ et al. Report from the National Transplanation Pregnancy Registry: outcomes of pregancy after transplanation. *Clin. Transplant* 2000; 123-134.

[68] Pergola PE, Kancharla A, Riley DJ. Kidney transplantation during the first trimester of pregancy: immunosuppression with mycophenolate mofetil, tacrolimus, and prednisolone. *Transplantation* 2001; 71:994-7.

In: Progress in Cystic Fibrosis Research
Editor: Margaret A. Harrison, pp. 171-183
ISBN 1-59454-232-5

Chapter IX

Interleukin-8 in Sputum from Cystic Fibrosis Patients during Ibuprofen Treatment

Ferenc Karpati [1,3,*], Lennart Meurling[2], Bengt Wretlind [3] and Lena Hjelte [1]

[1] Stockholm Cystic Fibrosis Centre, Division of Paediatrics,
[2] Department of Clinical Pharmacology,
[3] Division of Clinical Bacteriology, Karolinska Institutet, Karolinska University Hospital, Huddinge S-141 86 Stockholm, Sweden

Abstract

Background

To evaluate the effect of short-term ibuprofen therapy on interleukin-8 (IL-8) cytokine levels in sputum-producing patients with cystic fibrosis (CF), a double-blinded, placebo-controlled study was performed in a crossover manner, consisting of two 14-day periods.

Methods

Pharmacokinetic analysis was done by high-performance liquid chromatography before start. Nineteen patients completed the study (7 females, median age 30 (16-56) years). Serial sputum samples were analysed for IL-8 by enzyme immunoassay.

* Dr. Ferenc Karpati, Department of Paediatrics, B 57, Karolinska University Hospital, Huddinge S-141 86 Stockholm, Sweden Tel: +46 8 58581656, Fax: +46 8 58587310, E-Mail: Ferenc.Karpati@klinvet.ki.se Dr. Ferenc Karpati Department of Paediatrics, B 57, Karolinska University Hospital, Huddinge S-141 86 Stockholm, Sweden Tel: +46 8 58581656, Fax: +46 8 58587310, E-Mail: Ferenc.Karpati@klinvet.ki.se

Results

The median value of the IL-8 concentration in sputum was 88 (quartile range 118) μg/L during ibuprofen treatment and 87 (quartile range 254) μg/L during treatment with placebo (n. s., p=0.31). No treatment-by-time interaction could be demonstrated (p=0.38). No significant changes in forced vital capacity or forced expiratory volume in one second (% predicted) were found after ibuprofen treatment compared to placebo. Most of the patients did not experience any effect of the treatment. None of them discontinued treatment due to side effects: nasal congestion (3/19), transient diarrhoea (1/19) and dry mouth (1/19). Four patients had occult blood in stool during the ibuprofen period in contrast to two during placebo administration.

Conclusion

Short-term high-dose ibuprofen treatment did not result in significantly decreased IL-8 concentration in sputum of CF patients with relatively advanced pulmonary disease. Slightly lower levels during day 8-14 of ibuprofen therapy were seen. A multicenter approach may be necessary for further evaluation of the place of ibuprofen in the anti-inflammatory treatment of CF patients.

Key words: IL-8; NSAID; pharmacokinetics; sputum.

Introduction

Cystic fibrosis (CF) is one of the most common progressive, autosomal recessive hereditary diseases in Caucasian populations. Inflammation in the airways occurs early [1] and a pathological high concentration of the proinflammatory cytokine interleukin-8 (IL-8) has been detected with or without the presence of colonising bacteria [2]. IL-8 is a potent neutrophil chemoattractive agent produced in epithelial cells and fibroblasts in response to tumour necrosis factor alpha (TNF-α and interleukin-1 beta (IL-1β) after bacterial and viral challenges. It has proved to be an important marker of the inflammatory activity in the sputum of CF patients [3]. Lung infections and chronic inflammation in the CF lung demand early and aggressive treatment with antibiotics. Great interest has been focused also on anti-inflammatory agents as adjuvant. Ibuprofen has proved useful in slowing the progression of the lung disease in CF, administered in high dose over four years by Konstan et al [4] with the best outcome in patients younger than 13 years. The exact mechanism of this effect has not been proven [5]. Pulmonary exacerbations lead to significantly increased IL-8 concentrations [6] which decrease after antibiotic treatment [1] according to earlier observations. We have published similar results [7].

The aim of this study was to evaluate the effect of short-term ibuprofen therapy with special regard to the IL-8 cytokine levels in sputum of CF patients in clinically stable condition.

Materials and Methods

Patient Selection

All eligible chronic sputum producers attending the Stockholm Cystic Fibrosis Center (approximately 60 of a total of 190 during the study period 1998-2000) were invited to participate in the study. The diagnosis of CF was based on standard criteria, including sweat chloride determinations (>80 mmol Cl -/L) and mutation analysis of the CF gene. The inclusion criteria were ability to expectorate sputum specimens daily even in stable clinical condition and presumptive good compliance. Exacerbations were treated prior to start by 10-days intravenous courses with antibiotics directed against the bacteria present in current sputum cultures. Exclusion criteria were age over 60 years, renal insufficiency, liver cirrhosis, possible pregnancy and recurrent hemoptysis.

Study Design

The study was double-blinded, placebo-controlled in a crossover manner. Pharmacokinetic analysis was performed to determine dose regimen. Thereafter, the patients were randomised.

The study consisted of two 14-day periods with a 7-day washout in between. Every patient received both ibuprofen and placebo randomly beginning either with ibuprofen or placebo.

A series of sputum specimens was collected and frozen during both periods. Dynamic lung function parameters were measured after both periods.

The study design was approved by the Ethics Committee of Huddinge University Hospital and the Medical Products Agency, Sweden. Consent of the patients or their parents was obtained before enrolment.

Determination of Ibuprofen in Plasma

To determine the anti-inflammatory dose of ibuprofen needed, blood samples were drawn before and every 30 minutes for 2 hours after a single oral dose of ibuprofen. Two additional samples were taken at 3 and 4 hours after intake. The patients were asked not to eat or take pancreatic enzymes within two hours before and during the procedure. The test dose was calculated between 20 and 30 mg/kg body weight, maximum 1200 mg.

Ibuprofen concentrations were determined by an in-house high-performance liquid chromatography (HPLC) procedure developed and modified by Jan-Olof Svensson [8]. In brief, plasma samples, calibrators or controls, 50 μL, were pipetted into auto injector vials. A 100 μL aliquot of 0.1 M formic acid in acetonitrile was added to each vial and the contents were vortex mixed for 30 seconds and centrifuged at 3000 g for 5 minutes. A 5 μL aliquot was injected on the column. The chromatography system consisted of a Gilson 231 sample injector, a Zorbax SB C18 column, 7.5x0.46 cm, and a Milton-Roy Spectromonitor 3100, operating at 220 nm. The eluent was a mixture of 10 mM phosphate buffer pH 7.1 and methanol/acetonitrile, 60/30/10, with a flow of 1.5 mL/minute. Under these conditions the retention time of ibuprofen was 6.9 minutes.

Peak concentration values should be between 50 and 100 µg/mL. After analysis, the test dose was either accepted or a higher, calculated dose was given, if necessary, up to a maximum of 2400 mg/day, the highest recommended by the manufacturer (Knoll, Sweden), divided in two doses.

Randomising and Manufacturing of Ibuprofen/Placebo

The randomising of the patients was done by Programmet Design©software, used exclusively for clinical trials. The ibuprofen and the placebo (cellulose) were filled into identical gelatin capsules (each containing 200 mg ibuprofen/placebo) by the Production and Laboratory Department of Apoteket AB (APL Stockholm, Sweden) that also performed the randomization. The pharmacist, who recorded the randomisation codes, dispensed the test drug.

Analysis of IL-8 Concentration in Sputum

All patients were asked to save a morning sputum sample daily during both treatment periods (ibuprofen/placebo). The samples taken in the patients' homes were stored at -20^{0}C until transported frozen to the hospital. All of the samples were homogenized and diluted with one volume of dithiothreitol (Sputolysin® prior to analysis. Enzyme immunoassay for IL-8 was performed according to the manufacturer's instructions by a kit from R&D Systems (Abingdon, UK). The detection limit of the assay was 31.2 ng/L.

Biochemical and Immunological Analyses

White blood cell count (WBC), thrombocyte count, C-reactive protein (CRP), erythrocyte sedimentation rate (ESR), serum protein electrophoresis, serum creatinine and the liver transaminases alanine aminotransferase (ALT) and aspartate aminotransferase (AST) were analyzed by routine laboratory methods. Serial test (Hemoccult II® was used for routine screening for faecal occult blood (SmithKline Diagnostics, Inc. San Jose CA, USA). Antibodies to staphylococcal teichoic acid and alpha toxin and *Pseudomonas aeruginosa* exotoxin A in serum were determined by enzyme-linked immunosorbent assay (ELISA) [9,10].

Pulmonary Function Tests

Pulmonary function was evaluated by forced expirograms (Vitalograph Ltd., Buckingham, England and Sensor Medics Corporation, Anaheim, CA, USA) giving forced vital capacity (FVC) and forced expiratory volume in one second (FEV_1). Data were expressed as percentage of the reference data [11,12].

Assessment of Clinical Status

All the patients were thoroughly investigated by a physician of the centre before the start of the study. The results of the physical examination, current therapy, dose of the test medicine, as well as specific questions regarding symptoms of ongoing exacerbation were registered before and after the two-week periods. The patients were informed about possible adverse effects of ibuprofen and a questionnaire was filled in at each visit during the study. The investigated safety parameters and markers of inflammation in blood samples were monitored every fifth day and evaluated continuously to avoid hazards.

Statistical Analysis

Pearson's correlation coefficient, Student's t-test, repeated measures analysis of variance (ANOVA) and the non-parametric Wilcoxon matched pairs test were used for statistical evaluation (Statistica® software).

Results

The HPLC Procedure

The assay was linear between 4.5 to 146 µg/mL. The low limit of quantitation (LOQ) and the limit of detection (LOD) were found to be 4.5 µg/mL and 0.5 µg/mL, respectively. Intra-assay precision and accuracy was determined to 4.7% and 6.2 %, respectively, at the low control level concentration of 7.34 µg/mL (n=5). Inter-assay precision and accuracy was found to be 4.6 and 2.3 % respectively at the same level.

Pharmacokinetics of Ibuprofen

One analysis per patient was performed. Peak concentrations after administration of a calculated 20-30 mg/kg body weight single dose of ibuprofen were reached within 120 minutes in 14 patients; the remaining 9 patients had their maximums at 180 minutes. At 240 minutes, all patients' ibuprofen concentration decreased. Eight patients needed the recommended maximal dose of the study medicine, 2400 mg/day.

Patient Results

Twenty-three patients signed up and entered the study after determination of the necessary dose of ibuprofen. Two of them dropped out after the first 14 days, one of them due to pulmonary exacerbation during the second 14 days, while the other refused to continue the study because of supposed excellent effect of the study medicine during the first 14 days. One patient had to be excluded due to bad compliance ascertained by counting the rest of the administered capsules by the conducting pharmacist. Values of IL-8 determinations in sputum were not reproducible in the case of one patient, probably because of technical factors like repeated freezing and thawing of the samples. Thus, the data of 19 patients (intention-to-treat group) were included in the evaluation (7 females, 12 males, median age 30 years, range: 16-56). Genetically, 7 patients were homozygous and 9 heterozygous for the most common CF mutation, ΔF508 (Table 1). All but one of the 19 patients harboured *P. aeruginosa* in sputum or had chronically elevated titres of *P. aeruginosa* anti-exotoxin A in serum as a sign of chronic colonization with this bacterium, even if it was not detected during the study. Three patients had positive sputum cultures for *Staphylococcus aureus*, while five patients had elevated titres of the staphylococcal antibodies alpha toxin or teichoic acid.

Table 1. Basic clinical characteristics of 19 CF patients

Patient no.	Age (y)	Gender	Genotype	Current colonisation in sputum during treatment		FVC (%predicted) after treatment		FEV_1 (%predicted) after treatment	
				Ibu-profen	placebo	Ibu-profen	placebo	Ibu-profen	placebo
1	37	m[1]	ΔF508/394delTT	Pa[3]	Pa	57	60	43	43
2	31	f[2]	ΔF508/ΔF508	Pa	Pa, Hi[4]	56	56	42	41
3	28	f	ΔF508/394delTT	Pa	Pa	48	n. d.	37	n. d.
4	18	m	3659delC/394delTT	normal flora	normal flora	115	107	90	85
5	16	m	ΔF508/2183AA—G	Pa	Pa	66	70	49	49
6	16	m	ΔF508/2183AA--G	Pa	Pa	72	77	52	55
7	17	f	ΔF508/2183AA--G	Pa	Pa	62	64	57	55
8	30	m	3659delC/394delTT	Pa, Sa[5]	Pa, Sa	56	n. d.	46	n. d.
9	22	m	3659delC/3659delC	Pa, Ma[6]	Pa, Ma	86	89	89	90
10	25	m	ΔF508/3659delC	Pa, Sa	Pa, Sa	57	60	47	42
11	19	f	ΔF508/394delTT	Sa	Sa	87	89	75	74
12	56	m	ΔF508/R75Q-N1088D	Pa	Pa	77	80	77	51
13	35	f	ΔF508/3659delC	Pa	Pa	97	91	97	75
14	34	m	ΔF508/ΔF508	Sa, Hi	Sa, Hi	74	73	50	49
15	34	m	ΔF508/ΔF508	Pa	Pa	75	74	46	45
16	17	f	ΔF508/ΔF508	Pa	Pa	44	65	21	29
17	40	f	ΔF508/ΔF508	Pa	Pa	69	68	60	57
18	34	m	ΔF508/ΔF508	Pa, Sm[7]	Pa	56	58	29	33
19	36	m	ΔF508/ΔF508	Pa	Pa	61	61	54	50

[1] male, [2] female, [3] Pseudomonas aeruginosa, [4] Haemophilus influenzae, [5] Staphylococcus aureus, [6] Mycobacterium avium, [7] Stenotrophomonas maltophilia

Other bacteria (*Stenotrophomonas maltophilia* or *Haemophilus influenzae*) were found in single patients during the study together with *P. aeruginosa* or *S. aureus*, respectively. FVC (% of predicted) (median 66 after ibuprofen, 72 after placebo) and FEV_1 (% of predicted) (median 52 after ibuprofen, 51 after placebo) were also registered (Table 1). Chest radiographs showed major changes including peribronchial infiltrates, bronchiectasis in all except an 18-year old male patient at the time of the closest available yearly check-up. Four patients had elevated values of CRP together with signs of inflammatory activity detected by protein electrophoresis without reporting exacerbation during treatment with ibuprofen; these patients were withdrawn in the by-protocol analysis, since the primary aim of the study was to perform IL-8 measurements in clinically stable patients.

Prolonged washout period (i. e. more than 7 days) was not regarded as an excluding factor. To assure optimal clinical status during the study, five of 19 patients received a 10-day on-demand intravenous antibiotic treatment course between the two 14-day treatment periods according to the general treatment policy of our centre [13].

Analysis of the IL-8 Levels During Therapy

The randomisation codes were opened after the completion of all sputum cytokine analyses. Most of the patients were able to save consecutive sputum samples during the study (Table 2). A few specimens had to be excluded due to unspecified date of sampling. The overall median value of the IL-8 concentration in sputum was 88 μg/L (quartile range 118) during ibuprofen treatment and 87 μg/L (quartile range 254) during treatment with placebo. The Wilcoxon matched pairs test showed no significant difference between these values (p-level: 0.31). The IL-8 concentrations tended to be lower within a narrower range during the second week of ibuprofen treatment compared to the placebo period (Figure 1), but this difference was not significant. There was no difference between the intention-to-treat and the by-protocol group in this regard. Grouping of the patients by age did not affect these results. No treatment-by sequence group interaction could be demonstrated between those who started the study with ibuprofen and those with placebo, suggesting no 'period or carry-over effect' (two-way repeated ANOVA, log-transformed data). To study repeated measures within subjects with regard to periods of treatment, ANOVA was performed including IL-8 concentrations of week 1 and 2 as shown in Table 2. No treatment-by-time interaction could be demonstrated ($p=0.38$).

Analysis of Biochemical Variables

Pearson's product-moment correlation was calculated between logarithmically transformed IL-8 concentrations and median WBC, thrombocyte count, CRP, ESR, immunoglobulin G, ALT, AST and serum creatinine levels. No correlation was found in either the intention-to-treat or the by-protocol group of the patients during ibuprofen treatment. There was no significant difference between values of liver transaminases or creatinine in serum with respect to ibuprofen or placebo period either, as calculated by paired t-test (not shown).

Analysis of Grouping Variables

The possible influence of the CF genotype was evaluated by repeated measures ANOVA between homozygotes for the ΔF508 mutation ($n=7$) and the patients with other mutations ($n=12$) - the overall median levels of IL-8 were higher in the first group ($p=0.03$) but no effect of the treatment could be demonstrated ($p=0.16$). Neither elevated levels of staphylococcal antibodies, nor ongoing long-term oral antibiotic treatment against *S. aureus* (in five of 19 patients) affected the IL-8 levels during the study, as analysed by ANOVA (not shown). One of the patients received treatment against *Mycobacterium avium*, another long-term azithromycin therapy, which were considered not to influence the outcome of this short-term study.

Table 2. IL-8 concentrations of 19 CF patients during ibuprofen/placebo treatment

Patient no.	Sputum samples (n) during treatment		IL-8 (median) (μg/L) 1st week		IL-8 (median) (μg/L) 2nd week		Overall median IL-8 (μg/L)	
	ibuprofen	placebo	ibuprofen	placebo	ibuprofen	Placebo	ibuprofen	placebo
1	14	13	215	83	56	107	112	87
2	14	13	108	429	203	172	163	298
3	12	9	12	3	3	3	8	3
4	14	13	17	28	17	27	19	27
5	13	9	54	44	59	38	57	43
6	12	8	65	162	66	50	66	131
7	14	13	40	28	60	29	35	28
8	14	14	28	75	136	61	88	73
9	14	13	148	382	173	249	136	344
10	14	14	45	54	208	36	92	41
11	13	14	80	70	62	77	80	74
12	14	14	31	61	46	66	32	63
13	12	13	234	615	178	333	194	347
14	13	14	316	754	37	576	46	595
15	12	14	265	217	116	210	183	211
16	14	12	451	342	373	294	409	318
17	14	13	148	134	137	48	143	75
18	9	14	208	281	201	135	201	195
19	10	8	18	120	36	131	21	131

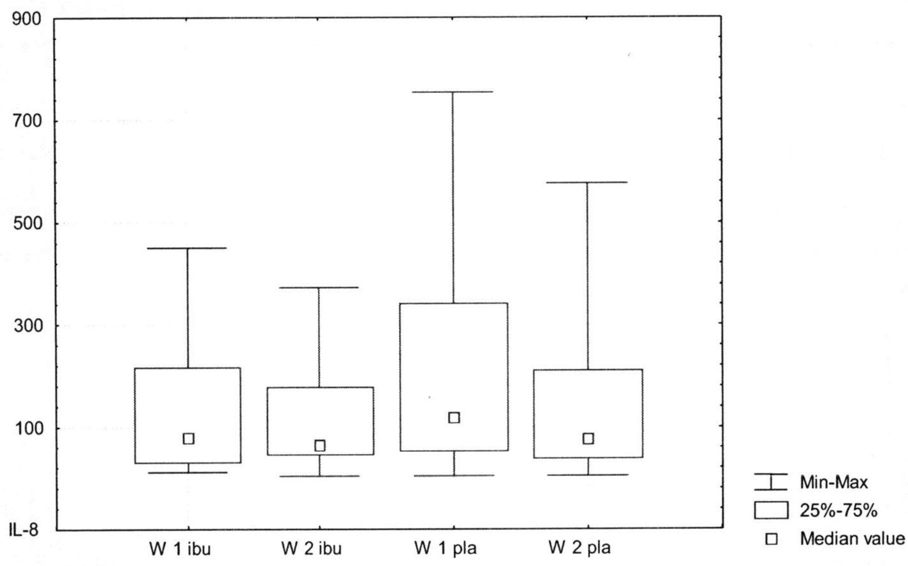

Figure 1. Box and whisker plot of IL-8 concentrations (median values). *y* axis: IL-8 (μg/L). W 1 ibu and W 2 ibu: median values during week 1 and 2 of ibuprofen treatment, W 1 pla and W 2 pla: median values during week 1 and 2 of placebo administration.

Lung Function Measurements

There was a negative correlation between FVC after ibuprofen therapy and the values of IL-8 during day 8-14 (Pearson's coefficient, r= -0.48; p=0.048) in the intention-to-treat group, but not in the by-protocol group (r= -0.32; p=0.28). Paired t-test revealed no significant changes in FVC or FEV_1 after ibuprofen treatment compared to placebo. There was no other correlation between the outcome of FVC and FEV_1 measurements and the found IL-8 concentrations.

Clinical Effect and Side Effects

Most of the patients did not experience any effect of the ibuprofen/placebo treatment. Three patients reported better general condition during the treatment with ibuprofen and placebo, respectively. An additional patient, who refused to complete the study because of well being during the first period, and dropped out, was later found out to have received placebo. Less expectoration did not differentiate between the two periods. One patient reported increasing expectoration during the placebo period. Nasal congestion (slight symptoms of upper airway infection) was reported in four patients during the ibuprofen treatment. The only patient having similar symptoms during the placebo treatment had elevated CRP, ESR and signs of inflammatory activity in the serum protein electrophoresis, while the other three had not. Two patients having crackles at physical examination during both periods had signs of exacerbation seen also in biochemical markers. Two patients reported decreasing cough frequency during the ibuprofen treatment; one of them and additional two experienced more cough during the treatment with placebo. Transient diarrhoea lasting two days or dry mouth during the ibuprofen treatment occurred in single patients. The occurrence of blood in the stool differed in the two periods: four patients had positive Hemoccult® test during the ibuprofen period in contrast to two during the placebo administration. The latter two began the study with the placebo period. None of the patients discontinued the treatment due to side effects.

Discussion

The need for anti-inflammatory treatment of the CF lung evoked controlled studies with oral glucocorticoids. Significant adverse effects have been reported [14] hampering the long-term use of this option. Recently, azithromycin has been reported to reduce the inflammatory activity in the CF lung of both children [15] and adults [16]. Ibuprofen as a non-steroid anti-inflammatory drug (NSAID) is an inhibitor of the enzyme cyclooxygenase resulting in the reduction of prostaglandin synthesis and also inhibits the migration of polymorphonuclear leukocytes [17]. It is regarded safe in most clinical situations including long-term administration to CF patients [4]. There is however concern for serious side effects. The risk of renal damage has been reviewed [18], cases of renal insufficiency occurred in patients receiving ibuprofen together with tobramycin [19,20] and intestinal ulceration was described in a rat model using high doses of ibuprofen in combination with pancreatic enzyme preparation [21], beyond numerous reports on gastrointestinal ulcerations due to inhibition of protective prostaglandin products [22]. The ulcerogenic potential of ibuprofen is regarded lower than that of older NSAIDs [23], but higher doses seemed to be associated with similar risks in a meta-analysis of Henry et al [24]. Gastrointestinal and renal side effects leading to discontinuation of ibuprofen therapy were reported in five of 81 CF patients in the study of Oermann [25]. Concern over safety was the highest ranked reason for not prescribing ibuprofen to CF patients in the survey of Oermann et al [26].

For anti-inflammatory effect in CF patients high doses are required and determination of the pharmacokinetics of ibuprofen is mandatory [27-30]. The HPLC quantitation method used in this study was validated according to standards [31]. Similar methods have previously been used for the determination of ibuprofen in serum [28, 30].

Absorption of single ibuprofen doses may be delayed [32], as was seen in 9 of our 23 patients tested. There is a considerable variation in gastric emptying between patients [32], but accelerated gastric transit seems to occur more often [33].

As most patients reach adulthood in the Swedish CF population, our study was orientated to young adult sputum-producing patients and both the effect of ibuprofen and security aspects were considered. Observations in the patient population of the Stockholm CF Centre [7] revealed fluctuations in sputum cytokine concentrations both in optimal condition and during exacerbation, probably due to regional variability of lung inflammation as seen in another study [34]. Serial sampling and stable experimental conditions were therefore attempted but proved difficult in this group of patients with relatively frequent pulmonary exacerbations. In the statistical analysis, median values were used and changes over 7-day periods were evaluated. However, there was no difference between the results of the intention-to-treat and the by-protocol group: IL-8 levels were not significantly lower in sputum after ibuprofen treatment in 14 days. The sample size in this study would have demanded a high effect size (0.68) to have 80% power. The standard deviation of the IL-8 values was also difficult to estimate in advance. There was a difference between patients with ΔF508/ΔF508 mutation and all others during both periods, which was significant. Higher IL-8 values may be interpreted as sign of constitutional over-production in these patients, as described by Tabary et al [35]. For possible confirmation of this finding, IL-8 data of 48 patients at our centre in optimal clinical condition [7] were re-evaluated regarding a correlation between IL-8 values and genotype. There was however no significant difference found in that population.

As to the monitored safety parameters, no serious side effect was observed, but a tendency of more frequent occult blood in stool was found and nasal congestion occurred during ibuprofen therapy. Regarding distinct pulmonary symptoms, less frequent cough was mentioned by two of 19 patients as a positive effect during the ibuprofen period, to be compared with three patients experiencing more cough during the placebo period. The crossover design of the study did not permit longer therapy, implying an additional limitation of the outcome. There was also a placebo effect to be considered: an equal number of the study subjects assessed themselves feeling better during the ibuprofen or placebo period, respectively.

In conclusion, short-term high-dose ibuprofen treatment did not result in significantly decreased IL-8 concentration in sputum of CF patients with relatively advanced pulmonary disease [36]. However, a tendency of slightly lower levels during the second 7-day period of ibuprofen therapy was seen. This fact is in contrast to our experience regarding 10-day intravenous antibiotic treatment courses that resulted in decreasing IL-8 in sputum already within a few days [7]. Prescribing ibuprofen treatment for this group of CF patients needs individual evaluation, but can be an alternative mainly when aminogycosides are not used at the same time. This conclusion is in concordance with the recommendation of the Cochrane review on the same topic [37]. A multicenter approach may be necessary for further evaluation of the place of ibuprofen in the anti-inflammatory treatment of CF patients.

Acknowledgements

The authors thank Elisabeth Berg statistician, Department of Humanities, Informatics and Social Sciences, Karolinska Institutet, for thoroughly revising the statistical calculations and Dr. Jon Jonasson for the revision of the chapter.

References

[1] Armstrong DS, Grimwood K, Carlin JB et al.. Lower airway inflammation in infants and young children with cystic fibrosis. *Am J Respir Crit Care Med* 1997; 156: 1197-1204.

[2] Khan TZ, Wagener JS, Bost T, Martinez J, Accurso FJ, Riches DW. Early pulmonary inflammation in infants with cystic fibrosis. *Am J Respir Crit Care Med* 1995;151:1075-1082.

[3] Richman-Eisenstat JB, Jorens PG, Hebert CA, Ueki I, Nadel JA. Interleukin-8: an important chemoattractant in sputum of patients with chronic inflammatory airway diseases. *Am J Physiol* 1993;264:L413-418.

[4] Konstan MW, Byard PJ, Hoppel CL, Davis PB. Effect of high-dose ibuprofen in patients with cystic fibrosis. *N Engl J Med* 1995;332:848-854.

[5] Konstan MW, Davis PB. Pharmacologic approaches for the discovery and development of new anti-inflammatory agents for the treatment of cystic fibrosis. *Adv Drug Deliv Rev* 2002;54:1409-1423.

[6] Koller DY, Nething, I, Otto J, Urbanek R, Eichler I. Cytokine concentrations in sputum from patients with cystic fibrosis and their relation to eosinophilic activity. *Am J Respir Crit Care Med* 1997;155:1050-1054.

[7] Karpati F, Hjelte L, Wretlind B. TNF-α and IL-8 in consecutive sputum samples from cystic fibrosis patients during antibiotic treatment. Scand J Infect Dis 2000;32:75-79.

[8] Svensson JO. Simple HPLC method for determination of antiepileptic drugs in plasa. *Ther Drug Monit* 1995;17:408.

[9] Ericsson A, Granström M, Möllby R, Strandvik B. Antibodies to staphylococcal teichoic acid and alpha toxin in patients with cystic fibrosis. *Acta Ped Scand* 1986;75:139-144.

[10] Granström M, Ericsson A, Strandvik B et al. Relation between antibody response to *Pseudomonas aeruginosa* exoproteins and colonization/infection in patients with cystic fibrosis. *Acta Ped Scand* 1984;73:772-777.

[11] Solymar L, Aronsson PH, Bake B, Bjure J. Nitrogen single breath test, flow volume curves and spirometry in healthy children, 7-18 years of age. *Eur J Respir Dis* 1980;61:275-286.

[12] Quanjer PhH. Standardized lung function testing. *Bull Eur Physiopathol Respir* 1983;19(Suppl 5):45-51.

[13] Strandvik B. Antibiotic therapy of pulmonary infections in cystic fibrosis. *Chest* 1988;94:146-149.

[14] Eigen H, Rosenstein BJ, FitzSimmons S, Schidlow DV. A multicenter study of alternate-day prednisone therapy in patients with cystic fibrosis. Cystic Fibrosis Foundation Prednisone Trial Group. *J Pediatr* 1995;126:515-523.

[15] Equi A, Balfour-Lynn M, Bush A, Rosenthal M. Long term azithromycin in children with cystic fibrosis: a randomised, placebo-controlled crossover trial. *Lancet* 2002;360:978-984.

[16] Wolter J, Seeney S, Bell S, Bowler S, Masel P, McCormack J. Effect of long term treatment with azithromycin on disease parameters in cystic fibrosis: a randomised trial. *Thorax* 2002;57:212-216.

[17] Ibuprofen. In: *Dollery C Sir, ed. Therapeutic Drugs*. 2nd ed. Edinburgh: Churchill Livingstone; 1999. p. I 1-3.

[18] Clive DM, Stoff JS. Renal syndroms associated with nonsteroidal anti-inflammatory drugs. *N Engl J Med* 1984;310:563-572.

[19] Kovesi TA, Swartz R, MacDonald, N. Transient renal failure due to simultaneous ibuprofen and aminoglycoside therapy in children with cystic fibrosis. *N Engl J Med* 1998;338:65-66.

[20] Scott CS, Retsch-Bogart GZ, Henry MM. Renal failure and vestibular toxicity in an adolescent with cystic fibrosis receiving gentamycin and standard-dose ibuprofen. *Pediatr Pulmonol* 2001;31:314-316.

[21] Kimura RE, Dy SAD, Uhing MR, Beno DWA, Jiyamapa VA, Lloyd-Still JD. The effects of high-dose ibuprofen and pancreatic enzymes on the intestine of the rat. *J Ped Gastroenterol Nutr* 1999;29:178-183.

[22] Hawkey CJ. Non-steroidal anti-inflammatory drug gastropathy: causes and treatment. *Scand J Gastroenterol (Suppl)* 1996;220:124-127.

[23] Taha AS, Dahill S, Sturrock RD, Lee FD, Russell RI. Predicting NSAID related ulcers--assessment of clinical and pathological risk factors and importance of differences in NSAID. *Gut* 1994;35:891-895.

[24] Henry D, Lim LL, Garcia Rodriguez LA et al. Variability in risk of gastrointestinal complications with individual non-steroidal anti-inflammatory drugs: results of a collaborative meta-analysis. *Br Med J* 1996;312:1563-1566.

[25] Oermann CM, Sockrider MM, Murry DJ. One year's experience with high dose ibuprofen therapy in cystic fibrosis. *Pediatr Pulmonol* 1996;13(suppl):281-282.

[26] Oermann CM, Sockrider MM, Konstan MW. The use of anti-inflammatory medications in cystic fibrosis: trends and physician attitudes. *Chest* 1999;115:1053-1058.

[27] Konstan MW, Hoppel CL, Chai BL, Davis PB. Ibuprofen in children with cystic fibrosis: pharmacokinetics and adverse effects. *J Pediatr* 1991;118:956-964.

[28] Rifai N, Sakamoto M, Law T, Galpchian V, Harris N, Colin AA. Use of a rapid HPLC assay for determination of pharmacokinetic parameters of ibuprofen in patients with cystic fibrosis. *Clin Chem* 1996;42:1812-1816.

[29] Scott CS, Retsch-Bogart GZ, Kustra RP, Graham KM, Glasscock BJ, Smith PC. The pharmacokinetics of ibuprofen suspension, chewable tablets, and tablets in children with cystic fibrosis. *J Pediatr* 1999;134:58-63.

[30] Murry DJ, Oermann CM, Ou CN, Rognerud C, Seilheimer DK, Sockrider MM. Pharmacokinetics of ibuprofen in patients with cystic fibrosis. *Pharmacotherapy* 1999;19:340-345.

[31] Shah VP, Midha KK, Dighe Set al. Analytical methods validation: bioavailability, bioequivalence and pharmacokinetic studies. Conference report. *Eur J Drug Metab Pharmacokinet* 1991;16:249-255.

[32] Taylor CJ, Hillel PG, Ghosal S, Frier MS, Tindale WB, Read N. Gastric emptying and intestinal transit of pancreatic enzyme supplements in cystic fibrosis. *Arch Dis Child* 1999;80:149-152.

[33] Collins CE, Francis JL, Thomas P, Henry RL, O'Loughlin EV. Gastric emptying time is faster in cystic fibrosis. *J Pediatr Gastroenterol Nutr* 1997;25:492-498.

[34] Meyer KC, Sharma A, Rosenthal NS, Peterson K, Brennan L. Regional variability of lung inflammation in cystic fibrosis. *Am J Respir Crit Care Med* 1997;156:1536-1540.

[35] Tabary O, Zahm JM, Hinnrasky J et al.Selective up-regulation of chemokine IL-8 expression in cystic fibrosis bronchial gland cells in vivo and in vitro. *Am J Pathol* 1998;153:921-930.

[36] Karpati F, Meurling L, Wretlind B, Hjelte L. Interleukin-8 in sputum from cystic fibrosis patients during ibuprofen treatment. *24th European Cystic Fibrosis Conference*, 6-9 June 2001, Vienna, Austria (P169).

[37] Dezateux C, Crighton A. *Oral non-steroidal anti-inflammatory drug therapy for cystic fibrosis* (Cochrane Review). In: The Cochrane Library, Issue 3, 2001. Oxford: Update Software.

In: Progress in Cystic Fibrosis Research
Editor: Margaret A. Harrison, pp. 185-213
ISBN 1-59454-232-5

Chapter X

Improving Survival as a Result of Modern Preventative Care: An Ageing Swedish Cystic Fibrosis Population

L. Lannefors

Lund Cystic Fibrosis Centre, Department of Respiratory Medicine, Lund University Hospital, Lund, Sweden

Abstract

Cystic fibrosis (CF) used to be considered a paediatric disease, as most patients died before school age. However, factors such as diagnosing at an earlier age, improved nutritional treatment, and more effective early use of anti-obstructive and antimicrobial therapy have resulted in improved clinical status and survival. The improved survival during the last decades, especially among the very young patients with CF, has totally changed the attitude towards the disease. But, the fact that fewer CF patients die early in life make long time survival predictions more and more difficult to carry out. Modern CF care emphasises preventative care to further improve survival and quality of life for individuals diagnosed with CF. In order to maintain adherence with life long treatment, patients may need support to build up self-esteem to stand up to the fact of being different, having to carry out daily treatment and take enzymes with every meal. Assessing the results of the offered CF care and estimating the future population and its demography are important in order to evaluate treatment regimens and to calculate future needs of health care resources. It is of great importance that resources match the growing adult population, otherwise the improving survival rate can not be expected to continue.

Keywords: cystic fibrosis, survival, centralized care, team-work, treatment regimen

Cystic fibrosis (CF) used to be considered a paediatric disease, as most patients died before school age. However, factors such as diagnosing at an earlier age, improved nutritional treatment, and more effective early use of anti-obstructive and antimicrobial therapy have resulted in improved clinical status and survival [1-9]. The improved survival during the last decades, especially among the very young patients with CF [10], has totally changed the attitude towards the disease [11]. Modern CF care emphasises preventative care to further improve survival and quality of life for individuals diagnosed with CF [4,9,12]. In order to maintain adherence with life long treatment, patients may need support to build up self-esteem to stand up to the fact of being different, having to carry out daily treatment and take enzymes with every meal. But, the fact that fewer CF patients die early in life make long time survival predictions more and more difficult to carry out [13]. Assessing the results of the offered CF care and estimating the future population and its demography are important in order to evaluate treatment regimens and to calculate future needs of health care resources [14,15]. It is of great importance that resources match the growing adult population, otherwise the improvement in survival can not be expected to continue [3,14,15].

Symptoms

CF typically produces malnutrition and chronic infections in the respiratory system. However, symptoms from the upper respiratory tract and the intestinal organs are common. As concomitants of increasing age, CF adults will experience additional health challenges like the population in general [11]. Added to that, what CF itself and the treatment do to the body in the long run still remains to be seen [11]. CF related diabetes is a known complication that needs to be screened for regularly and treated in an adequate way to avoid unnecessary nutritional and lung function decline [9,11,16,17] and other effects. Osteoporosis has been shown to be another long-term problem that must be prevented, if possible, not to cause severe complications or irreparable damages [11,18,19]. Joint disease and chronic pain have been reported. Depression among adults with a chronic disease is a known complication from other diagnosis and has been shown to appear in the CF population as well. Depression must be defined and taken care of in an adequate way [9]. But, a continuously decreasing lung function eventually leading to respiratory insufficiency is the most common reason to premature death among the CF population [12]. Therefore, this chapter goes a little more into detail on the lung disease.

Lung Disease

Over 97% of the CF population is reported as having lung symptoms [20]. Due to impaired mucociliary transport, the increasing amounts of viscous secretions plug the small airways which contribute to the bio-chemical environment that allows anaerobic micro-organisms (common around us and harmless for healthy lungs) to settle and grow [21,22]. An intense airway mucosal inflammation is activated, which becomes chronic and gradually destroys the lung tissue [22,23]. The damaged respiratory epithelium results in further impairment of mucociliary transport, causing increasing retention of infected secretions [24]. Larger sputum volumes are correlated with a greater degree of inflammation and hence a greater degree of lung obstruction and destruction. The more airway obstruction, the more the ventilation distribution and gas exchange is affected [25]. Study results show infection and inflammation within the airways in very young infants, prior to clinical manifestations in apparently asymptomatic children [26-32]. Airway dysfunction responding to bronchodilators already in young infants [33,34] has also been shown. The present clinical tools used to assess the degree of respiratory involvment in infants seem inadequate in detecting the underlying lung pathology [31,35,36]. Several studies have shown that most patients with CF begin to develop pulmonary obstruction during early childhood [33,34,37-42]. Colonization with Pseudomonas Aeruginosa (PsA) may be common already during the first months or year of life [43], a CF population was reported as being colonised with PsA to 97% before the age of 3 years [44]. It is shown that PsA may survive longer in airways abundantly filled with sputum [45]. If allowed to settle, the PsA can not be eradicated and reports say that the majority of CF adults are colonised with PsA [3,9,46]. The progressive lung destruction, due to the vicious cycle of chronic inflammation and infection, results in irreparable bronchiectasis, airway wall thickening, cysts and lung parenchyma damage [47-49]. Patients chronically infected with PsA have been shown to have a worse outcome than non-infected patients [50,51]. The objective of modern CF care is to prevent or postpone chronic colonisation with PsA and/or to suppress their growth, in order to minimise the chronic inflammation and its destructive effects on the lung parenchyma.

CF Care in General

Depending on intrinsic and individual variations of the underlying disorder, CF is a very heterogeneous disease. Consequently, there is not a standard treatment for all CF patients. However, there is a basic CF treatment package of which all parts always should be considered for each individual [4]. The basic package contains nutritional support, physiotherapy, antimicrobial therapy, psycho-social support and continuously ongoing education about the disease and its treatment, in order to motivate to adherence with treatment. Different CF centres have developed treatment regimens that may put a main focus on different parts of the treatment package [52].

Nutritional Support

Nutritional support as an early and continuous intervention is known to be essential in order to avoid malnutrition and negative effects such as growth retardation, puberty delay and increased lung function decline [53-56]. A balanced nutritional status is a known factor of great importance for growth, pulmonary function and suvival [3,9,57]. Therefore close monitoring of nutritional parameters resulting in early detection of negative trends and earlier intervention are recommended [3,12].

Antibitotic Therapy

Aggressive antibiotic treatment of the early lung infections have shown good results [19, 58,59] and is recommended in consensus documents [60,61]. But, side effects is a growing problem in an ageing population, the number of infections with resistant isolates is increasing [62,63] and response in more severe disease may be reduced [64]. Bacterial resistance against potent antibiotics is becoming common [60,65,66] and is an increasing problem. Whether frequent use of antibiotics can increase the incidence of PsA colonisation is discussed [50,67,68]. Newer CF pathogens like S. maltophilia, B. cepacia, non-tuberculous mycobacteria, Aspergillus fumigatus and respiratory viruses are considered to be of growing importance in the CF lung disease [69-76].

Pseudomonas aeruginosa may survive longer in airways filled with sputum [45] and airway plug formation is one factor reducing the eradication of pathogens from CF airways by antibiotic therapy [77]. It has been shown that mucus plugs may bind aminoglycosides, enlarge and cause further obstruction [77]. One factor causing the need for high doses of antibiotics is the inaccessibility of the bacteria in the plugs [60]. This may explain why increased effects of antibiotic therapy are achieved if they are combined with airway clearance therapy aimed at removing secretions and plugs [78]. Antibiotic therapy should always be combined with (intensified if needed) airway clearance therapy. Removing as much mucus and as many plugs as possible from the airways results in an improved ventilation distribution, which will influence the outcome of inhaled antibiotics too. This allows an improved breathing pattern and inhalation technique, which is likely to increase the intrapulmonary deposited dose and to give an improved deposition pattern resulting in an increased outcome of inhaled antibiotic therapy [77,79]. Therefore airway clearance therapy should always precede inhaled antibiotics in patients with hypersecretion problems.

Airway Clearance Therapy

Airway clearance therapy is an alternative and/or complementary way to decrease the amount of infected mucus and the effects of inflammation [12,80], and a way to compensate for the impaired mucociliary clearance. Most often patients are prescribed to carry out airway clearance therapy once or twice a day, making it one of the most frequently described parts of the basic CF treatment package. Until the beginning of the 1980:ies, most physiotherapists knew and used only one airway clearance technique; the postural drainage (PD) with percussion, vibrations and breathing exercises, which during the late 1970:ies was complemented with the forced expiration technique (FET) [81]. Patients were instructed to stay for a specified number of minutes in each of up to 12 positions, while an assisting person (e.g. physiotherapist, parent or partner) performed the percussion and vibrations on the chest. The aim with the therapy has been expressed as a way to remove excessive secretions thereby improving ventilation in the short term and, in the long term reduce elastase mediated damage to the airways to slow the progressive damage and impairment of the mucociliary clearance [82,83]. Many different airway clearance techniques have been developed, presented and studied during the last decades [81], and more will come as we keep learning how to use the tools; the lung volumes and the expiratory flow velocity. The new techniques emphasise an active patient participation in order to maintain good treatment quality and efficiency during every day life and to make the patient independent of daily assistance. The different techniques have repeatedly been shown to be equally effective, at least in short-term perspectives [84,85]. The collected wisdom of experienced physiotherapists based in clinical praxis is that no standard airway clearance technique will suit all patients. Physiotherapists are often of the opinion that having several techniques to choose from improves the chances of finding an airway clearance regimen that is effective for and suits the single individual. The more satisfied the patient is with the treatment programme, the better the adherence [86].

However, many CF centres chose not to introduce the new techniques, convinced that they would not add anything to the existing regimen. To continue using PD with percussion and vibration and, when >5 years old, combine it with the FET seemed optimal, since this regimen was well known to patients and caregivers. But, quite a few reports have shown that this airway clearance regimen is among the least performed components of CF care [87-90]. Patient adherence to the prescribed physiotherapy ranged from 26-47% [91-94]. Two studies showed that 53% and 74% respectively, performed their physiotherapy twice or fewer times per week [92,94]. Patients studied considered the airways clearance therapy described above to be too time consuming, uncomfortable, distasteful, unhygienic, painful, requiring reliable availability of highly skilled care givers, space, slant boards, pillows, wedges, comprising privacy, imposing on others and disrupting family life [95,96].

Although many centres have adopted the modern airway clearance techniques for older children, teenagers, adolescents and adults, they still consider PD with percussion and vibration the only possible alternative for small children, since they are unable to follow instructions. However, several reports about gastro-oesophageal reflux(GOR) during head down positions have been published [97-100]. Links between GOR and a declining lung function [100-105] have been shown. To be sure not to do any harm, an increasing number of CF centres have either changed the infant and small children treatment to modified PD (leaving out the head down positions) [99,104,106] or to a completely different airway clearance technique [107-110].

Preventative Rather Than Rehabilitative Care

An increasing number of infants have their CF diagnosis through screening, before lung symptoms are clinically detectable [111]. This makes early intervention possible, aiming at preventing negative development of environmental and mechanical changes in the peripheral airways. However, the effects of screening are dependent on the treatment offered [3], which may be dependent on expectations. Too many caregivers still seem to accept a gradual decline in lung function compared to predicted, it is considered "normal" since CF is a progressive lung disease. Such expectations are likely to lead to less aggressive therapy than if caregivers strive for a stable lung function, for no decline. International discussions often conclude that modern CF care is to be preventative rather than rehabilitative [85, 110,112,113].

Preventative nutritional care to avoid malnutrition is nowadays usually part of the treatment routines. Measurements of height (until growth is finished) and weight are routine and supplemental nutritional care is offered when needed. But, the term preventative care seems to be used in different ways when it comes to lung disease; everything from starting aerosol therapy and/or airway clearance therapy and/or antimicrobial therapy 1) at diagnosis, before symptoms have appeared, 2) when symptoms are being defined or 3) when lung function clearly has started to decline. Close monitoring of lung function in order to detect negative trends are advocated. Lung function tests carried out at least twice a year is recommended [9] and ways to carry out such tests in infants and small children are under development [31]. So far, the most important parameter is the FEV1.0, since it has been shown to be the strongest clinical predictor of mortality [114,115] and has therefore been used as the primary outcome measure in many clinical trials. Expiratory flow during the last part of a forced vital capacity manoeuvre can be of great value earlier in the disease progress.

Looking for evidence that physiotherapy improves impaired lung function still seem to be a major concern, although ongoing international discussions regarding preventative care in

CF aim at preserving lung function. Currently it is debated whether physiotherapy in order to prevent lung function decline should be started at diagnosis in the screened, apparently asympotmatic infants. Prophylactic PD with percussion and vibration places a great burden on the family, and adherence is known to be poor [83]. This airway clearance regimen is now being questioned, partly because head down positions have been found to cause or worsen GOR, but not the least because it may do more harm than good in affecting the relationship between parents and child when children are forced to do the treatment against their will (figure 1) [83,88,95].

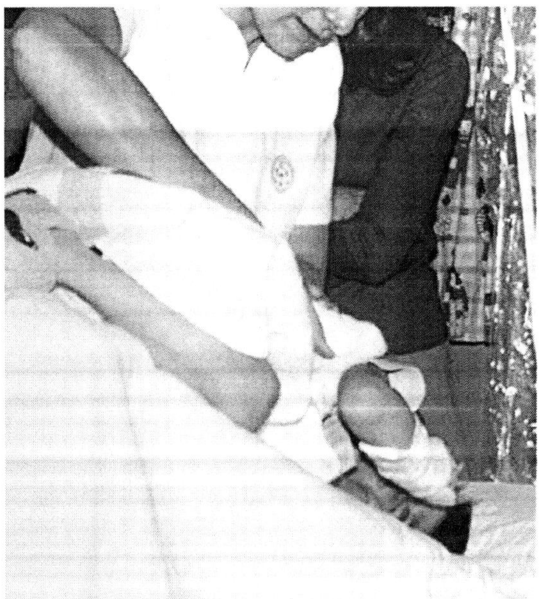

Fig. 1. A crying child placed in a 45 degree head down position during airway clearance therapy (reprinted with permission J R Soc Med 2004;97(Suppl.44):8-25).

If the lung disease can not be controlled and airway obstruction progresses, the human body defends itself by gradually increase the FRC-level in order to keep airways open (figure 2). This hyperinflation is not dependent on the CF diagnosis itself, but is secondary to the airway obstruction. The chest becomes gradually more hyperinflated as the FRC increases. But, the higher the FRC the more actively insufficient the inspiratory muscles become, since they are working on an increasingly unfavourable part of the length/tension curve. Accessory breathing muscles are activated in the struggle to maintain adequate ventilation [110,116]. If not stretched to its full range regularly the muscles and joint tissues in the hyperinflated chest will shorten, resulting in decreased mobility of the chest, elevated and protracted shoulders, thoracic kyphosis and cervical lordosis [117,118]. Many children, adolescents and young adults with CF are reported as having a stiff chest, bad posture, thoracic kyphosis and back pain [19,117,119-122]. A stiff chest makes efficient airway clearance therapy impossible and affects the deposition pattern of inhaled drugs in a negative way as ventilation distribution decreases. A vicious circle is started. The reported wedging or compression of vertebrae may be caused by the ergonomic burden of the thoracic kyphosis in combination with osteoporosis [19,123]. Bad posture, thoracic kyphosis and back pain are partly reversible [117,118,122,124], but trying to regain what has been lost can be difficult, time-consuming and uncomfortable. Vertebral fractures can not be rehabilitated. Instead, trying to prevent bad posture, musculoskeletal complications and back pain may be part of the treatment package.

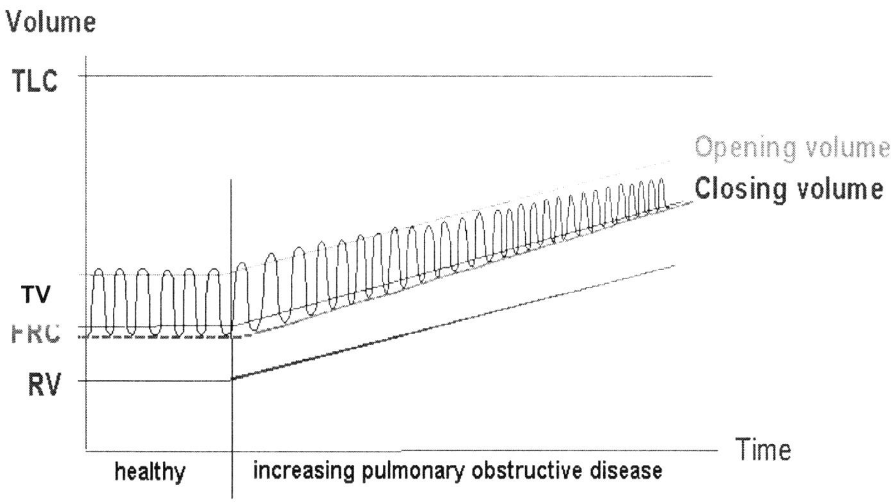

Fig. 2. Changes in lung volumes with progressing obstructive pulmonary disease. TLC=total lung capacity, FRC=functional residual capacity, RV=residual volume (reprinted with permission J R Soc Med 2004;97(Suppl.44):8-25).

Centralised Care

The importance of centralised and preventative, aggressive treatment in CF care is emphasised in discussions [1-4,13,14,125,126]. The CF team should be multidisciplinary and all members of the team must actively stay up-dated with the continuously developing multifaceted treatment [1-6,9,13,14,125,127,128]. However, the results of the care differs a lot from one country to another [6] and sometimes from centre to centre [4,126].

Results of Swedish CF Care

Data concerning all known dead and alive CF patients in Sweden were collected and summarised at the end of 1999 [8]. The total number of known CF patients in Sweden since 1971 was 628. Of these, 475 individuals were alive at the time of the study, 0-63 years old (51% male). CF is not being screened for in Sweden. The median age at diagnosis was 9 months (0-64 years) and 59% had their diagnosis by the age of one year. Of the whole population, 6% were diagnosed after age 18 years. Most patients with late diagnosis had a milder disease, but this was not always the case. There were patients who were diagnosed as respiratory insufficient adults. Continuous information and reminders about CF within adult health care of different disciplines remains important. Twenty-nine patients of the Swedish CF population had been transplanted; 24 lung, 4 heart-lung and 1 liver. Median age at the time for lung or heart-lung transplantation was 28 years (range 11-46). At the time for the study, three individuals were on the waiting list for lung transplantation.

Genetics

The ΔF508 is generally associated with a more aggressive disease. The frequency of ΔF508 mutations among CF alleles within the living Swedish CF population was 68%, 47% of the patients were homozygous for ΔF508 [129]. The ΔF508 was more frequent in the southern region of the country than in the north. Two other mutations were fairly common, 394delTT 8,5% and 3659delC 7,9% [129]. The ΔF508 frequency in the Swedish CF population was slightly lower but still comparable to that in other European populations studied, where the ΔF508 frequency has been reported to be 54 – 88% [130].

Pancreatic Dysfunction

Another factor associated with severe clinical disease is pancreatic dysfunction.

Of the Swedish CF-population 87% within the paediatric and 90% within the adult part received pancreatic enzyme substitution [national CF-registry, unpublished results]. This is comparable to most CF populations [46,130]. Data from the European Epidemiologic Registry of Cystic Fibrosis (ERCF) in 1997 including 11 749 CF-patients from 9 countries showed 97% of the <18 years old and 95% of the >18 years old to be treated with pancreatic enzymes [131].

Pseudomonas Aeruginosa Colonisation

Of the whole Swedish CF-population 48% was chronically colonised with PsA; 36% of the paediatric and 62% of the adult population [national CF-registry, unpublished results]. This is comparable to the reported 45% of a Danish CF-population [59]. A study including 63% of the whole North American CF-population reported 61% chronically colonised with PsA [46]. In the southern part of Sweden, 51% of the adult CF population was colonised with PsA in 2002 [132]. Of the adults taken care of at a CF-centre in the UK, 90% were reported being chronically colonised with PsA [3].

Survival and Estimated Population

Statistical methods used for the following parameters cumulated in a 1-year survival, logistic regression and Cox regression. Results from the study compiling all Swedish CF patients showed a mean annual mortality rate since 1991 in the Swedish CF population of 0,9% (±0,4), corresponding results specified for different periods are presented in figure 3 [8]. Similar results have been shown by Frederiksen et al, who reported an annual mortality rate of 0-1,2% during 1989-1993 among Danish CF patients treated at the Copenhagen CF-centre (75% of the whole Danish CF-population) [2]. Data from 114 accredited CF-centres in the USA in 1990 showed a mortality rate of 2,3% [127] and the mortality rate for the UK CF population was 2,1% during 1995 [13].

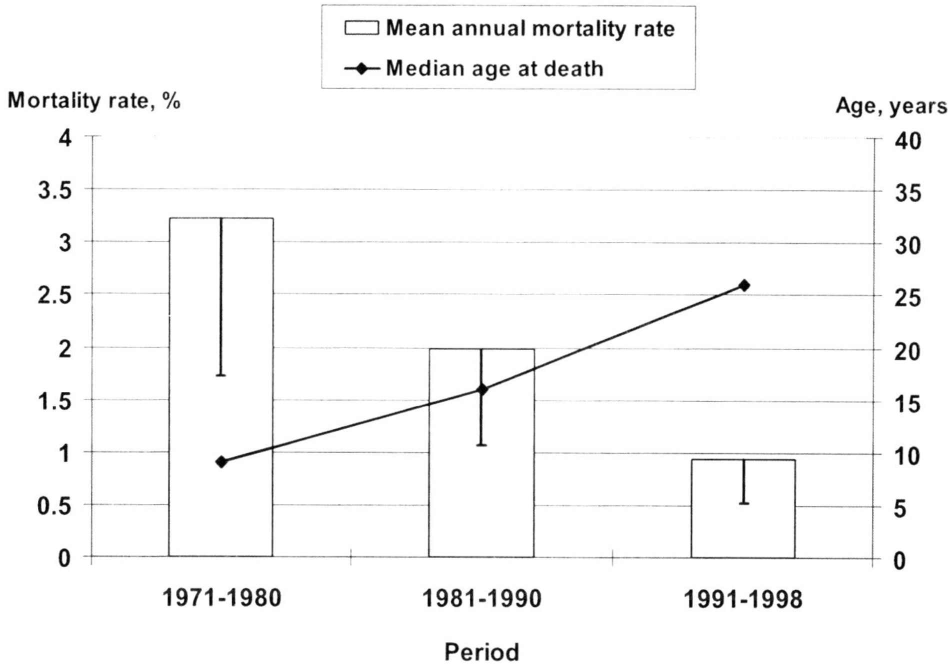

Fig. 3. Mean annual mortality rate/period ± sd and median age at death/period in the Swedish CF-population (reprinted with permission Respir Med 2002;96:681-5)

Another parameter of interest when assessing treatment effects for a whole population is the median age at death [6]. The median age at death in the Swedish CF population since 1991 was 26 years (range 0-72) (figure 3), which is relatively high in comparison to other reports [2,5,6,13,127,128].

Median survival was not possible to estimate in the Swedish CF population, since only a few patients <18 years old had died during the last decade. Instead survival was expressed as predicted survival above a certain age. Since the Swedish CF population is small, only a short survival prediction to 2016 was considered reliable. The predicted survival for the different groups until year 2016 are shown in figure 4; 95% of the patients born in 1991 or later were predicted to become 25 years old or older. The survival probability in Denmark for a child born with CF 1989-93 and treated at a CF centre was estimated to be 80% reaching its 45th birthday [2]. For patients included in the US Cystic Fibrosis Foundation registry in the year 2002, median survival was predicted into the early 30s [9]. Canadian data from 1998 showed predicted survival till adulthood of 80% [133]. The largest difference and improvement in the Swedish study was seen during the first year of life (figure 4), as has been shown by others as well [14]. This difference is probably due to the modern CF care dealing with meconium ileus and malnutrition in a more effective way [12]. Survival rate after the first year(s) of life or in different age cohorts during the last ten years may be more informative when it comes to evaluating standards for CF treatment (figure 4) [10]. Comparable differences may then be focusing on the modern CF care dealing with long term nutritional factors, pulmonary hyper-secretion, pulmonary infections and on adequate measurements of pulmonary function, physical capacity and quality of life.

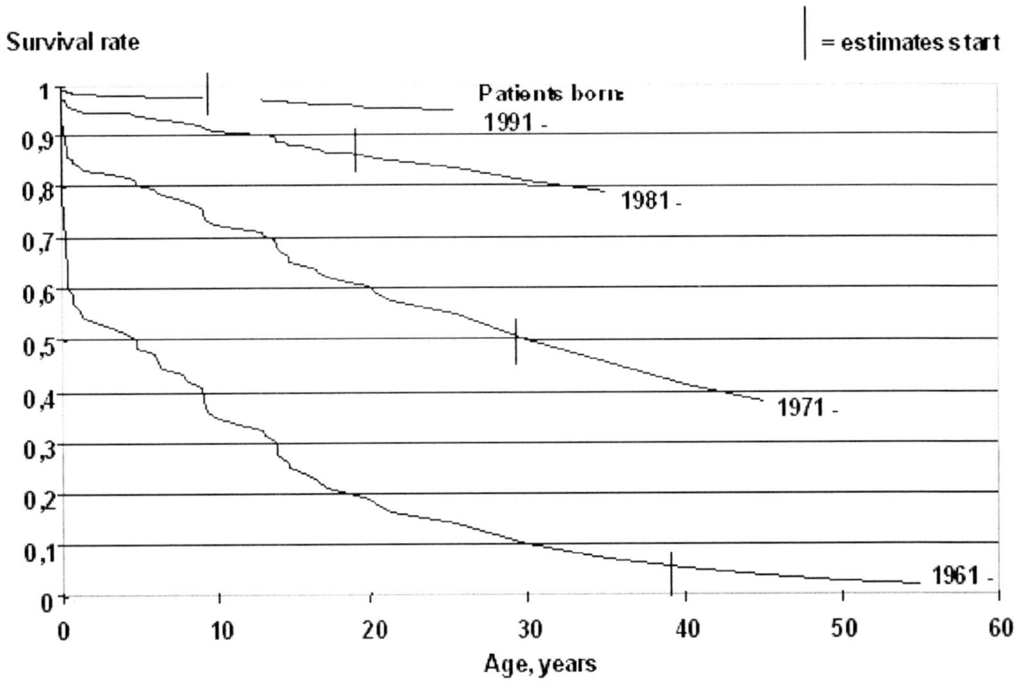

Fig. 4. Current and estimated survival rate of four different cohorts of Swedish CF patients (reprinted with permission Respir Med 2002;96:681-5)

Lung Function

Median lung function for the different age groups 7-12, 13-17, 18-29, 30+ years old in the entire Swedish CF population 2001 was FEV1.0: 93, 88, 84 and 67% of predicted values respectively and VC: 98, 97, 94 and 90% of predicted values. The mean annual change in FEV1.0 from 1998 to 2001 was between ±0.0 and minus 0.6% in the different age groups [134].

Centralised Care

Of all the 475 CF patients alive in Sweden at the time of the study, 97% were in contact with a CF centre, 54% solely with a CF centre while 43% had their care shared between their home hospital and a CF centre. The remaining 3% were seen at their home hospital only. Shared care is usually appreciated by both the patients living far from a CF-centre and by their home hospital staff, but requires "maintenance work" to function properly. Consulting clinics at the local hospitals are carried out regularly in parts of the country and/or home hospital staff are stimulated to regularly visit the CF centre together with their patients. A big effort is put into functioning communication routines between home hospitals and the CF centres and education days for home hospital staff are organised annually by the centres.

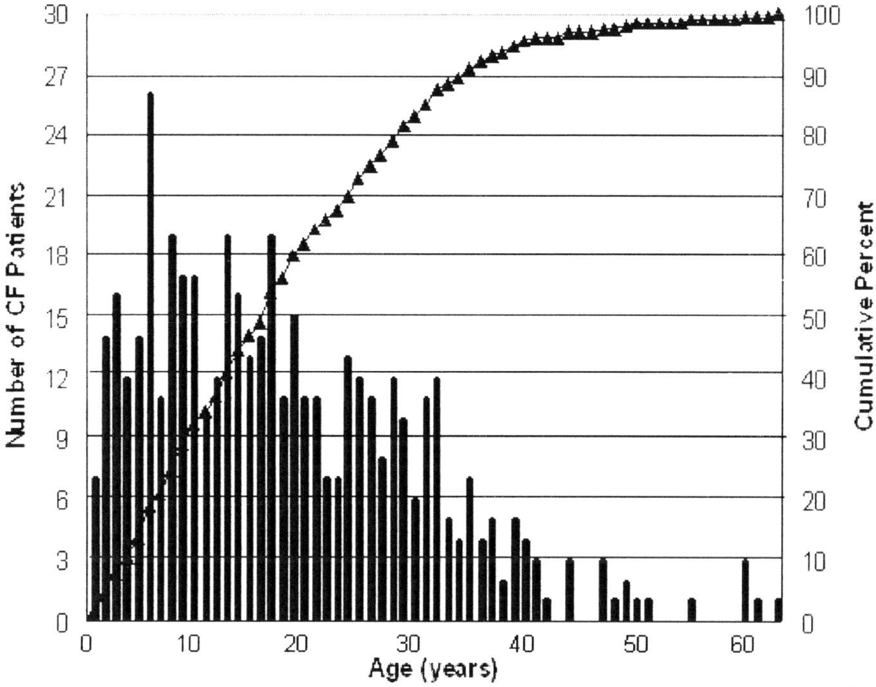

Fig. 5. Age distribution of the Swedish CF population of 1999 (reprinted with permission Respir Med 2002;96:681-5)

Ageing CF Population

Considering the high median age at death, the size of the paediatric group will stabilize while the major future increase of the CF-population will be within the adult population (≥18 years). The proportion adults (≥18 years old) within the Swedish CF population at the time for the study was 45% (figure 5) [8], compared to 32% in 1986 [135]. Data from the European CF registry 1997 including 12 447 individuals with CF (from Austria, Belgium, Denmark, France, Germany, Ireland, Netherlands, Sweden and United Kingdom) showed 29% of the population to be ≥18 years old [5]. Among the CF patients included in the US Cystic Fibrosis Foundation Registry 2002, 40% were 18 years old or older [9]. At the Lund CF centre, which is responsible for the care of all CF patients in the south of Sweden, the median age of the CF population at the end of 2002 was 20 years [unpublished data from Lund CF-centre registry]. Increasing health challenges and progressing CF lung disease in the ageing CF population will require increased resources as the number of CF adults grows [11,13].

In the same way as any child or youngster, patients with CF need to be psychosocially prepared for an adult life. Many need support to build self-confidence, finish an education, get a job, a relation and a family. Among all the Swedish CF adults at the time of the study, 22% (31 females and 17 males) had children, of whom 5 had adopted their child(ren). Of the adults who had finished school/education, 75% were working part or full time [8].

Potential Reasons for the Good Results of Swedish CF Care

Knowing that the progressing chronic lung destruction is the main reason for the premature death in most cases, it seems relevant to try to prevent or at least retard the irreparable damage to the lung parenchyma. The CF care in Sweden has since at least mid 70s/early 80s focused upon preventative care. Resources have been put into outpatient care, focusing on an optimal, individually tailored basic, preventive, daily treatment that is possible for patients/families to adhere to during every day life.

CF care in the whole country has for a long time been organised into centralised care. The four existing CF centres have multidisciplinary teams working in a flat organisation with a good communication, where each discipline's specific expert knowledge is fully utilised. The centres are responsible for the care of almost all known patients in the country. Almost half of them live that far away from the CF centre that they also see a team at the local hospital in between the check-ups at the CF centre, so called shared care. Patients are in frequent contact with their caregivers, intense during the time after diagnosis and thereafter depending on needs. Most commonly, patients have an appointment for check-up every 6th-8th week, either with the CF centre team or with the local hospital team in an agreement with the CF-centre. If/when needed, patients have appointments more often. Many patients living far away still see the CF centre team 2-4 times/year. At each check-up patients see their doctor and nurse, and they carry out a full physiotherapy treatment session together with their physiotherapist. At each visit height (until growth is completed) and weight is measured, a physical examination as well as a lung function test is carried out and sputum cultures obtained and specific blood samples are collected if/when necessary. Regularly (often if needed) patients see their dietician, social worker and psychologist. Patients and physiotherapist meet either at the clinic or in patients' home in between the check-ups when needed, to carry out a treatment session often including physical exercise. The aim is to continuously educate patients and to motivate adherence with the treatment, to optimise every day routines and treatment quality. Most of the patients who are prescribed intravenous antibiotic courses, are being trained to administer the treatment themselves at home, supported by their nurse when needed.

All patients carry out an extended annual check-up at the CF-centre. The extended annual check up is scheduled for 2-3 days to allow patients to find time during these days to carry out their daily treatment. What is included and how things are carried out varies a little from center to center. But, apart from what is carried out at each check-up, the annual review may include lung mechanics, working capacity test, pulmonary X-ray, pulmonary HRCT, ultra-sound liver, liver biopsy and blood samples for numerous analyses. Every, or every second year review includes an oral glucose tolerance and bone mineral density test for adolescents and adults. Patients carry out the daily inhalation therapy, airway clearance and the physical exercise together with their physiotherapist during these days, in order to re-assess and optimise the techniques used. The days for the expanded annual check up are also used for continued education.

Preventative Care

The goal has been to prevent airway or lung tissue damage by retarding lung disease and limiting the number and degree of exacerbations. The basic preventive CF care package is usually based upon: nutritional support, airway clearance therapy, physical exercise, antibiotic therapy, psychosocial support and continuously ongoing education, some centers use intravenous fat solutions. Aggressive nutritional care as an important part of the early intervention is probably an important factor for the good results. Nutritional parameters are plotted in curves, in order to detect early negative trends, which allows early intervention with an adequate nutritional support. Modern, active, individualised physiotherapy including physical activity is introduced at the time of diagnosis and is continuously optimised, re-tailored to be efficient and to fit as well as possible into patients' every day life. Small pulmonary signs of infection are treated with appropriate antibiotics in adequate dose and duration. All parents/patients are offered psychosocial support to build positive life long relations, to have a normal psychosocial development and to be stable individuals prepared to stand having a progressing disease requiring a lot of daily treatment. All patients are continuously educated about CF and its treatment, individually as well as in groups and camps.

No treatment is successful unless it is carried out. The treatment quality and the adherence with the treatment are essential for the results and the parts considered of importance for the single individual are continuously re-assessed, discussed and optimised if needed. Patients/parents are working partners and are always fully involved in discussions and in decisions/agreements relating to their treatment regimen, in order to stimulate adherence.

Most parts of the Swedish CF care have been following international guidelines. But, the airway clearance therapy, especially among infants, toddlers and small children has differed since the early 80:ies and preventative use of physical activity/exercise has been part of the basic therapy for a long time. The definition of the term "modern physiotherapy in CF" is wide in Sweden. It involves the whole individual in a long-term perspective and includes inhalation therapy, airway clearance therapy, physical exercise and education [81,110]. The primary goal with the physiotherapy is to preserve a good ventilation distribution and avoid development of non-ventilated anaerobic intrapulmonary environment (such as clogged and plugged airways, trapped gas or microathelectasis) where pathogens are attracted to grow. The immediate aims with the therapy cycles carried out at each physiotherapy session are

(1) to open up and get air behind secretions,
(2) to optimise the expiratory flow velocity at functional residual capacity (FRC) and residual volume (RV) levels in order to mobilise secretions from the small airways,
(3) to transport secretions to the bigger airways and
(4) from where they can be coughed up.

This concept, to preserve ventilation distribution, is part of the treatment from the very beginning, commencing at diagnosis. Combining physical exercise with FET was shown in a small but long time study to be equally effective as PD with percussion [136]. Therefore, no patients have used postural drainage or percussion in any form, regardless of age, since the beginning of the 80:ies.

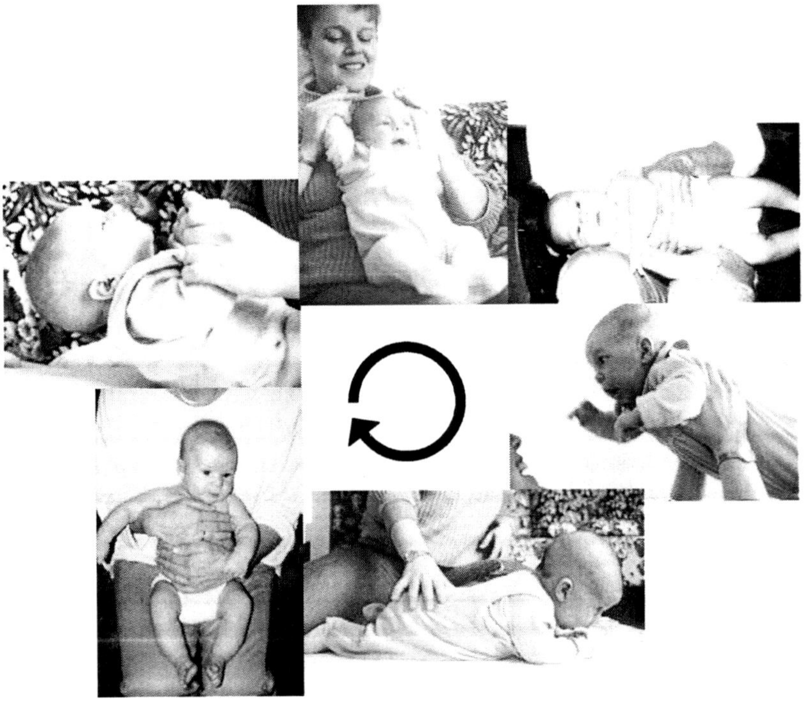

Fig. 6. An example of an airway clearance therapy cycle carried out with CF infants. The cycles consist of physical exercises and Assisted Autogenic Drainage manoeuvres (AADs)

Airway Clearance Therapy the Swedish Approach

The airway clearance therapy in infants and young children is based upon a combination of physical exercises/activities/playing and Assisted Autogenic Drainage manoeuvres (AADs) (figure 6) [107,110,137]. The fact that physical exercise has a positive effect on mucus clearance has been known for a long time [136,138-140]. The physiological theory that this way of working is based upon is to use the effects of an altered breathing pattern and increased minute ventilation caused by the physical activity to get air behind secretions [81,110]. The more active the children get, the more effects the physical exercise may have on sputum viscosity (figure 7a-h) [141]. The exercises are interspersed with AADs in the infants and toddlers, aiming at prolonging the expirations towards RV and to optimise the expiratory flow velocity at low lung volumes to mobilise and transport secretions [107]. Parents are carefully taught how to carry out the AADs in a correct and gentle way, not to use violence to make the child feel uncomfortable or the treatment to be frightening. Physiotherapy is always carried out in a way that makes future co-operation possible. At about the age of 2 years patients start to learn how to increase the expiratory flow themselves (figure 8). As patients get older, other airway clearance techniques such as PEP, HiPEP, AD or FET or individually tailored combinations of these techniques are introduced since that may be found to be more efficient. Physical activity interspersed with AADs is combined with positioning (figure 7a-h) and airway clearance therapy of other kind is often carried out in upright sitting as well as in bilateral horizontal side lying to utilise the effects that gravity has on regional FRC and on regional ventilation [35,142-145]. As soon as possible patients are taught how to master the cough and to use "controlled coughing" at low lung volumes as part of the airway clearance therapy.

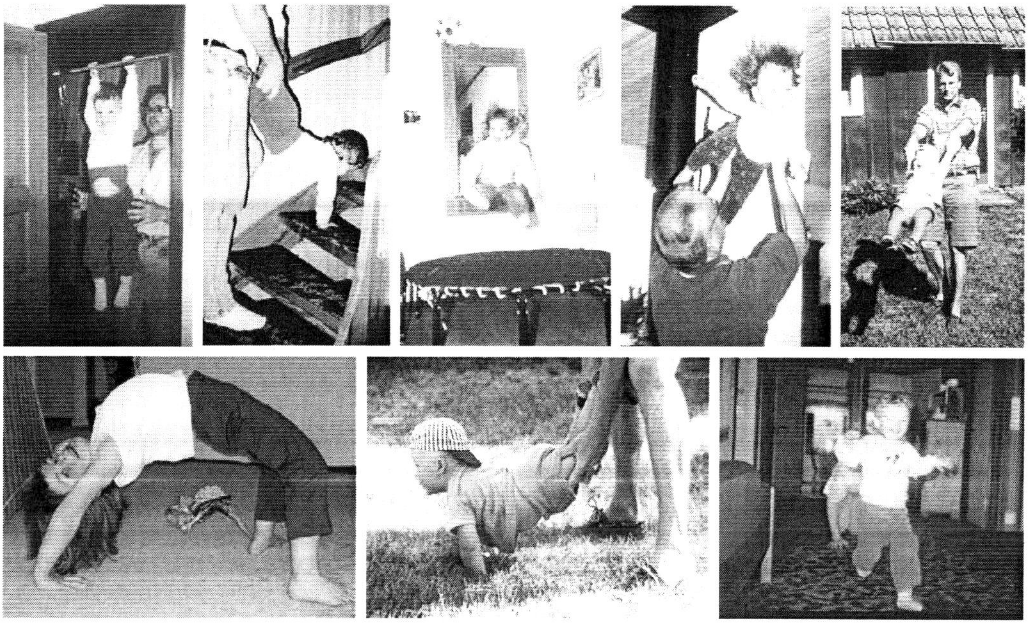

Fig. 7a-h. Examples of physical exercises used as part of the airway clearance therapy for toddlers. These active physical exercises are experienced as play, but parents are educated in what to include and regularly provided with up-dated "exercise banks" that are adapted to age and needs of the child.

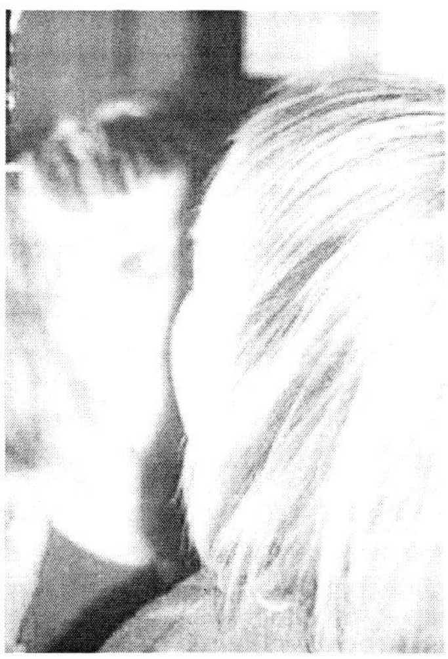

Fig. 8. At about the age of 2 years children start to learn how to force expirations by misting a mirror or a window. As soon as a child masters the technique, it gradually replaces the AADs that intersperse the physical activity during the airway clearance therapy.

Inhalation Therapy

Aerosol therapy is becoming increasingly important in CF care, but large differences in practices occur throughout the world [146]. Within the Swedish CF population, inhaled bronchodilators, DNase, hypertonic saline, antibiotics, antifungals and anti-inflammatory agents are being used when indicated and/or of benefit. Patients are carefully selected and the treatment is closely followed up [147,148]. Bronchodilators are increasingly often administrated through a powder inhaler (a MDI with a spacer in the youngest or most severely ill), not to be unnecessarily time consuming, anti-inflammatory agents are always administrated by the help of a powder inhaler or a MDI with a spacer in the youngest and the more severely ill patients. Other inhaled drugs are administrated via a high capacity nebulizer system that delivers an aerosol with a low mass median aerodynamic diameter (MMAD) and has a high output rate to be effective and make the therapy fit into every day life. Patients are adequately trained in how to use it and the inhalation technique is regularly re-assessed. In order to get the most out of the inhalation therapy, a treatment strategy is made up for each patient. One important factor considered is the aim with the different agents prescribed, is it 1) to optimise ventilation distribution and/or avoid bronchospasm by inhaling a bronchodilator prior to inhaling other agents or to physical exercise, or 2) to affect the viscosity of the pulmonary secretions that is difficult to evacuate, by inhaling a mucolytic either before or after airway clearance depending on how much there is and how easy it is evacuated, or 3) to inhale anti-microbials and anti-inflammatory agents after airway clearance therapy when as much as possible of the obstructing secretions are evacuated? If patients are prescribed nebulization therapy, they bring their equipment for service at the time for their annual check up. While admitted or staying at the patients' hotel patients have access to another nebulizer system of the same kind.

Physical Exercise

The positive effects of physical exercise on CF patients' clinical status are well known [74, 136,149-151]. But it has been shown that children with CF, although having good lung function, are less spontaneously active than their peers [152]. Since only recommending physical exercise is not known to be enough, many patients in the Swedish CF population are actively assisted by their physiotherapist to find routines for this. If physical activity/exercise is not part of the airway clearance therapy, it is recommended to be carried out as a complementary part of the treatment provided patients are in a stable nutritional status [81,110,137]. The physically active part of the treatment is appreciated by parents and by siblings, who usually take part in the activities. Preserving good chest mobility is essential to allow efficient airway clearance therapy (figure 9a-d) and a good posture is preserved even in severely ill patients (figure 10a-d) in order to look like others and to avoid musculo-skeletal back/neck complications and pain [22,81,110]. Working capacity is trained (figure 11a-b) and a good physical capacity is preserved in order to be able to live an active life with a good quality. Even severely ill patients carry out physical exercise, adapted to their current condition and with oxygen supplementation when desaturating in order to keep them above SpO2 90% (figure 12).

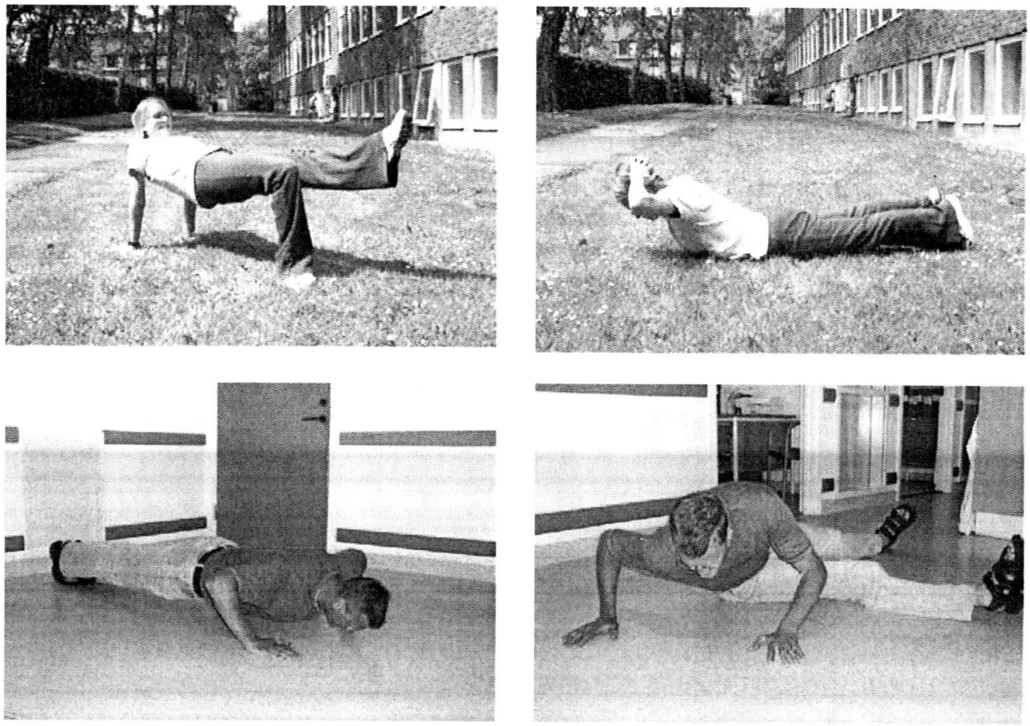

Fig. 9a-d. Examples of chest mobility and postural muscle strengthening exercises. A preserved chest mobility and posture is essential and therefore the exercises are part of the preventative treatment.

Experience from many years show several positive side-benefits from the use of a physically active physiotherapy regimen:

- Daily, regular episodes with increased minute-ventilation and improved ventilation distribution in all parts of the lungs may reduce the hypoxia in the otherwise not ventilated parts of the lungs, which may affect the bio-chemical environment where anaerobic pathogens are known to settle and grow
- Apart from looking like others having adequate muscle mass and a preserved posture, patients get to know their body very well. Knowing their body well helps patients to learn new airway clearance techniques properly and to maintain a good treatment quality that makes every day care efficient.
- Good body knowledge is being used to detect exacerbations at an early stage. Simple every day activities can be used as functional references; playing and running during school breaks like skip rope and sports, laughing without coughing, speaking long sentences while walking, walking up the stairs, etc, (depending on lung function status). Detecting an exacerbation early makes an early intervention possible, before it is settled and risking a permanent damage to the airway or the lung tissue.
- Long-term complications like osteoporosis may be less frequent with an appropriate nutritional therapy and physically active loading of the skeleton.
- Long-term complications like thoracic kyphosis, back pain and vertebral fractures, may be less frequent if chest mobility and muscle strengthening exercises, especially for the postural muscles, are included from the very beginning.

- The positive treatment atmosphere and the physically active physiotherapy is often reported as being enjoyable for patients, parents and for siblings who can participate to a great extent during early life. This allows development of positive relations between child, siblings and parents. Non-adherence with the treatment seems to be less of a problem than what has been reported in discussions and studies.
- Patients develop an optimal physical capacity which often makes them excel at gymnastics in pre-school and school, giving them an unshakeable self-esteem that is positive for the rest of their lives.

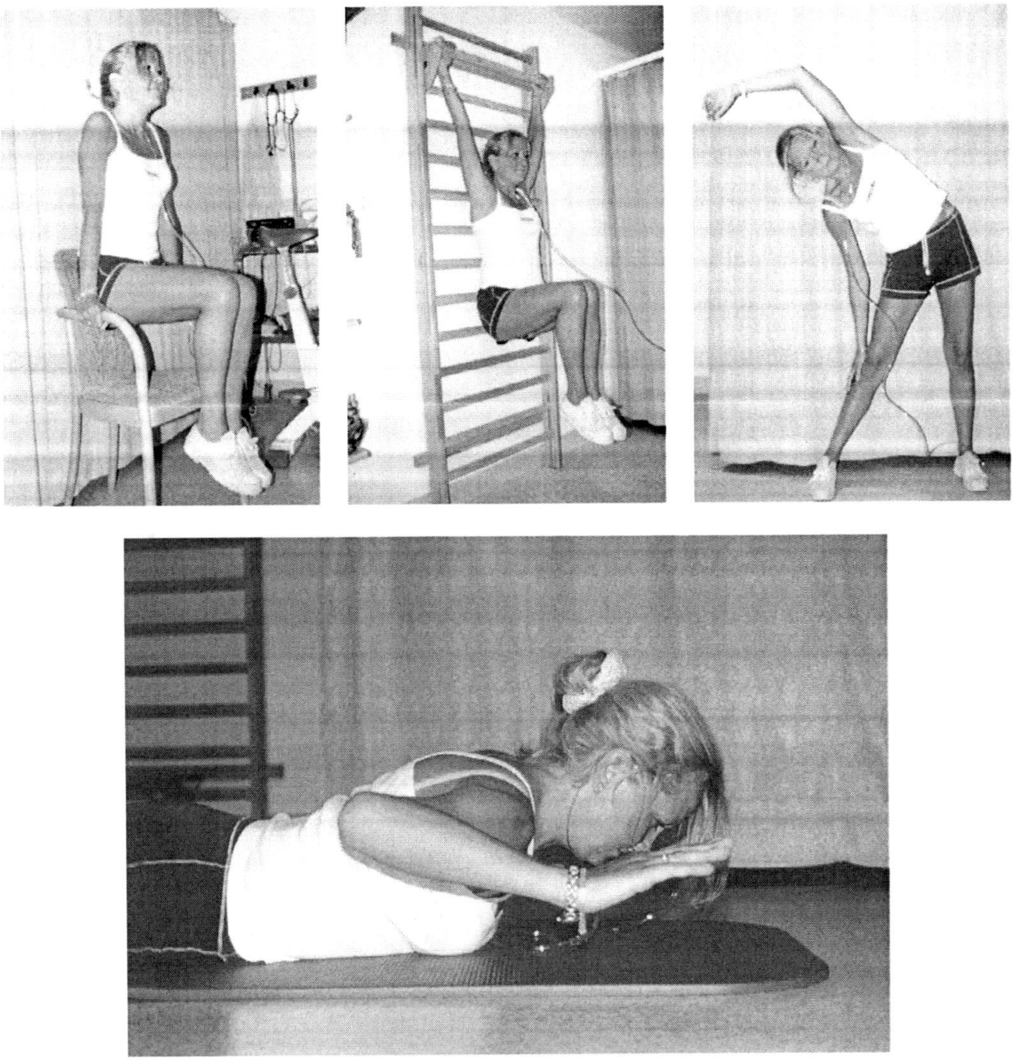

Fig. 10a-d. Even severely ill patients can have a good posture and few or no musculo-skeletal problems, as this young CF woman on the transplant list. Chest mobility and postural exercises have been carried out since diagnosis, here with supplemental oxygen to keep her saturation above 90%.

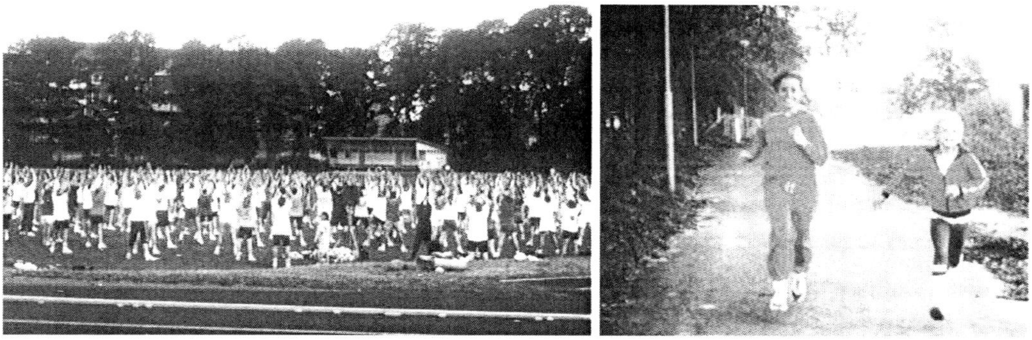

Fig. 11a-b. Working capacity training is part of the treatment package from the beginning in order to preserve a good physical capacity. Depending on what suits the individual for the moment, they may train either individually or in aerobic groups together with friends or in public.

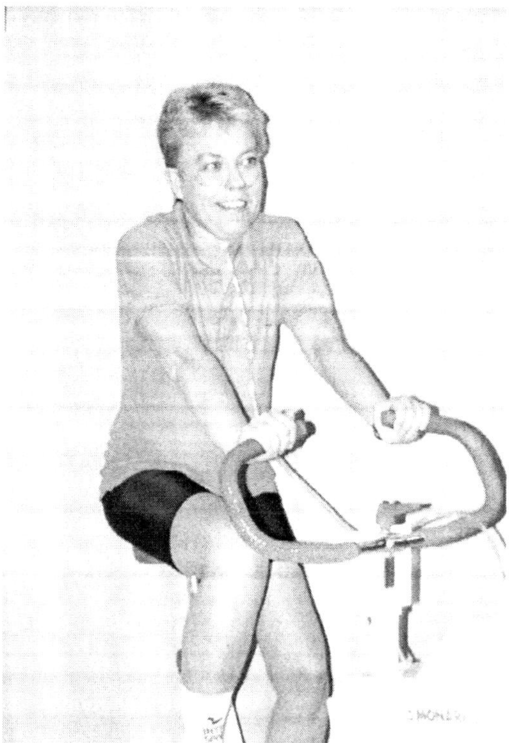

Fig. 12. Severely ill patients like this CF woman on the transplant list carry out working capacity training with oxygen supplement to keep their saturation above 90%.

Evaluation of Outcomes of and Agreements About the Treatment Regimen

The evaluation of the treatment is always carried out together with patients and parents, although children most often get a little time on their own with the different caregivers. With increasing age, evaluation of and agreements about the treatment are carried out to a gradually larger extent with the adolescent patient him/herself, in order to help them manage the responsibility for the treatment themselves once being an adult. Parents are gradually getting the role as a background support resource. Patients are in frequent contact with the CF team and physical condition is closely monitored and plotted in curves. Treatment adherence is continuously assessed, inhalation and airway techniques used are continuously re-assessed and optimised at each physiotherapy appointment.

The information evaluated at check ups involves not only clinical data, but also number of days off from school/work, degree of spontaneous physical activity during every day life, coughing pattern, sleeping quality, and functional physical every day references as discussed above. At each check up a dynamic lung function test is carried out, measuring expiratory flow parameters, FEV1.0 and FVC. The mid and end expiratory flow in relation to FVC are sensitive to early changes in the peripheral airways and are therefore considered important information and are being used when evaluating the preventative care. If needed, additional lung function tests are carried out in between check ups, when patients see the physiotherapist.

In Summary

Several basic factors in the Swedish holistic approach to CF care have probably contributed to the good results. Such factors are frequent contacts with the caregivers and striving for patients seeing the same team members to ensure continuity. The aim with this is to make it possible to build a co-operation situation with the patient/parents where they feel they are working partners who have an input in their care, being involved in discussions, evaluations and agreements concerning their daily treatment. This way of working gives a possibility to detect deteriorating trends early, which allows for an early intervention. Added to these factors are an active nutritional therapy, an aggressive antibiotic therapy, an individually tailored active physiotherapy regimen that involves physical exercise from the very beginning, an active psychosocial support and continuously ongoing education. When care is shared, communication with caregivers at local hospitals is kept active, caregivers are invited to visit the centre together with their patients and education days are regularly organised. When admitted to the hospital, patients still see their CF team caregivers to as large an extent as possible, regardless of what ward is involved. These situations are used for intense training of treatment quality, but also for further education in order to improve adherence with the preventative every day care. Patients and local caregivers always have access to the CF-centre for emergencies or other consultations and written guidelines for the treatment of complications are available and regularly up-dated.

Patients have frequent appointments with their physiotherapist, where the prescribed inhalation therapy, airway clearance and physical exercise are carried out together with the physiotherapist. This gives an opportunity to train and maintain good treatment quality and to stimulate good adherence with the treatment. The delicate but time-consuming physiotherapy part of the treatment that is recommended is thereby often re-considered, optimised or modified to be a positive experience and to be ensured as not being too big a burden on the patient, parents, siblings or partner. A strategic plan is made up for inhalation therapy, especially if inhaling corticosteroids or antimicrobials. These agents are inhaled after airway clearance therapy, as well as DNase is in patients with large amounts of secretions. A good airway clearance is a good base for effective antibiotic therapy it is either administered intravenously or inhaled.

The preventative every day treatment is considered essential for the results, it is therefore optimised frequently. Patients/parents are usually prepared to dedicate a limited amount of time to treatment each day, which is why our struggle as caregivers is to use that limited time as efficiently as possible in order to achieve good adherence with the daily care.

Acknowledgements

The author wishes to thank A. Lindgren, Dept. Mathematical Statistics, Centre for Mathematical Sciences, Lund University, for her invaluable help with the statistical analyzes.

References

[1] Dankert-Roelse JE, te Meerman GJ. Long term prognosis of patients with cystic fibrosis in relation to early detection by neonatal screening and treatment in a cystic fibrosis centre. *Thorax* 1995;50:712-718.

[2] Frederiksen B, Lanng S, Koch C, Høiby N. Improved survival in the Danish center-treated cystic fibrosis patients: results of aggressive treatment. *Pediatr Pulmonol* 1996;21:153-158.

[3] Mahadeva R, Webb K, Westerbeek RC, Carroll NR, Dodd ME, Bilton D, Lomas DA. Clinical outcome in relation to care in centres specialising in cystic fibrosis: cross sectional study. *BMJ* 1998;316:1771-5.

[4] Marshall BC, Samuelsson WM. Basic therapies in cystic fibrosis. Does standard therapy work? *Clin Chest Med* 1998;19/3:487-504.

[5] Hodson ME, Rainisio M, McKezie S, Harms HK, Koch C, Mastella G, Navarro J. The European Epidemiologic Registry of Cystic Fibrosis (ERCF). *In 1998 – where are we? 22nd European CF Conference*, Berlin 1998; S6-1, Book of Abstract page 65.

[6] Fogarty A, Hubbard R, Britton J. International comparison of median age at death from cystic fibrosis. *Chest* 2000;117:1656-1660.

[7] Jaffe A, Bush A. Cystic fibrosis: review of the decade. *Monaldi Arch Chest Dis* 2001;56:240-7.

[8] Lannefors L, Lindgren A. Demographic transition of the Swedish cystic fibrosis community – results of modern care. *Respir Med* 2002;96:681-5.

[9] Cystic Fibrosis Foundation (CFF) *National Patient Registry, Annual Data Report.* 2002, Bethesda, Maryland, USA, 2003. www.CFF.org

[10] Kulich M, Rosenfeld M, Goss CH, Wilmott R. Improved survival among young patients with cystic fibrosis. *J Pediatr* 2003;142(6):631-6.

[11] Dobbin CJ, Bye PTP. Clinical perspectives. Adults with cystic fibrosis: meeting the challenge! *Intern Med J* 2003;33:593-7.

[12] Wagener JS, Headley AA. Cystic fibrosis: current trends in respiratory care. *Respir Care* 2003;48(3):246-7.

[13] Dodge JA, Morison S, Lewis PA, Coles EC, Geddes D, Russell G, Littlewood JM, Scott MT. Incidence, population, and survival of cystic fibrosis in the UK, 1968-95. *Arch Dis Child* 1997; 77:493-496.

[14] Elborn JS, Shale DJ, Britton JR. Cystic fibrosis: current survival and population estimates to the year 2000. *Thorax* 1991;46:881-885.

[15] Conway SP, Stableforth DE, Webb AK. The failing health care system for adult patients with cystic fibrosis. *Thorax* 1998;53:3-4.

[16] Mackie ADR, Thornton SJ, Edenborough FP. Cystic fibrosis-related diabetes. *Diabet Med* 2003;20:425-36.

[17] Koch C, Rainiso M, Madessani U, Harms HK, Hodson ME, Mastella F, McKenzie SG, Navarro J, Strandvik B; Investigators of the European Epidemiologic Registry of Cystic Fibrosis. Presence of cystic fibrosis-related diabetes mellitus is tightly linked to poor lung function in patients with cystic fibrosis: data from the European Epidemiologic Registry of Cystic Fibrosis. *Pediatr Pulmonol* 2001;32(5):343-50.

[18] Conway SP, Morton AM, Oldroyd B, Truscott JG, White H, Smith AH, Haigh I. Osteoporosis and osteopenia in adults and adolescents with cystic fibrosis: prevalence and associated factors. *Thorax* 2000;55:798-804.

[19] Elkin SL, Fairney A, Burnett S, Kemp M, Kyd P, Burgess J, Compston JE, Hodson ME. Vertebral deformities and low bone mineral density in adults with cystic fibrosis: a cross-sectional study. *Osteoporos Int* 2001;12(5):366-72.

[20] Cystic Fibrosis Foundation (CFF) *National Patient Registry, Annual Data Report.* 2000, Bethesda, Maryland, USA, 2001. www.CFF.org

[21] Worlitzsch D, Tarran R, Ulrich M, Schwab U, Cekici A, Meyer KC, Birrer P, Bellon G, Berger J, Weiß T, Botzenhart K, Yankaskas JR, Randell S, Boucher RC, Döring G. Reduced oxygen concentrations in airway mucus contribute to the early and late pathogenesis of Pseudomonas aeruginosa cystic fibrosis airways infection. *J Clin Invest* 2002; 109:317-25.

[22] Boucher RC. New concepts of the pathogenesis of cystic fibrosis lung disease. *Eur Resp J* 2004;23(1):146-58.

[23] Demko CA, Byard PJ, David PB. Gender differences in cystic fibrosis: Pseudomonas aeruginosa infection. *J Clin Epidemiol* 1995; 48:1041-9.

[24] Amitani R, Wilson R, Rutman A, Reed R, Ward C, Burnett D, Stockley RA, Cole PJ. Effects of human neutrophil elastase and Pseudomonas aeruginosa on human respiratory epithelium. *Am J Respir Cell Mol Biol* 1991;4:26-32.

[25] Hart N, Polkey MI, Clement A, Boule M, Moxham J, Lofaso F, Fauroux B. Changes in pulmonary mechanics with increasing disease severity in children and young adults with cystic fibrosis. *Am J Respir Crit Care Med* 2002;166(1):61-6.

[26] Birrer P, McElvaney NG, Rudeberg A, Sommer CW, Liechti Gallati S, Kraemer R, Hubbard R, Crystal RG. Protease antiprotease imbalance in the lungs of children with cystic fibrosis. *Am J Respir Crit Care Med* 1994; 150:207 13.

[27] Armstrong DS, Grimwood K, Carzino R, Carlin JB, Olinsky A, Phelan PD. Lower respiratory infection and inflammation in infants with newly diagnosed cystic fibrosis. *BMJ* 1995;310:1571-2.

[28] Cantin, A. Cystic fibrosis lung inflammation: early, sustained and severe. *Am J Respir Crit Care Med* 1995; 151:939 41.

[29] Khan TZ, Wagener JS, Bost T, Martinez J, Accurso FJ, Riches DWH. Early pulmonary inflammation in infants with cystic fibrosis. *Am J Respir Crit Care Med* 1995;151:1075-82.

[30] Armstrong DS, Grimwood K, Carlin JB, Carzino R, Gutierrez JP, Hull J, Olinsky A, Phelan EM, Robertson CF, Pheland PD. Lower airway inflammation in infants and young children with cystic fibrosis. *Am J Respir Crit Care Med* 1997;156:1197-204.

[31] Tepper RS. Assessment of the respiratory status of infants and toddlers with cystic fibrosis. *J Pediatr* 1998;132:380-1.

[32] Nixon GM, Armstrong DS, Carzino R, Carlin JB, Olinsky A, Robertson CF, Grimwood F. Early airway infection, inflammation, and lung function in cystic fibrosis. *Arch Dis Child* 2002;87:306-11.

[33] Hardy KA, Wolfson MR, Schidlow DV, Shaffer TH. Mechanics and energetics of breathing in newly diagnosed infants with cystic fibrosis: effect of combined bronchodilator and chest physical therapy. *Pediatr Pulmonol* 1989;6(2):103-8.

[34] Ranganathan SC, Bush A, Dezateux C, Carr SB, Hoo AF, Lum S, Madge S, Price J, Stroobant J, Wade A, Wallis C, Wyatt H, Stocks J. Relative ability of full and partial forced expiratory maneuvers to identify diminished airway function in infants with cystic fibrosis. *Am J Respir Crit Care Med* 2002;166:1350-7.

[35] Phelan PD, Olinsky A, Robertson CF. *Lung growth and development. In: Respiratory illness in children*. 4th edn. Oxford: Blackwell, 1994;1:1-7.

[36] Maffessanti M, Candusso M, Brizzi F, Piovesana F. Cystic fibrosis in children: HRCT findings and distribution of disease. *J Thorac Imag* 1996;11:27-38.

[37] Bedrossian CW, Greenberg SD, Singer DB, Hansen JJ, Rosenberg HS. The lung in cystic fibrosis. A quantitative study including prevalence of pathologic findings among different age groups. *Hum Pathol* 1976;7:195-204.

[38] Tepper RS, Hiatt PW, Eigen H, Smith J. Total respiratory system compliance in asymptomatic infants with cystic fibrosis. Am Rev Respir Dis 1987;135(5):1075-9.

[39] Beardsmore CS. Lung function from infancy to school age in cystic fibrosis. *Arch Dis Child* 1995;73(6):519-23.

[40] Dakin CJ, Numa AH, Wang H, Morton JR, Vertzyas CC, Henry RL. Inflammation, infection, and pulmonary function in infants and young children with cystic fibrosis. *Am J Respir Crit Care Med* 2002;165(7):904-10.

[41] Tiddens HA. Detecting early structural lung damage in cystic fibrosis. *Pediatr Pulmonol* 2002;34(3):228-31.

[42] Frederick R, Long MD, Roger S, Williams BS, Robert G, Castle MD. Structural airway abnormalities in infants and young children with cystic fibrosis. *J Pediatr* 2004;144:154-61.

[43] Saiman L. Microbiology of early CF lung disease. *Paediatr Respir Rev* 2004;5 Suppl A:S367-9.

[44] Burns JL, Gibson RL, McNamara S, Yim D, Emerson J, Rosenfeld M, Hiatt P, McCoy K, Castile R, Smith AL, Ramsey BW. Longitudinal assessment of Pseudomonas aeruginosa in young children with cystic fibrosis. *J Infect Dis*. 2001; 183:444-52.

[45] Döring G, Jansen S, Noll J, Grupp H, Frank F, Botzenhart K, Magdorf K, Wahn U. Distribution and transmission of Pseudomonas aeruginosa and Burkholderia Cepacia in a hospital ward. *Pediatr Pulmonol* 1996;21:90-100.

[46] Morgan WJ, Butler SM, Johnson CA, Colin AA, Fitzsimmons SC, Geller DE, Konstan MW, Light MJ, Rabin HR, Regelmann WE, Schidlow DV, Stokes DC, Wohl ME, Kaplowitz H, Wyatt MM, Stryker S. Epidemiologic Study of Cystic Fibrosis Design and Implementation of a Prospective, Multicenter, observational study of patients with cystic fibrosis in the U.S. and Canada. *Pediatr Pulmonol* 1999;28:231-241.

[47] Tepper RS, Montgomery GL, Ackerman V, Eigen H. Longitudinal evaluation of pulmonary function in infants and very young children with cystic fibrosis. *Pediatr Pulmonol* 1993;16(2):96-100.

[48] Hamutcu R, Rowland JM, Horn MV, Kaminsky C, MacLaughlin EF, Starnes VA, Woo MS. Clinical findings and lung pathology in children with cystic fibrosis. *Am J Respir Crit Care Med* 2002;164(8):1172-5.

[49] Gibson RL, Burns JL, Ramsey BW. Pathophysiology and management of pulmonary infections in cystic fibrosis. *Am J Respir Crit Care Med* 2003;168:918-51.

[50] Kosorok MR, Zeng L, West SE, Rock MJ, Splaingard ML, Laxova A, Green CG, Collins J, Farrell PM. Acceleration of lung disease in children with cystic fibrosis after Pseudomonas aeruginosa acquisition. *Pediatr Pulmonol* 2001; 32:277-87.

[51] Emerson J, Rosenfeld M, McNamara S Ramsey B, Gibson RL. Pseudomonas aeruginosa and other predictors of mortality in young children with cystic fibrosis. *Pediatr Pulmonol* 2002;34:91-100.

[52] Koch C, McKenzie S, Kaplowitz H, Hodson M.E, Harms H.K, Navarro J, Mastella G. International Practice Patterns by Age and Severity of Lung Disease in Cystic Fibrosis: Data From the Epidemiologic Registry of Cystic Fibrosis (ERCF). *Pediatr Pulmonol* 1997;24:147-154.

[53] Ramsey BW, Farrell PM, Pencharz P. Nutritional assessment and management in cystic fibrosis: a consensus report. *Am J Clin Nutr* 1992;55:108-16.

[54] Sinaasappel M, Stern M, Littlewood J, Wolfe S, Steinkamp G, Heijerman HGM, Robberecht E, Doring G. Nutrition in patients with cystic fibrosis: a European Consensus. *J Cystic Fibrosis* 2002;1:51-75.

[55] Steinkamp G, Wiedermann B. On behalf of the German CFQA Group. Reslationship between nutritional status and lung function in cystic fibrosis: cross sectional and longitudinal analyses from the German Quality Assurance Project. *Thorax* 2002;57:596-601.

[56] Borowitz D, Baker RD, Stalling V. Consensus report on nutrition for pediatric patients with cystic fibrosis. *J Pediatr Gastroenterol Nutr* 2002;35(3):246-59.

[57] Corey M, McLaughlin FJ, Williams M, Levison H. A comparison of survival, growth and pulmonary function in patients with cystic fibrosis in Boston and Toronto. *J Clin Epidemiol* 1988;4:588-91.

[58] Frederiksen B, Koch C, Hoiby N. Antibiotic treatment of initial colonization with Pseudomonas aeruginosa postpones chronic infection and prevents deterioration of pulmonary function in cystic fibrosis. *Pediatr Pulmonol* 1997;23(5):330-5.

[59] Frederiksen B, Koch C, Høiby N. Changing epidemiology of Pseudomonas aeruginosa infection in Danish CF patients (1974-1995). *Pediatr Pulmonol* 1999;28:159-166.

[60] Döring G, Conway SP, Heijerman HGM, Hodson ME, Høiby N, Smyth A, Touw DJ, for the Consensus Committee. Antibiotic therapy against Pseudomonas aeruginosa in cystic fibrosis: a European consensus. *Eur Respir J* 2000; 16:749-67.

[61] Antibiotic Treatment for Cystic Fibrosis. *Report of the UK Cystic Fibrosis Trust Antibiotic Group*. Second edition. Cystic Fibrosis Trust, London, UK, 2002.

[62] Conway SP, Brownlee KG, Denton M, Peckham DG. Antibiotic treatment of mulitdrug-resistant organisms in cystic fibrosis. *Am J Respir Med* 2003;2(4):321-32.

[63] Chernish RN, Aaron SD. Approach to resistant gram-negative bacterial pulmonary infections in patients with cystic fibrosis. *Curr Opin Pulm Med* 2003;9:509-15.

[64] Jensen T, Pedersen SS, Hoiby N, Koch C, Flensborg EW. Use of antibiotics in cystic fibrosis. The Danish approach. *Antibiot Chemother* 1989;42:237-46.

[65] Saiman L, Mehar F, Niu WW, Neu HC, Shaw KJ, Miller G, Prince A. Antibiotic susceptibility of multiply resistant Pseudomonas aeruginosa isolated from patients with cystic fibrosis, including candidates for transplantation. *Clinical Infectious Diseases* 1996;23:532-7.

[66] Miall LS, McGinley NT, Brownlee KG, Conway SP. Methicillin resistant Staphylococcus aureus (MRSA) infection in cystic fibrosis. *Arch Dis Child* 2001; 84:160-2.

[67] Ratjen F, Comes G, Paul K, Posselt HG, Wagner TO, Harms K. Effect of continuous anti-staphylococcal therapy on the rate of P. aeruginosa acquisition in patients with cystic fibrosis. *Pediatr Pulmonol* 2001; 31:13-6.

[68] Stutman HR, Lieberman JM, Nussbaum E, Marks MI. Antibiotic prophylaxis in infants and young children with cystic fibrosis: a randomized controlled trial. *J Pediatr* 2002; 140:299-305.

[69] Demko CA, Stern RC, Doershuk CF. Stenotrophomonas maltophilia in cystic fibrosis: incidence and prevalence. *Pediatr Pulmonol* 1998; 25:304-8.

[70] Denton M, Kerr KG. Microbiological and clinical aspects of infection associated with Stenotrophomonas maltophilia. *Clin Microbiol Rev* 1998; 11:57-80.

[71] Armstrong D, Grimwood K, Carlin JB, Carzino R, Hull J, Olinsky A, Phelan PD. Severe viral respiratory infections in infants with cystic fibrosis. *Pediatr Pulmonol* 1998; 26:371-9.

[72] Hiatt PW, Grace SC, Kozinetz CA, Raboudi SH, Treece DG, Taber LH, Piedra PA. Effects of viral lower respiratory tract infection on lung function in infants with cystic fibrosis. *Pediatrics* 1999; 103:619-26.

[73] Mastella G, Rainisio M, Harms HK, Hodson ME, Koch C, Navarro J, Strandvik B, McKenzie SG. Allergic bronchopulmonary aspergillosis in cystic fibrosis. A European epidemiological study. Epidemiologic Registry of Cystic Fibrosis. *Eur Respir J* 2000; 16:464-71.

[74] Navarro J, Rainisio M, Harms HK, Hodson ME, Koch C, Mastella G, Strandvik B, McKenzie SG. Factors associated with poor pulmonary function: cross-sectional analysis of data from the ERCF. *European Epidemiologic Registry of Cystic Fibrosis.* Eur Respir J 2001; 18:298-305.

[75] Liou TG, Adler FR, FitzSimmons SC, Cahill BC, Hibbs JR, Marshall BC: Predictive 5-year survivorship model of cystic fibrosis. *Am J Epidemiol* 2001; 153:345-52.

[76] Olivier KN, Weber DJ, Lee JH, Handker A, Tudor G, Molina PL, Tomashefski J. Knowles MR. Nontuberculous mycobacteria. *Amer J Respir Crit Care Med* 2003;167:835-40.

[77] Levy J. Antibiotic activity in sputum. *J Pediatr* 1986;108:841-6.

[78] Bosworth DG, Nielson DW. Effectiveness of home versus hospital care in the routine treatment of cystic fibrosis. *Pediatr Pulmonol* 1997;24:42-7.

[79] Ilowite JS, Gorvoy JD, Smaldone GC. Quantitative deposition of aerosolized gentamicin in cystic fibrosis. *Am Rev Respir Dis* 1987; 136:1445-9.

[80] Zach MS, Oberwaldner B. Chest physiotherapy: the mechanical approach to anti-infective therapy in cystic fibrosis. *Infection* 1987;15:381-4.

[81] International Physiotherapy Group for Cystic Fibrosis (IPG/CF). *Physiotherapy in the treatment of cystic fibrosis*. 3rd version, 2002. www.cfww.org

[82] Zach MS. Lung disease in cystic fibrosis – an updated concept. *Pediatr Pulmonol* 1990;8:188-202.

[83] Wallis C, Prasad A. Who needs chest physiotherapy? Moving from anecdote to evidence. *Arch Dis Child* 1999;80(4):393–7.

[84] Thomas J, Cook DJ, Brooks D. Chest physiotherapy management of patients with cystic fibrosis: a meta-analysis. *Am J Respir Crit Care Med* 1995;151:846-50.

[85] Goss CH. Airway clearance in cystic fibrosis. *Respir Care* 2003;48:20-21.

[86] Oermann CM, Swank PR, Sockrider MM. Validation of an instrument measuring patient satisfaction with chest physiotherapy techniques in Cystic fibrosis. *Chest* 2000;118:92-7.

[87] Passero MA, Remor B, Salomon J. Patient-reported compliance with cystic fibrosis therapy. *Clin Pediatr* 1981,20(4):264-8.

[88] Geiss SK, Hobbs SA, Hammersley-Maercklein G, Kramer JC, Henley M. Psychosocial factors related to perceived compliance with cystic fibrosis treatment. *J Clin Psychol* 1992;48:99-103.

[89] Abbott J, Dodd M, Bilton D, Webb AK. Treatment compliance in adults with cystic fibrosis. *Thorax* 1994;49(2):115-20.

[90] Chappell F, Williams B. Rates and reasons for non-adherence to home physiotherapy in paediatrics. *Physiotherapy* 2002;88(3):138-47.

[91] Currie DC, Munro C, Gaskill D, Cole PJ. Practice, problems, and compliance with postural drainage: a survey of chronic sputum producers. *Br J Dis Chest* 1986;80:249-53.

[92] Davids LM, Heneley LD. Investigation into the compliance with and effectiveness of physiotherapy regimen in CF. *S Afr J Physioth* 1990;46:7-10.

[93] Muszynski-Kwan AT, Perlman R, Rivington-Law B. Compliance with and effectiveness of chest physiotherapy in CF. *Physiother Can* 1988;40:28-32.

[94] Fong S, Dales R, Tierney M. Compliance among adults with cystic fibrosis. *Pediatr Pulmonol* 1988;5(Suppl 120):140.

[95] Prasad SA, Main E. Finding evidence to support airway clearance techniques in cystic fibrosis. *Disabil Rehabil* 1998;20(6/7):235-46.

[96] Coyle J, Williams B. Adherence to physiotherapy among children with cystic fibrosis: a qualitative investigation. *J Cystic Fibrosis* 2003;2(Suppl 2):A242.

[97] Foster AC, Voyles JB, Murphy SA. Twenty four hour pH monitoring in children with cystic fibrosis: association of chest physiotherapy to gastro-esophageal reflux. *Paediatr Res* 1983;17:A188.

[98] Newell SJ, Booth IW, Morgan MEI, McNeish AS. Gastro-esophageal reflux in the preterm infant. *Pediatr Res* 1987;22:A104.

[99] Button BM, Heine RG, Catto-Smith AG, Phelan PD, Olinsky A. Postural drainage and gastro-oesophageal reflux in infants with cystic fibrosis. *Arch of Dis in Child* 1997;76:148-50.
[100] Button BM, Heine RG, Catto-Smith AG, Olinsky A, Phelan PD. Postural drainage in cystic fibrosis: is there a link with gastro-oesophageal reflux? *J Paediatr Child Health* 1998;34:330-4.
[101] Vinocur CD, Marmon L, Schidlow DV, Weintraub WH. Gastroesophageal reflux in the infant with cystic fibrosis. *Am J Surg* 1985;149:182-6.
[102] Stringer DA, Sprigg A, Juodis E, Corey M, Daneman A, Levison HJ, Durie PR. The association of cystic fibrosis, gastroesophageal reflux, and reduced pulmonary function. *Can Assoc Radiol J* 1988;39:100-2.
[103] Munck A, Castaing M, Faure C, Viarme F, Gerardin M, Ajzenman C, Navaroo J. Acquisition of P Aeruginosa (PA) in CF children under 3 years: potential role of gastro esophageal reflux (GER). *J Cystic Fibrosis* 2001:Book of abstracts:A122.
[104] Button BM, Heine RG, Catto-Smith AG, Olinsky A, Phelan PD, Ditchfield MR, Story I. Chest physiotherapy in infants with cystic fibrosis: To tip or not? A five year study. *Pediatr Pulmonol* 2003;35:208-13.
[105] Button BM, Heine RG, Catto-Smith AG, Phelan PD, Olinsky A. Chest physiotherapy, *gastro-oesophageal reflux and arousal in infants with cystic fibrosis.* Arch Dis Child, in press.
[106] Orenstein DM. Heads up! clear those airways! *Pediatr Pulmonol* 2003;35(3):160-1.
[107] Van Ginderdeuren F, Malfroot A, Verdonk J, Vanlaethem S, Vandenpals Y. Influence of asssisted autogenic drainage (AAD) and AAD combined with bouncing on gastro-oesophageal reflux (GOR) in infants under the age of 5 months. *J Cystic Fibrosis* 2003;2(Suppl1):A251.
[108] Button BM, Oberwaldner B, Carr M, Story I. The development of international guidelines for the physiotherapy management of infants with CF; results of a worldwide survey forming the foundations of the project. A European Respiratory Society taskforce project endorsed by the IPG. *Pediatr Pulmonol* 2001;Suppl 22:A399.
[109] Lannefors L, Dennersten U, Theander K, Mårtensson J, Kornfält R. Successful treatment of infants and small children with cystic fibrosis. *J Cystic Fibrosis* 2003;2(Suppl1):A250.
[110] Lannefors L, Button B, McIlwaine M. Physiotherapy in infants and young children with cystic fibrosis: current practice and future developments. *J R Soc Med* 2004;97(Suppl.44):8-25..
[111] Southern KW, Littlewood JM. Newborn screening programmes for cystic fibrosis. *Paediatr Respir Rev* 2003;4(4):299-305.
[112] Weller P. Implications of early inflammation and infection in cystic fibrosis: a review of new and potential interventions. *Pediatr Pulmonol* 1997;24:143-6.
[113] Wang SS, O'Leary LA, FitzSimmons SC, Khoury MJ. The impact of early cystic fibrosis diagnosis on pulmonary function in children. *J Pediatr* 2002; 141:804-10.
[114] Ramsey BW, Boat TF. Outcome measures for clinical trials in CF: summary of a Cystic Fibrosis Conference. *J Pediatr* 1994;124:177-92.
[115] Kerem E, Reisman J, Corey M, Canny GJ, Levison H. Prediction of mortality in patients with cystic fibrosis. *N Engl J Med* 1992;326:1187-91.

[116] O'Neill S, McCarthy DS. Postural relief of dyspnoea in severe chronic airflow limitation: relationship to respiratory muscle strength. *Thorax* 1983;38:595-600.

[117] Rose J, Gamble J, Schultz A, Lewiston N. Back pain and spinal deformity in cystic fibrosis. *AJDC* 1987;141:1313-6.

[118] Pryor JA, Webber BA. Physiotherapy techniques. In: Pryor JA, Prasad SA, eds. *Physiotherapy for respiratory and cardiac problems*. 3rd edn. Edinburgh: Churchill Livingstone. 2002:161-242.

[119] Henderson RC, Specter BB. Kyphosis and fractures in children and young adults with cystic fibrosis. *J Pediatr* 1994 Aug;125(2):208-12.

[120] Aris RM, Renner JB, Winders AD, Buell HE, Riggs DB, Lester GE, Ontjes DA. Increased rate of fractures and severe kyphosis: sequelae of living into adulthood with cystic fibrosis. *Ann Intern Med* 1998 Feb 1;128(3):186-93.

[121] Parasa RB, Maffulli N. Musculoskeletal involvement in cystic fibrosis. *Bull Hosp Jt Dis* 1999;58(1):37-44.

[122] Tattersall R, Walshaw MJ. Posture and cystic fibrosis. *J R Soc Med* 2003;96(Suppl43):18-22.

[123] Conway SP. Impact on lung inflammation on bone metabolism in adolescents with cystic fibrosis. *Paediatr Respir Rev* 2001;2(4):324-31.

[124] Vibekk P. *Chest mobilization and respiratory function*. In: Pryor JA, ed. Respiratory Care. Edinburgh: Churchill Livingstone. 1991:103-19.

[125] Dodge JA. Why screen for cystic fibrosis? A clinician's view. *Acta Paediatr Suppl* 1999;432:28-32.

[126] Johnson C, Butler SM, Konstan MW Morgan W, Wohl ME. Factors influencing outcomes in cystic fibrosis. A center based analysis. *Chest* 2003;123:20-7.

[127] FitzSimmons SC. The changing epidemiology of cystic fibrosis. *J Pediatr* 1993;122:1-9.

[128] Wiedemann B, Sens B, Stern M. *CF quality management in Germany*. 22nd European CF Conference, Berlin 1998; S3-3, Book of Abstracts page 13.

[129] Schaedel C, Hjelte L, de Monestrol I, Johannesson M, Kollberg H, Kornfält R, Holmberg L. Three common CFTR mutations should be included in a neonatal screening programme for cystic fibrosis in Sweden. *Clin Genet* 1999;56:318-22.

[130] Tsui L-C, Markiewicz D, Zielinski J, Corey M, Durie P. *Mutation analysis in cystic fibrosis*. In: Dodge JA, Brock DJH, Widdicombe JH, ed. Cystic fibrosis - current topics. Chichester, England: John Wiley & Sons Ltd, 1993:27-44.

[131] Koch C, Cuppens H, Rainisio M, Madessani U, Harms H.K, Hodson M.E, Mastella G, Navarro J, Strandvik B, McKenzie S.G. European Epidemiologic Registry of Cystic Fibrosis (ERCF): Comparison of Major Disease Manifestations Between Patients With Different Classes of Mutations. *Pediatr Pulmonol* 2001;31:1-12.

[132] Lannefors L, Dennersten U, Eriksson L, Mared L. Functional status of an adult CF population. *J Cystic Fibrosis* 2003;2(Suppl1):A195.

[133] Corey M. *Epidemiology and outcome*; Canadian data. 22nd European CF Conference, Berlin 1998; S3-3, Book of Abstracts page 11.

[134] Dennersten U, Lannefors L, Andersson M, Lagerkvist AL, Johansson H, Sahlberg M, Sellberg M, Theander K. Lung function and working capacity in the entire Swedish

cystic fibrosis population ≥7 years old over a three years period. *Pediatr Pulmonol* 2003;Suppl 25:A411.

[135] Kollberg H. Increasing survival of Swedish patients with CF. *Acta Univ Carol Med* 1990;36;213-214.

[136] Andreasson B, Jonsson B, Kornfalt R, Nordmark E, Sandstrom S. Long-term effects of physical exercise on working capacity and pulmonary function in cystic fibrosis. *Acta Pediatr Scand* 1987;76:70-5.

[137] *Lund Cystic Fibrosis Centre. Staying ahead – modern chest physiotherapy.* [Video]. Address: Sjukgymnasterna, Lungmott, Universitetssjukhuset, 221 85 Lund, Sweden.

[138] Zach M, Oberwaldner B, Hausler F. Cystic fibrosis: physical exercise versus chest physiotherapy. *Arch Dis Child* 1982;57(8):587-9.

[139] Kruhlak RT, Jones R, Brown NE. Regional airtrapping before and after exercise in young adults with cystic fibrosis. *West J Med* 1986;145:196-9.

[140] Sahl W, Bilton D, Dodd M, Webb AK. Effect of exercise and physiotherapy in aiding sputum expectoration in adults with cystic fibrosis. *Thorax* 1989;44:1006-8.

[141] Hebestreit A, Kersting U, Basler B, Jeschke R, Hebestreit H. Exercise inhibits epithelial sodium channels in patients with Cystic fibrosis. *Am J Respir Crit Care Med* 2001;164(3):443-6.

[142] Menkes H, Britt J. Physical therapy rationale for physical therapy. *Am Rev Respir Dis* 1980;122(suppl 2):127-31.

[143] Oberwaldner B. Physiotherapy for airway clearance in paediatrics. *Eur Respir J* 2000;15:196-204.

[144] Lannefors L, Wollmer P. Mucus clearance with three chest physiotherapy regimes in cystic fibrosis. A comparison between postural drainage, positive expiratory pressure and physical exercise. *Eur Resp J* 1992;5:748-53.

[145] West JB. *Respiration.* In: Physiological basis of Medical Practise, 12th edn. West JB, ed. Baltimore: Williams & Wilkins. 1990.

[146] Borsje P, de Jongste JC, Mouton JW, Tiddens HAWM. Aerosol therapy in cystic fibrosis: a survey of 54 CF centres. *Pediatr Pulmonol* 2000;30:368-76.

[147] Boe J, Dennis JH, O'Driscoll BR, Bauer TT, Carone M, Dautzenberg B, Diot P, Heslop K, Lannefors L. European Respiratory Society Task Force on the use of nebulizzers. European Respiratory Society Guidelines on the use of nebulizers. *Eur Respir J* 2001;18:228-42.

[148] Bush A, Bisgaard H, Geddes D, Lannefors L. Nebulizers in cystic fibrosis. *Eur Respir Rev* 2000;10:76,552-7.

[149] Rose J, Jay S. A comprehensive exercise program for persons with cystic fibrosis. *J Pediatr Nurs* 1986;1:323-34.

[150] Stanghelle JK, Skyberg D, Haanaes OC. Eight-year follow-up of pulmonary function and oxygen uptake during exercise in 16 year old males with cystic fibrosis. *Acta Paediatr* 1992;81(6-7);527-31.

[151] Schneiderman-Walker J, Pollock SL, Corey M, Wilkes DD, Canny GJ, Pedder L, Reisman JJ. A randomised controlled trial of a 3-year home exercise program in cystic fibrosis. *J Pediatr* 2000;136(3):304-10.

[152] Nixon PA, Orenstein DM, Kelsey SF. Habitual physical activity in children and adolescents with cystic fibrosis. *Med Sci Sports Exerc* 2001;33(1):30-5.

Index

A

B

C

D

E

F

G

H

I

J

K

L

M

N

S

T

U

V

W

Y

Z